# HIGH DENSITY LIPOPROTEINS
# AND ATHEROSCLEROSIS III

# HIGH DENSITY LIPOPROTEINS AND ATHEROSCLEROSIS III

Proceedings of the 3rd International Symposium on Plasma High Density Lipoproteins and Atherosclerosis, San Antonio, 4–6 March 1992.

*Editors:*

**Norman E. Miller**

Department of Medicine,
Bowman Gray School of Medicine,
Winston-Salem, NC, U.S.A.

**Alan R. Tall**

Department of Medicine,
Columbia University College of Physicians and Surgeons,
New York, U.S.A.

 1992

**EXCERPTA MEDICA, Amsterdam - London - New York - Tokyo**

International Congress Series No. 1001
ISBN 0 444 81442 6

*This book is printed on acid-free paper.*

*Published by:*
Elsevier Science Publishers B.V.
P.O. Box 211
1000 AE Amsterdam
The Netherlands

*Library of Congress Cataloging in Publication Data:*

```
International Symposium on Plasma High Density Lipoproteins and
   Atherosclerosis (3rd : 1992 : San Antonio, Tex.)
   High density lipoproteins and atherosclerosis III : proceedings of
the 3rd International Symposium on Plasma High Density Lipoproteins
and Atherosclerosis, San Antonio, 4-6 March 1992 / editors Norman E.
Miller, Alan R. Tall.
      p.   cm.
   Includes index.
   ISBN 0-444-81442-6 (alk. paper)
   1. Atherosclerosis--Pathophysiology--Congresses.  2. High density
lipoproteins--Pathophysiology--Congresses.  3. High density
lipoproteins--Metabolism--Congresses.   I. Title.
   [DNLM: 1. Atherosclerosis--etiology--congresses.  2. Lipoproteins,
HDL--metabolism--congresses.   W3 EX89 no.1001 / QU 85 I619 1992h]
RC692.I547   1992
616.1'36071--dc20
DNLM/DLC
for Library of Congress                          92-49651
                                                     CIP
```

Printed in The Netherlands

# FOREWORD

In 1988 the Second International Symposium on HDL and Atherosclerosis was held in Leeds Castle, England. On that occasion epidemiologists, biochemists, cell biologists and cardiologists met to discuss recent important progress that had been made in this field. Since then there has been a movement in HDL research towards molecular biology and experimental models of atherosclerosis. Important new findings have emerged on the biochemistry of reverse cholesterol transport and on the relationship of HDL metabolism to triglyceride transport. In clinical studies new genetic disorders of HDL have been discovered. And more evidence that HDL-raising agents can help to reduce the progression of coronary artery disease in hypercholesterolaemic subjects with low initial HDL levels has been presented. These new developments were the subject of the third symposium in the series, held in San Antonio in 1992. As on previous occasions, it was a stimulating event. The papers that were presented are summarised in this volume.

**Norman E Miller**
**Alan R Tall**

# ACKNOWLEDGEMENT

The 3rd International Symposium on Plasma High Density Lipoproteins and Atherosclerosis was sponsored by the Council on Arteriosclerosis of the American Heart Association, and was made possible by a grant from Parke-Davis, a Division of Warner Lambert Company.

# CONTENTS

## HUMAN HDL METABOLISM AND GENETICS

## DRUGS, HORMONES AND EPIDEMIOLOGY

**HIGH DENSITY LIPOPROTEIN
GENE REGULATION**

High density lipoproteins and atherosclerosis III.
N.E. Miller and A.R. Tall, editors.

Identification of Genetic Loci Contributing to High Density Lipoprotein
Metabolism and Early Atherosclerosis in a Mouse Model

Craig H. Warden[1], Margarete Mehrabian[1], Yu-Rong Xia[1], Kong-Yuan He[1], Ping-Zi Wen[1], Jian-Hua Qiao[1], Anh Diep[1], Diane Ruddle[2], Craig Laughton[2], and Aldons J. Lusis[1].

[1]Department of Medicine and Department of Microbiology and Molecular Genetics, University of California at Los Angeles, Los Angeles, CA 90024

[2]Syntex Corporation, 3401 Hillview Avenue, Palo Alto, CA 90024

## INTRODUCTION

High density lipoprotein metabolism is complex, with numerous genetic and environmental contributions. As discussed below the genetic analysis of such complex traits is difficult or impossible directly in humans. However, methods for the analysis of polygenic traits have recently been developed for animal models (reviewed in 1). We describe here preliminary results utilizing these methods to clarify the genetic control of HDL metabolism in the mouse animal model.

## DIFFICULTIES OF GENETIC ANALYSIS IN HUMANS

Family studies have demonstrated that a large proportion of the variance of high density lipoprotein (HDL) levels is due to genetic influences, but the mode of inheritance and the identity of the genes responsible remain largely unknown. Information concerning the genes likely to be important in HDL metabolism has been derived largely from biochemical studies and from studies of rare genetic syndromes affecting HDL metabolism (Figure 1). Thus, biochemical studies have identified the major apolipoproteins of HDL and the primary enzymes mediating HDL metabolism in the circulation, and studies of familial syndromes have revealed that mutations of the genes for apolipoprotein AI (apoAI), lecithin:cholesterol acyl transferase (LCAT) and cholesteryl ester transfer protein (CETP) can dramatically influence HDL levels and structures (reviewed 2,3). However, such monogenic syndromes explain only a small fraction of the variation in HDL metabolism in the population.

Whether the "candidate genes" revealed through studies of HDL biochemistry and genetic syndromes contribute to the population variation in HDL metabolism can be tested by "molecular epidemiology." This involves studies of populations or families to determine whether polymorphisms of the various candidate genes are statistically associated with differences in HDL levels or structures. Such studies have provided suggestive, but not definitive, evidence for the involvement of certain genes, such as lipoprotein lipase (4) and the apoAI/CIII/AIV gene cluster (reviewed in 5) in the controlling of HDL levels. The role of these genes in HDL metabolism can also be tested in animal models, for example, through studies with transgenic mice, gene targeting, or naturally occurring genetic variations (Fig. 1).

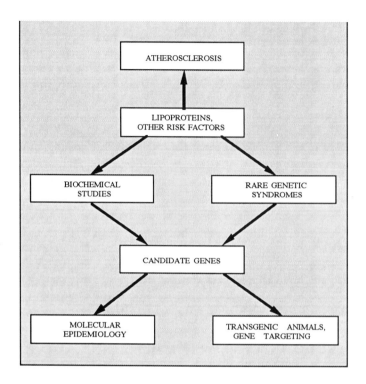

Figure 1. Approaches for studying the genetic control of HDL levels and structures.

Efforts to understand the genetic factors contributing to plasma HDL levels are complicated by multiple genetic and environmental influences and by genetic heterogeneity. Both population and family studies are greatly complicated by genetic heterogeneity since differences in HDL levels and structures among individuals can be due to differing genetic factors. (Fig. 2). Thus HDL cholesterol may appear to be linked to one gene in one family, but may appear to be unlinked to that same gene in a different family. Moreover, the metabolic complexity and structural heterogeneity of HDL have also made biochemical approaches difficult and it is likely that at present we have knowledge of only a subset of the genes which underlie HDL cholesterol levels.

## ADVANTAGES OF STUDIES WITH ANIMAL MODELS

We have studied the mouse animal model because of the difficulties in the analysis of complex genetic traits such as HDL levels directly in humans. Animal models provide important advantages for genetic as well as biochemical studies of complex traits, and genetic variations affecting lipoprotein metabolism and early atherosclerosis have been identified among inbred strains of mice (reviewed 1,6). Most importantly for the problem of HDL metabolism, the methods for analysis for multigenic traits have recently been developed for inbred animal models (7). In particular, the problem of genetic heterogeneity is avoided by the use of inbred strains of animals. Thus, in a genetic cross constructed from two different inbred parental strains, all of the progeny will differ from one another in HDL metabolism due to the same set of genetic factors differing between the two parental strains. The experimental design for mapping of genetic loci for multigenic traits in animal models is summarized in Figure 3.

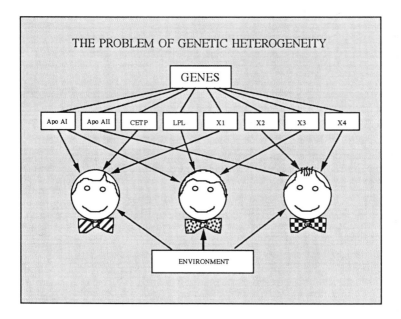

Figure 2. The problem of genetic heterogeneity. HDL levels and structures are determined by multiple genetic and environmental influences. In most cases, the genetic factors contributing to HDL metabolism in one individual will differ from those contributing to HDL metabolism in another individual. In the hypothetical example shown, individual 1 exhibits altered HDL levels due to genetic variations of the genes for apolipoprotein AI (apoAI), cholesteryl ester transfer protein (CETP) and an as yet unidentified gene (X1). Individual 2, on the other hand, exhibits altered HDL levels due to genetic variations of the genes for apoAI, lipoprotein lipase (LPL) and an as yet unknown gene (X3).

6

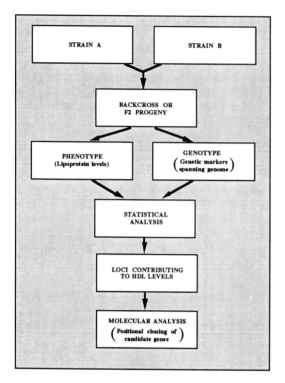

Figure 3. Identification of genes contributing to polygenic traits (such as HDL metabolism). Using animal models, the experimental design is as follows. First, the inbred strains of animals (designated "A" and "B") differing for the trait of interest are crossed to produce a large number of backcross or F2 progeny. Second, the individual progeny are typed for the trait of interest (HDL levels or structures). Third, the individual progeny are typed for genetic markers that span the genome at intervals of about 20 centimorgans (cM). Fourth, statistical analyses are performed to test for significant associations between the trait and individual genetic markers. Statistically significant associations provide evidence for the identity of loci containing genes controlling the trait. Finally, the gene responsible for the trait must be identified. This can be approached by transferring the individual loci onto a common genetic background by a series of backcrosses, thereby reducing the polygenic trait to a monogenic trait. Following this, "positional cloning" can be used to identify the relevant gene. Alternatively, any "candidate gene" residing at the locus can be tested for effects on HDL metabolism.

Within the past year, the method has been applied successfully to the analysis of several risk factors associated with atherosclerosis, including obesity, diabetes, and hypertension (reviewed in 1). Importantly, the approach does not require any knowledge of the molecular basis of the traits. It therefore has the potential of identifying new genes or pathways not previously revealed using biochemical approaches. There has been rapid progress in the development of useful genetic markers in several mammalian species. The most useful of these are "microsatellites" or "simple sequence repeats" that are highly polymorphic and can be rapidly assayed by the polymerase chain reaction (for example, 8).

## HDL METABOLISM IN THE MOUSE MODEL

Inbred strains of mice differ widely in the levels and structures of HDL (6). Previous genetic studies have revealed two important genes contributing to HDL metabolism in mice. One of these is the apoAII gene located in the distal region of mouse chromosome one. Genetic variations of the human apoAII gene affect the size and apolipoprotein composition of HDL (2). More recently, we have also demonstrated that the apoAII gene contributes importantly to variations of HDL levels among inbred strains of mice (Mehrabian, M., Qiao, J.-H., Ruddle, D., Laughton, C., Lusis, A., unpublished) Previous studies have also revealed a gene designated Ath-1, that determines development of early atherosclerotic lesions in response to a high fat, high cholesterol diet containing bile acids. The gene appears to act by determining HDL levels in response to the diet. The identity of the Ath-1 gene is unknown but it appears to be closely linked to the apoAII gene on mouse chromosome one (10). Efforts to identify other genetic variations contributing to HDL metabolism, have, however, been frustrated by multigenic inheritance.

## GENETIC CROSS: PHENOTYPES AND GENOTYPES

In order to identify additional genetic loci controlling HDL metabolism, we have applied the methodology described in Figure 3.
The genetic cross initially utilized for these studies was constructed from the parental strains C57BL/6J and M. spretus. These two strains were selected for two reasons. First, the inbred strain C57BL/6J is susceptible to early atherosclerosis and HDL cholesterol levels are reduced when maintained on a high fat, high cholesterol diet (10). Second, the inbred strain M. spretus differs greatly from most other laboratory strains of mice in terms of its genetic constitution (it has been estimated that M. spretus mice diverged from laboratory mice (M. musculus) several million years ago). Because of the evolutionary divergence, it is relatively straightforward to identify polymorphisms that serve as genetic markers. The two parental strains were crossed to produce F1 progeny, and the F1 Females were then backcrossed to C57BL/6J males. For any genetic locus, about half of the resulting backcross progeny would be homozygous for the C57BL/6J allele, and about half would be heterozygous (containing one allele from C57BL/6J and one allele from M. spretus). About 250 such backcross animals were studied when the mice in each subgroup are added together.
The levels of HDL in the backcross mice, maintained either on a chow diet or a high fat, high cholesterol diet containing bile acids (high fat diet), are shown in Figure 4. Considerable variability was observed. Thus, HDL-cholesterol levels on the chow diet ranged from about 20 mg/dL to over 100 mg/dL whereas on the high fat diet they range from about 10 mg/dL to over 100 mg/dL. In contrast the

parental strain C57BL/6 exhibited an HDL cholesterol level of about 60 mg/dL on the chow diet and about 30 mg/dL on a high fat diet. <u>M. spretus</u> mice have somewhat higher levels of HDL cholesterol and the levels are not significantly reduced when maintained on a high fat diet (data not shown).

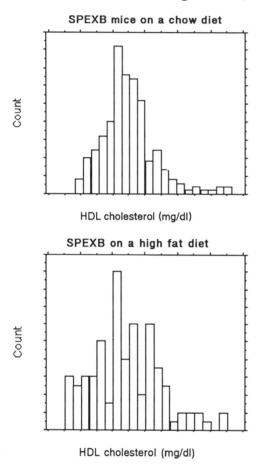

Figure 4. HDL-cholesterol levels among backcross progeny from a genetic cross between inbred strains C57BL/6J (designated "B") and <u>M. spretus</u> (designated "S"). The two strains were crossed to produce F1 animals, which were then backcrossed to the C57BL/6J parental strain. Backcross progeny were then tested for plasma HDL-cholesterol levels on a chow diet or a high fat, high cholesterol diet containing bile acids (HF) (10). HDL was separated from plasma low density and very low density lipoproteins by precipitating the latter with phosphotungstic acid and magnesium chloride. Cholesterol was then determined using an enzymatic procedure.

The backcross mice were individually typed for a large set of genetic markers. Initially they were scored using restriction fragment length polymorphisms identified using cDNA probes for various previously mapped "anchor genes". They were then typed for a new set of genetic markers identified using random mouse liver cDNA clones. We partially sequenced these random cDNA clones and compared the sequences to those in GenBank (70.0). About 30% of the clones proved to correspond to previously identified genes in the mouse or another species. Finally, the mice were typed for a number of "microsatellite" polymorphisms by polymerase chain reaction amplification using appropriate oligonucleotide primers. Thus far, about 188 such genetic markers have been typed among a subset of about 67 C57BL/6J x M. spretus backcross mice (SPEXB mice). We estimate that these markers sweep about 80% of the mouse genome with an interval of 20 centimorgans (cM) or less, although there are a number of clear gaps in which no markers occur.

Among the loci typed were those corresponding to various "candidate genes" that are likely to be involved in HDL metabolism (Figure 5) These include the genes for various apolipoproteins, enzymes involved in plasma cholesterol metabolism, and lipoprotein receptors. Because of accumulating evidence that certain cytokines may influence HDL metabolism, we also typed the genes for interleukin 1 (Il-1) macrophage colony stimulating factor (*Csfm*) and tumor necrosis factor a (*Tnfa*).


## IDENTIFICATION OF POSSIBLE LOCI CONTROLLING HDL LEVELS

Statistical methods were used to identify genetic loci underlying HDL cholesterol levels. In particular, the MAPMAKER-QUANTITATIVE TRAIT LOCUS (QTL) program developed by Lander, Lincoln and colleagues (11) provides a powerful method to identify associations. The program uses the method of maximum likelihood to calculate a probability of the existence of a quantitative trait locus at 2 cM intervals between linked genetic markers. The probability is expressed as a LOD score, which is the $\log_{10}$ of the ratio of the maximum likelihood for an association between the phenotype and the predicted genotype to the maximum likelihood for no association. In the mouse, a LOD score of about 3 is considered significant at the p<0.05 level. The program also provides an estimate of the total variance of the phenotype that is determined by the locus.

Figure 6 shows the results for 3 possible loci contributing to HDL levels found in a survey of the first 67 SPEXB mice. The Chr. 1 locus, with a maximal LOD score of 3.0, appears to determine HDL-cholesterol levels on high fat diet but not a chow diet. (Figure 6a). It is noteworthy that HDL-cholesterol levels in the C57BL/6J parent but not the M. spretus parent decrease about two-fold in response to the high fat diet challenge. Previous studies with recombinant inbred mice suggested that a single major gene (designated *Ath-1*) residing near the gene for apoAII on mouse chromosome 1 determined this trait. However, the locus revealed in C57BL/6J x M. spretus cross appears to be considerably more proximal (to the centromere) than the putative *Ath-1* gene.

10

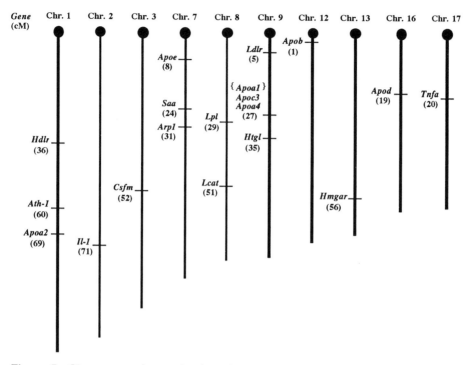

Figure 5. Chromosomal organization of "candidate genes" for HDL metabolism on mouse chromosomes. The positions of the genes are indicated by the gene symbols with the distance (in cM) from the centromere given in parentheses. Beginning with Chr.1, the gene symbols correspond to the following genes: High density lipoprotein receptor (Hdlr); atherosclerosis 1 (Ath-1), apoAII (Apoa2); interleukin 1 (Il-1), macrophage colony stimulating factor (Csfm); apoE (Apoe); serum amyloid A (Saa); apoAl regulatory protein-1 (Arp1); lipoprotein lipase (Lpl); lecithin:cholesterol acyl transferase (Lcat); low density lipoprotein receptor (Ldlr); the apoAl-CIII-AIV gene cluster (Apoa1, Apoc3, Apoa4); hepatic triglyceride lipase (Htgl); apoB (Apob); hydroxymethyl glutaryl Coenzyme A reductase (Hmgar); apoD (Apod); tumor necrosis factor a (Tnfa).

The most striking association was observed with a region of mouse Chr. 2 containing the interleukin 1 (Il-1a) candidate gene (Figure 6b). Maximum LOD scores greater than 4.3 were observed for both total cholesterol and HDL-cholesterol on a chow diet. It should be noted that in most strains of mice maintained on a chow diet, HDL represents by far the major cholesterol carrying particle. Thus, the association with total cholesterol is probably a reflection of HDL-cholesterol.

Finally, a possible association between the fold change of HDL cholesterol (that is, the ratio of HDL levels on the chow diet divided by HDL levels on the high fat diet) was observed with genetic markers on mouse Chr. 15 (Fig. 6c). Chromosome 15 does not contain any obvious candidate genes.

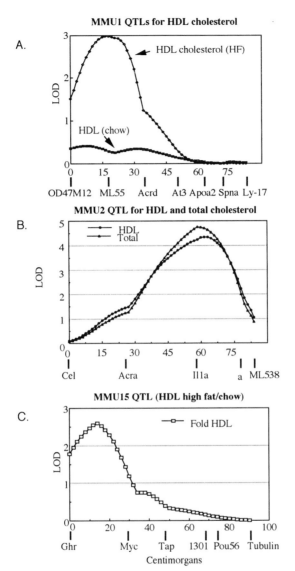

Figure 6. Possible associations between loci on mouse Chr. 1 (a), 2 (b) and 15 (c) and HDL cholesterol levels in C57BL/6J x M. Spretus backcross mice. Plotted on the X axis are the LOD scores for the associations and shown along the Y axis are the locations (in cM) of genetic markers typed among the backcross mice. The results represent analyses of a subset of about 70 mice maintained on a chow diet and then challenged for five weeks with a high fat (HF) diet. The LOD scores were estimated using the MAPMAKER/QTL program.

We have also determined the levels of apoAI, the major protein of HDL, in a subset of backcross mice (data not shown).  As expected, HDL-cholesterol levels (chow) were strongly correlated with serum apoAI levels (chow) (p<0.001).  Also as expected, some of the genetic loci identified for HDL-cholesterol levels were also associated with plasma apoAI levels.  Thus, plasma apoAI levels correlated with the Il-1a gene locus on Chr. 2 (p<0.006), using the non-parametric Mann-Whitney U test).

These results must be considered preliminary since the number of animals examined thus far is relatively small and the LOD scores barely exceed statistical significance.  Experiments are now in progress to extend the studies to the additional C57BL/6J x M. spretus backcross mice and to crosses with other inbred strains of mice.

## ARTERIAL LESIONS

Studies with inbred strains of mice may also allow analysis of the contributions of HDL to fatty streak development.  We scored a subset of backcross mice (maintained on a high fat diet for 15 weeks) for fatty streak formation in the aortic sinus using previously described procedures (12).  When maintained on the high fat diet, strain C57BL/6J mice develop fatty streaks in the aortic sinus whereas M. spretus mice appear to be relatively resistant to lesion development.  C56BL/6J mice also exhibit much lower levels of HDL cholesterol that M. spretus mice when maintained on the high fat diet.

Our survey of the mouse genome revealed an association between aortic fatty streaks and a mouse chromosome 10 cDNA marker ML36 (p<.005, non-parametric Mann-Whitney U test).  ML36 is a randomly isolated mouse liver cDNA clone isolated as a part of the SPEXB mapping effort.  Lesions at the ML36 locus were predominantly found in females with the "BB" C57B46J/C57B46J) genotype.  No lesions were found in "SB" genotype males or females at the ML36 locus.  While this data suggests the existence of a new locus for fatty streak formation, the "n" of 36 animals scored for fatty streaks is too low to allow any definite conclusions about the presence of a fatty streak locus on mouse chromosome 10.  Inbred strains of mice also exhibit genetic differences in the development of lipofuscin pigment in the aortic and mitral valves, with strain C57BL/6J mice being particularly susceptible (12).  Lipofuscin formation may involve processes related to those determining fatty streak development, including lipid oxidation and intimal macrophage accumulation.  A strong correlation (p<0.0001) was observed between aortic and mitral valve lipofuscin, suggesting that common genetic factors control pigment deposition at the two sites.  A possible association between aortic valve lipofuscin and a polymorphism of the apoE gene on Chr. 7 (p<0.008, in females tested by non-parametric Mann-Whitney U) was observed.  This is of potential interest since it has been suggested a gene in the proximal region of Chr. 7 may contribute to fatty streak development in mice (13).

## CONCLUSIONS

Animal models are likely to be of great utility in efforts to understand complex traits such as HDL metabolism. Because of problems resulting from genetic heterogeneity and environmental influences, it is likely that only a subset of the genes important in HDL metabolism can be identified directly through human studies. Our results are preliminary, as only a small number of animals from genetic crosses have been studied thus far. However, the overall approach is clearly feasible and has already been profitably used for studies of complex traits such as diabetes, obesity and hypertension (reviewed in 1). Once the animal loci are identified, it will of course be necessary to isolate and study the responsible genes. This can be approached by "positional cloning", which is at present a very formidable undertaking. Alternatively, it may be possible to identify candidate genes mapping to some of the relevant genetic loci. The results will also be of immediate relevance to human genetic studies in providing "candidate loci" (based on syntenic relationships between animal and human chromosome) for human genetic studies.

## ACKNOWLEDGMENTS

This work was supported by USPHS grants HL42488 and HL28481.

## REFERENCES

1. Lusis AJ, Castellani LW, Fisler J. Curr Opin Lipidol 1992; in press.

2. Breslow JL. In: Schriver, et al., eds. The Metabolic Basis of Inherited Disease. New York: McGraw-Hill, 1989; 6th ed, 1: 1251-1264.

3. Tall A. J Clin Investig 1990; 86: 379-384.

4. Heinzmann C, Kirchgessner T, Kwiterovich PO, Ladias JA, Derby C, Antonarakis SE, Lusis AJ. Hum Genet 1991; 86: 578-584.

5. Humphries SE. Atherosclerosis 1988; 72: 89-108.

6. Ishida BY, Paigen B. In: Lusis AJ, Sparkes RS eds. Genetic Factors in Atherosclerosis: Approaches and Model Systems. Basel, Switzerland: S. Karger AG, 1989; 189-222.

7. Lander ES and Botstein D. 1989. Genetics 121:185-199.

8. Hearne CM, McAleer MA, Love JM, Aitman TJ, Cornall RJ, Ghosh S, Knight AM, Prins J-B, Todd JA. Mammalian Genome 1991; 1: 273-282.

9. Doolittle MH, LeBoeuf RC, Warden CH, Bee LM, Lusis AJ. 1990. J Biol Chem 265:10380-10388.

10. Paigen BD, Mitchell K, Reue K, Morrow A, Lusis AJ, LeBoeuf RC.  Proc Natl Acad Sci USA 1987; 84: 3763-3767.

11. Paterson AH, Lander ES, Hewitt JD, Peterson S, Linsoln SE, Tanksley SD. Science 1988; 335: 721-726.

12. Mehrabian M, Demer LL, Lusis AJ. 1991.  Arteroscl. Thromb. 11: 947-957.

13. Paigen B, Nesbitt MN, Mitchell D, Albee D, LeBoeuf RC.  Genetics 1989; 122: 163-168.

**CORRESPONDENCE**

Aldons J. Lusis
Department of Medicine
University of California
Los Angeles, CA 90024
Phone:  (310) 825-1359
FAX:  (310) 794-7345

High density lipoproteins and atherosclerosis III.
N.E. Miller and A.R. Tall, editors.

Genetics of the lipoprotein lipase/apolipoprotein C-II lipolytic system: insight from structural and evolutionary considerations

L. Chan

Department of Cell Biology, Baylor College of Medicine, One Baylor Plaza, Houston TX 77030

## INTRODUCTION

The metabolism of the triglyceride-rich lipoproteins requires a functional lipoprotein lipase (LPL). A disruption of this process results in elevated chylomicrons and very low density lipoproteins (VLDL) and other indirect consequences. A total absence of LPL function can be inherited in the form of LPL deficiency or apolipoprotein (apo) C-II deficiency, apoC-II being a necessary cofactor for LPL action. It is known that heterozygous LPL deficiency is a cause of familial combined hyperlipidemia, the most common form of genetically transmitted hyperlipidemia [1]. In contrast, the phenotype for heterozygous apoC-II deficiency is not well established because the number of such individuals is still quite small. Most of them have been reported to have normal lipid values, though as a group their triglycerides may be slightly elevated.

## LIPOPROTEIN LIPASE

Lipoprotein lipase belongs to the lipase super-family which includes LPL, hepatic lipase (HL) pancreatic lipase (PL) and Drosophila vitellogenins [2,3]. The three vertebrate lipases share considerable sequence homology. LPL and HL are more similar to each other than either is to PL. Evolutionarily LPL and HL probably came from a common ancestor which had previously diverged from PL. Among the three lipase genes, LPL is evolutionarily the most conservative [3].

The similarity in structure among LPL, HL and PL indicates that they have similar mechanism of action. The crystal structure of PL was recently published by Winkler et al. [4]. PL active center was found to consist of a serine protease-like catalytic Asp-His-Ser triad. Sequence alignment with LPL indicates that a similar triad exists in LPL which maps to residues $Asp^{156}$, $His^{241}$ and $Ser^{132}$. The high degree of sequence conservation between LPL and PL and the site-dependent variation in the enzymatic activities of a large number of site-specific LPL mutants strongly suggest that LPL has a three-dimensional structure very similar to that of PL.

Lipoprotein lipase contains 10 exons and 9 introns [2,5]. Exons 2 - 9 cover all the coding regions of LPL. Intron 9 splits the termination codon and exons 1 and 10 encompass a large part of the 5' untranslated region and all the 3' untranslated region of LPL, respectively. The catalytic residues, $Ser^{132}$, $Asp^{156}$ and $His^{241}$ are located within exon 4, 5 and 6 respectively.

A large number of mutations affecting LPL activity have been described (Table 1). These include major disruptions of the gene such as deletions, rearrangements, splice mutations, nonsense and frameshift mutations, as well as a large number of missense mutations. It is reasonable to expect that LPL catalytic function will be lost or grossly impaired with the first two major groups of gene disruptions shown in Table 1. Some of these mutations are also associated with an absence of detectable LPL mRNA or protein presumably caused by highly unstable transcripts or translation products. In addition to such major defects, LPL deficiency has also been reported to result from a large number of point mutations causing single amino acid substitutions which have been grouped under missense mutations in Table 1. Most of these missense mutations are located in exons 4, 5 and 6 which contain the catalytic triad residues. One of the triad residues, Asp[156], has actually been reported to be mutated in 2 unrelated families with the syndrome of familial chylomicronemia, to a Gly residue in one case, and an Asn residue in another. One case of an exon 3 mutation, Trp[86]→Arg, has been reported recently [6].

Table 1.
Mutations in the LPL Gene Causing Familial Chylomicronemia

---

1. Deletions, Rearrangements, and Splice Mutations
   6 kb deletion → missing exons 3, 4 and 5
   2 kb duplication → disrupted exon 6
   Splice mutants: intron 2 (donor Ggt→Gat, acceptor gG→aG)

2. Nonsense and Frameshift Mutations
   Tyr 61   → Stop
   Gln 106  → Stop
   Tyr 262  → Stop
   Trp 382  → Stop
   5 bp insertion in exon 3

3. Missense Mutations
   Exon 3:  Trp 86   →  Arg
   Exon 4:  Gly 142  →  Glu
   Exon 5:  Asp 156  →  Gly
            Asp 156  →  Asn
            Pro 157  →  Arg
            Ala 176  →  Thr
            Gly 188  →  Glu
            Ile 194  →  Thr
            Asp 204  →  Glu
            Pro 207  →  Leu
            Cys 216  →  Ser
   Exon 6:  Arg 243  →  His
            Ser 244  →  Thr

---

Most of these mutations have been summarized by Hayden et al. [7]. Some of these not included in the review were reported by Faustinella et al. [8], Gotoda et al. [9], and Ishimura-Oka [6,10].

The occurrence of a large number of missense mutations in LPL deficiency is quite consistent with out understanding of the structural requirement for LPL function. For example, Faustinella et al. [11] have studied the functional activities of a large number of mutants involving 8 different Ser residues in LPL. They found that many of the mutations inactivated the enzyme, although only in the case of Ser[132] were all the mutant LPLs involving the same site completely inactive. The evolutionarily highly conserved structure of LPL suggests that deviations from the conserved residues are not well tolerated. Therefore, the large number of inactive Ser mutants reported by Faustinella et al. [11] and the numerous missense mutations shown in Table 1 are quite consistent with this interpretation.

The true prevalence of LPL deficiency is unknown [12]. It has been assumed that homozygous LPL deficiency is a relatively rare disease, occurring perhaps one in a million. However, this presumed prevalence rate does not take into consideration patients with less severe disorders who exhibit reduced but detectable postheparin LPL activity. Furthermore, unless there are clearly symptomatic homozygous relatives, we will easily miss patients with heterozygous LPL deficiency. Since the heterozygote state is a major cause of combined familial hyperlipidemia [1] and possibly of other forms of mild hypertriglyceridemia, heterozygous LPL deficiency is probably much more common than the one in five hundred as projected from the conservative estimate of one in a million homozygous rate.

## APOLIPOPROTEIN C-II

Apolipoprotein C-II is a 79-amino acid polypeptide. It is part of the apolipoprotein multigene family. In common with the other soluble apolipoprotein genes, it has a 3-intron, 4-exon genomic organization [13]. Moreover, apoC-II contains 11- and 22-amino acid repeats; 3 of the 11-amino acid repeats comprise the common 33-codon block in exon 3 found in all the soluble apolipoproteins [14].

ApoC-II is a cofactor for LPL; the activity of the enzyme is stimulated 5-10 fold in the presence of apoC-II. The structural requirement for apoC-II function has been investigated by synthetic peptide fragments or proteolytic fragments of apoC-II. The carboxy-terminal half of apoC-II appears to be much more important that the amino-terminal half for LPL activation. The minimal fragment that is active contains residues 61-79 [15,16]. Using monolayer techniques, Balasubramaniam et al. [17] found that at high surface pressure, fragment 56-79 was inactive. Attachment of an N-α-palmitoyl group to the amino-terminus of this fragment restored activity suggesting that the amphipathic helical segments predicted from amino-terminal sequences missing in this segment were required for lipid binding. Six vertebrate apoC-II sequences have been reported. Sequence alignment of these sequences indicates that apoC-II is not a conservative protein; substantial change in the primary structure has occurred with evolution (Fig. 1). Furthermore, it is apparent that the carboxy-terminal region is better conserved than the amino-terminal region of the molecule [18]. The region encoded by the 33-codon block in exon 3 is usually one of the best conserved regions when multiple sequences for individual soluble apolipoproteins are analyzed. In the case of apoC-II, this region is not as well conserved as the 22-residue repeat in exon 4 (Fig. 1) [18]. Synthetic peptide experiments suggested that the carboxy-terminal tripeptide Gly-Glu-Glu is essential for LPL activation [15]. It is evident from sequence comparison that only the Gly residue is conserved among the three residues. The penultimate residue is a charged residue among all vertebrate species examined (Fig. 1). Therefore the carboxy-terminal tripeptide has the consensus sequence Gly-X-Y where X is a charged residue.

```
                              33-codon block            C-II-4              79
        ##  ++++  +  #+      +#+ #+  #+##++  ++  #+  ##+  #+  +#+++##+#+#++#++#+++#  ##+ +
Hum  TQQPQQDEMPSPTFLTQ  VKESLSSYWESAKTAAQNLYEKTYLPAVDEKLR  DLYSKSTAAMSTYTGIFTDQVL  SVLKGEE
Chm  TQQPQQDEMPSPTFLTQ  VKESLSSYRESAKTAAQNLYEKTYLPAVDEKLR  DLYSKSTAAMSTYTGIFTDQVL  SVLKGEE
Mac  AQLPQQDEPPSPALLSR  VQESLSSYWESAKAAAQKLYEKTYLPAVDEKLR  DLYSKSTAAMSTYTGIFTDQVL  SVLKGEE
Cow  AHVPQQDEASSPALLTQ  VQESLLGYWDTAKAAAQKLYKKTYLPAVDEKIR  DIYSKSTAAVTTYAGIITDQVF  SVLSGKD
Dog  AHESQQDETTSSALLTQ  MQESLYSYWGTARSAAEDLYKKAYPTTMDEKIR  DIYSKSTAAVSTYAGIFTDQLL  SMLKGDS
Gpg  AHLTQQDEPTSPDLL--  --ETLSTYWDSAKAAAQGLYNNTYLPAVDETIR  DIYSKGSAAISTYTGILTDQIL  TMLQGKQ
```

Figure 1. Comparison of amino acid sequences of apoC-II. There is a common block of 33 residues at the end of exon 3, and the region encoded by exon 4 contains repeats of 11 or 22 residues, which are labeled as repeats E-4, E-5, etc. All these repeats are underlined. Residues identical among all the sequences aligned (+); residues that are similar in physiochemical properties (#). Hum, human; Chm, chimpanzee; Mac, Macaque (the cynomolgus monkey); Gpg, guinea pig. The sources of apoC-II sequences: human [13]; chimpanzee [19]; macaque [20]; cow [21], dog [22] and guinea pig [23].

The relatively rapid change in structure allowed in apoC-II evolution suggests that the structural requirement for apoC-II function is relatively lax. This conclusion is supported by observations on the genetic defects giving rise to apoC-II deficiency.

Familial apoC-II deficiency is a very rare autosomal recessive disorder [12]. It presents in the homozygous state as familial chylomicronemia. To date, only a handful of apoC-II deficiency alleles have been characterized (Table 2). The primary defect varies from splice junction mutations, frame-shift mutations, nonsense mutations to mutations affecting initiation codons and multiple mutations that appear to totally preclude the synthesis of any apoC-II-like proteins. In comparison with the mutations characterized in LPL deficiency (Table 1), conspicuously absent among the deleterious apoC-II mutations are missense mutations. Therefore, all mutations in the apoC-II gene described to date cause severe disruption of apoC-II protein structure or result in a total absence of circulating apoC-II. Since a highly conserved structure appears not to be required for apoC-II function, it is likely that many missense mutations in apoC-II are compatible with normal or only slightly impaired function. In other words, they are phenotypically silent and are routinely missed when we screen for patients with lipid disorders. It is probable that they occur fairly commonly.

Table 2.
Mutations in the ApoC-II Gene Causing Chylomicronemia

| Mutant Allele | Mutation | Consequence |
|---|---|---|
| ApoC-II$_{Hamburg}$ | G→C mutation at donor splice site of intron 2 | Abnormally spliced mRNA |
| ApoC-II$_{Nijmegen}$ | G deletion, exon 3 | Premature termination → ? 17 amino acid peptide (not detected) |
| ApoC-II$_{Padova}$ | C→A mutation, exon 3 | Premature termination → ? 36 amino acid peptide (8 kDa protein detected) |
| ApoC-II$_{Paris\ 1}$ | ATG→GUG, exon 2 | No apoC-II detected |
| ApoC-II$_{Paris\ 2}$ | T→C mutation, exon 2 | Premature termination at amino acid -19 of signal peptide → no apoC-II detected |
| ApoC-II$_{Toronto}$ | Deletion of a base at Thr$^{68}$ or Asp$^{69}$ | Abnormal sequence after Asp$^{69}$ terminating at residue 74 |
| ApoC-II$_{St.\ Michael}$ | Base insertion at Asp$^{69}$ or Gln$^{70}$ | Abnormal sequence after Asp$^{69}$ terminating at residue 96 |
| ApoC-II$_{Jap}$ | Multiple mutations, exons 3 & 4 | No apoC-II detected |
| ApoC-II$_{Ven}$ | Multiple mutations, exons 3 & 4 | No apoC-II detected |

The first 5 mutations were characterized by Fojo and associates [24-26]; the Canadian mutations were characterized by Connelly and associates [27,28]; the Japanese and Venezuelan mutations were reported by Xiong et al. [19].

## CONCLUSION

In conclusion, an evolutionary approach has led to predictions of the structural constraints that govern LPL and apoC-II function. The very stringent structural constraint for LPL action and the relatively lax sequence requirement for apoC-II function appear to be borne out by the molecular genetic defects in LPL and apoC-II deficiency. Further knowledge of apoC-II function can be achieved, as in the case of LPL, by additional functional studies on site-specific mutants. A more complete understanding of how these two proteins interact and function must await the determination of their three-dimensional structure.

## REFERENCES

1   Babirak SP, Iverius P-H, Fujimoto WY, Brunzell JD. Arteriosclerosis 1989; 9:326-334.
2   Kirchgessner TG, Chuat JC, Heinzman C, Etienne J, et al. Proc. Natl. Acad. Sci. USA 1989; 86: 9647-9651.
3   Hide WA, Chan L, Li W-H. J Lipid Res 1992; 33: 167-178.
4   Winkler FK, D'Arcy A, Hunziker W. Nature 1990; 343: 771-774.
5   Deeb SS, Peng R. Biochemistry 1989; 28: 4131-4135.
6   Ishimura-Oka K, Faustinella F, Kihara S, Smith LC, et al. Am J Hum Genet 1992; (in press).
7   Hayden MR, Ma Y, Brunzell JD, Henderson HE. Curr Opin Lipidol 1991; 2: 104-109.
8   Faustinella F, Chang A, Van Biervliet JP, Rosseneu M, et al. J Biol Chem 1991; 266:14418-14424.
9   Gotoda T, Yamada N, Kawamura M, Kozaiki K, et al. J Clin Invest 1991; 88: 1856-1864.
10  Ishimura-Oka K, Semenkovich CF, Faustinella F, Goldberg IJ, et al. J Lipid Res 1992; (in press).
11  Faustinella F, Smith LC, Semenkovich CF, Chan L. J Biol Chem 1991; 266: 9481-9485.
12  Brunzell JD (1989) In: Scriver CR, Beaudet AL, Sly WS, Valle D, eds. The Metabolic Basis of Inherited Disease, New York: McGraw-Hill, 1989; 1165-1180.
13  Wei CF, Tsao YK, Robberson DL, Gotto AM Jr, et al. J Biol Chem 1985; 260: 15211-15221.
14  Li W-H, Tanimura M, Luo C-C, Datta S, et al. J Lipid Res 1988; 29: 245-271.
15  Kinnunen PKJ, Jackson RL, Smith LC, Gotto AM, et al. Proc Natl Acad Sci USA 1977; 74: 4848-4851.
16  Vaino P, Virtanen JA, Kinnunen PKJ, Voyta JC, et al. Biochemistry 1983; 22: 2270-2275.
17  Balasubramaniam A, Rechtin A, McLean LR, Jackson RL. Biochem Biophys Res Commun 1986; 137: 1041-1048.
18  Chan L, Li W-H. In: Rosseneu M, ed. Structure and Function of Plasma Apolipoproteins. Boca Raton, Florida: CRC Press Inc., 1992 (in press).
19  Xiong W, Li W-H, Posner I, Yamamura T, et al. Am J Hum Genet 1991; 48:383-389.
20  Whitted BE, Castle CK, Polites HG, Melchior GW, et al. Molec Cell Biochem 1989; 90: 69-79.
21  Bengtsson-Olivecrona G, Sletten K. Eur J Biochem 1990; 192: 515-521.
22  Datta S, Li W-H, Ghosh I, Luo C-C, Chan L. J Biol Chem 1987; 262: 10588-10593.
23  Andersson Y, Thelander L, Bengtsson-Olivecrona G. J Biol Chem 1991; 266: 4074-4080.
24  Fojo SS, de Gennes J-L, Chapman J, Parrott C, et al. J Biol Chem 1989; 264: 20893-20842.

25  Fojo SS, Beisiegel U, Beil U, Higuchi K, et al. J Clin Invest 1988; 82: 1489-1494.
26  Fojo SS, Stalenhoef AFH, Marr K, Gregg RE, et al. J Biol Chem 1988; 263: 17913-17916.
27  Connelly PW, Maguire GF, Hoffman T, Little JA.  Proc Natl Acad Sci USA 1987; 84: 270-273.
28  Connelly PW, Maguire GF, Little AJ.  J Clin Invest 1987; 80: 1597-1606.

# Apolipoprotein AI Gene Regulation by Members of the Steroid/Thyroid Hormone Receptor Superfamily of Ligand Dependent Transcription Factors

## S.K. Karathanasis

## Department of Cardiovascular Molecular Biology, Lederle Laboratories, Pearl River, New York 10965

## INTRODUCTION

A large body of biochemical, nutritional and epidemiological observations suggest that apolipoprotein AI (apoAI) plasma levels are influenced by a diverse number of hormonal, dietary and various other environmental and physiological stimuli (for a recent review see ref. 1). Although intravascular metabolic events contribute significantly to the fluctuations of apoAI plasma levels in response to these stimuli, recent findings suggest that variations at the level of expression of the gene coding for apoAI may also contribute directly. For example, feeding of non-human primates with high amounts of polyunsaturated fat and cholesterol decreases hepatic apoAI mRNA and plasma apoAI levels (2), and hyperthyroidism, induced by administration of thyroid hormones to rats, increases hepatic apoAI gene transcription rates and plasma apoAI levels (3,4). These observations raise the possibility that the expression of the apoAI gene is regulated by signal transduction mechanisms responsive to these stimuli.

Recent progress in understanding transcriptional control in eukaryotes has revealed that the most common way to regulate gene expression in response to extracellular signals is by modulating the activity of transcription factors that recognize specific cis-acting elements in the regulatory regions of the genes, the transcription of which is affected by these signals (for recent reviews see refs. 5,6). It, therefore, follows that identification and characterization of transcriptional factors required for establishment and maintenance of gene expression could be instrumental in both the delineation of signal transduction pathways and the identification of relevant physiological signals involved in modulation of gene expression.

As summarized in the current communication, application of this principle in the case of the apoAI gene has led to the concept that apoAI gene expression is modulated by signal transduction mechanisms similar to those involved in modulation of expression of steroid/thyroid hormone responsive genes (reviewed in 7-9). These findings raise the possibility that upregulation of apoAI gene expression by manipulation of these signal transduction pathways may provide new pharmacological targets for sustained increase of plasma apoAI levels.

## RESULTS

1.  <u>Synergistic interactions between transcription factors control expression of the apoAI gene in liver cells.</u>
    Previous studies showed that in mammals, the apoAI gene is expressed predominantly in the liver and the intestine (see for example refs. 10, 11). Taking advantage of the observations that this pattern of expression is retained in various cell lines, for example the human hepatoma HepG2 and colon carcinoma Caco-2 cell lines (12), and that these cells can be easily

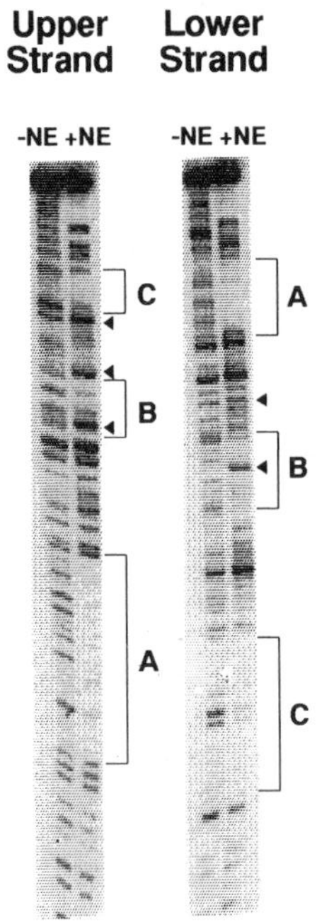

**Upper Lower**
**Strand Strand**

**Figure 1. Binding of nuclear proteins in HepG2 cells to three distinct sites within the apoAI gene enhancer.** A DNA fragment containing the -256 to -80 apoAI gene 5'-flanking sequences was labeled at the 5' end of either the coding (upper) or noncoding (lower) strand and used for DNase I protection experiments without (-NE) or with (+NE) HepG2 nuclear extracts as described in ref. 13. Sites protected by DNase I digestion (A, B, and C) are bracketed and DNase I sites induced by the extracts (DNase I-hypersensitive sites) are indicated by arrowheads.

transfected with plasmid DNA, we used various apoAI gene deletion plasmid constructs to delineate the cis-acting elements that control expression of the apoAI gene in liver and intestine (12,13). These studies revealed that different cis-acting elements control expression of the apoAI gene in liver and intestine (12) and that liver specific expression is controlled by a powerful liver-specific enhancer located between nucleotides -222 to -110 upstream of the apoAI gene transcription start site

(+1) (13). These findings raised the possibility that hepatocytes contain trans-acting factors that bind to cis-acting elements within this enhancer and stimulate transcription of the apoAI gene in liver.

A survey for such factors, carried out by DNase I protection experiments, revealed that indeed liver and HepG2 cells contain proteins that bind to three sites, sites A (-214 to -192), B (-169 to -146) and C (-134 to -119) within this enhancer and protect them from digestion by DNase I (Fig. 1 and refs 13,14). This , together with the observation that nuclei from several other tissues and cell lines that do not express apoAI contain proteins that bind to site A but not sites B and C (14) suggested that occupation of all three of these sites by nuclear factors is essential for expression of the apoAI gene in liver cells. This was further substantiated by site directed mutagenesis experiments indicating that prevention of binding of nuclear factors to a single site dramatically reduces expression of the apoAI gene in HepG2 cells while prevention of binding to two sites, in any combination, completely eliminates expression (13).

These findings and other relevant results detailed in ref. 13 established that maximal expression of the apoAI gene in liver cells is strongly dependent on synergistic interactions between transcription factors bound to all these sites A, B and C within the apoAI gene enhancer.

2.  ARP-1, a novel member of the steroid/thyroid receptor superfamily binds to site A and represses expression of the apoAI gene in liver cells.

To begin unravelling the molecular interactions between transcription factors involved in the control of expression of the apoAI gene in liver cells, we isolated the cDNA for a protein that binds to site A by screening a human placenta expression library for clones that produce proteins that bind to site A (14). Conceptual translation of this cDNA sequence and comparison of the resulting protein sequence with other proteins in various protein data banks revealed that this protein, which was named apolipoprotein AI regulatory protein 1 (ARP-1), is a novel member of the steroid/thyroid receptor superfamily of ligand dependent transcription factors (14, for reviews on steroid/thyroid receptor superfamily see refs. 7-9). The ability of ARP-1 to bind specifically and with high affinity (Kd=5nM) to site A was shown by DNase I protection, electrophoretic mobility shift, and methylation interference assays (14,15). These findings suggested that regulation of apoAI gene expression may be accomplished, at least in part, by signaling mechanisms similar to those regulating other genes responsive to these hormones (see refs. 7-9) and stimulated interest in the identification of signal(s) or ligand(s) to which ARP-1 responds. Although such signals or ligands have not yet been identified, transient transfection experiments indicated that ARP-1 influences apoAI gene expression. Specifically, cotransfection of HepG2 cells with constant amounts of a plasmid that expresses the bacterial chloramphenicol acetyl transferase (CAT) gene under the control of the apoAI gene enhancer and basal promoter (construct

-256AI.CAT ref. 12) and increasing amounts of a plasmid construct that expresses ARP-1 (construct pMT2-ARP-1 ref. 14, 16) resulted in a dramatic repression of the ability of -256AI.CAT to express CAT activity in these cells (Fig. 2, ref. 14). Although for this repression, ARP-1 must bind to site A because another apoAI gene construct that lacks site A (construct -192 AI.CAT ref. 12) is not repressed by ARP-1 (14), binding alone is not sufficient to repress expression of other basal promoters.

## -25GA1.CAT

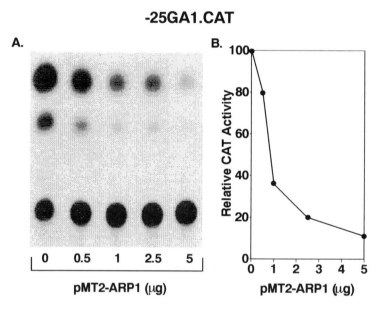

**Figure 2.  Repression of apoAI gene expression by ARP-1.** HepG2 cells were cotransfected with 10μg of the apoAI gene plasmid construct -256AI.CAT, 3μg of a control plasmid that expresses ß-galactosidase (ß-gal) under the control of the Rous Sarcoma Viral promoter, pRSV-ß-gal (see ref. 12) and the indicated amounts of the ARP-1 expression vector pMT2-ARP-1. The ß-gal activity in extracts prepared from these cells 48 hours after transfection was determined (see ref. 12) and used to normalize the amounts of extracts subsequently used for CAT assays (see ref. 12).  Panel A shows typical results from such an experiment.  Panel B shows normalized CAT activities expressed as percentages of the activity obtained with cells translated in the absence of pMT2-ARP-1 (Relative CAT Activity) averaged for three independent experiments.

For example, the presence of one or multiple copies of site A proximal to the simplex virus thymidine kinase (TK) gene promoter is not sufficient for repression of this promoter in response to increasing amounts of ARP-1 (unpublished data).

These observations suggested that ARP-1 by binding to site A, somehow interferes with the synergistic interactions between the transcription factors that bind to sites A, B and C in the apoAI gene enhancer, and thus represses apoAI gene expression in HepG2 cells. Furthermore, these observations suggested that either ARP-1 itself, in the presence of an appropriate ligand, or some other transcription factor that also binds to site A in liver cells participates in these synergistic interactions.

3.   Site A is a conditional retinoic acid response element.

Although, as mentioned above, the possibility that ARP-1, in the presence of an appropriate ligand, could activate apoAI gene expression has not been excluded, other evidence such as characterization of DNA-protein complexes formed with site A and liver nuclear proteins, using antibodies that immunoreact with ARP-1, have indicated that liver cells contain, in addition to ARP-1, other proteins that also bind to site A (unpublished observations).

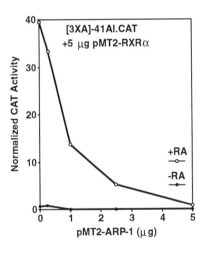

**Figure 3.   ARP-1 antagonizes RXRα and RA transactivation of the apoAI gene basal promoter.** The plasmid [3XA]-41AI.CAT was transiently transfected into HepG2 cells with 5μg of pMT2-RXRα and the indicated amounts of the ARP-1 expression vector pMT2-ARP-1 in the presence (open circles) or absence (filled circles) of $10^{-6}$M RA. Normalized CAT activity is defined in the legend to Fig. 2.

An attempt to clone cDNAs for such proteins by screening a human liver cDNA library with a DNA probe corresponding to the ARP-1 DNA binding domain led to the cloning of another member of the steroid/thyroid hormone receptor superfamily that functions as a transcriptional activator in the presence of retinoic acid (RXRα ref. 17). We have shown previously that RXRα binds to site A specifically and with high affinity (Kd=8.8nM) and activates nearby basal promoters, such as the TK promoter (construct [A] TK.CAT ref. 17) or the apoAI gene basal promoter (construct [A] -41A1.CAT ref. 15) in the presence of retinoic acid (RA).

The similarities of ARP-1 and RXRα in binding specificity and affinity for site A prompted the evaluation of their combined effects on the transcriptional activity of site A in the context of the basal apoAI gene promoter. Specifically, HepG2 cells were cotransfected with a constant amount of a plasmid construct containing three copies of site A inserted proximal to the apoAI gene basal promoter (construct [3XA]-41AI.CAT ref. 15), a constant amount of a vector that expresses RXRα (pMT2-RXRα ref. 17) and increasing amounts of a vector that expresses ARP-1 (pMT2-ARP-1 ref. 16) in the presence or absence of RA. As shown in Fig. 3, in the absence of RA, RXRα alone did not stimulate CAT expression, as expected, and the presence of increasing amounts of ARP-1 together with RXRα did not alter this pattern of expression (Fig 3A filled circles). However, the substantial stimulation of expression mediated by RXRα in the presence of RA was progressively inhibited by increasing amounts of ARP-1 (Fig.3A open circles). Control experiments showed that ARP-1 alone in the presence or absence of RA did not stimulate expression (15).

It is therefore concluded that the RXRα and RA mediated transcription activation of the apoAI basal promoter from site A is efficiently inhibited by ARP-1 and that the absolute level of RXRα and RA dependent transactivation is determined by the intracellular ratio of ARP-1 and RXRα. Thus, it appears that site A functions as a conditional retinoic acid response element; it responds to RXRα and RA when the intracellular ARP-1 concentration is low but loses responsiveness when the ARP-1 concentration is high.

4.   RXRα and RA alleviate ARP-1 mediated repression of the apoAI gene.

The ability of site A to function as a retinoic acid response element raised the possibility that signal transduction pathways relevant to RA signaling may regulate apoAI gene expression. To examine this possibility directly, HepG2 cells were cotransfected with the construct-256AI.CAT and the RXRα expressing vector pMT2-RXRα in the presence or absence of RA.

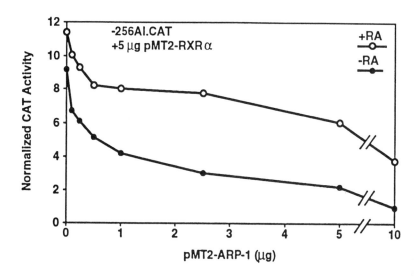

**Figure 4. RXR$\alpha$ and RA alleviate ARP-1 mediated repression of the apoAI gene.** The CAT reporter construct -256AI.CAT (10µg) was cotransfected into HepG2 cells with 5µg of pMT2-RXR$\alpha$ and increasing amounts of the ARP-1 expression vector pMT2-ARP-1 as indicated. Normalized CAT activity, defined in the legend to Fig. 2, is shown in the presence (open circles) or absence (filled circles) of $10^{-6}$M RA.

The CAT activities in these cells were subsequently determined and compared. As shown in Fig. 4 (15), there is only a small increase of CAT activity in the presence of RA compared to that in its absence. In contrast, when the same experiment was repeated in the presence of increasing amounts of the ARP-1 expression vector pMT2-ARP-1, the ARP-1 mediated repression of the activity of the -256 AI.CAT construct was almost completely alleviated in the presence, but not in the absence of RA (Fig. 4, ref. 15).

Based on these findings, we concluded that ARP-1 repression sensitizes transactivation of the apoAI gene by RXR$\alpha$ in the presence of RA and that the extent of this sensitization is controlled by the intracellular ratio of ARP-1 and RXR$\alpha$.

## DISCUSSION

Although several previous studies have shown that variations in apoAI gene expression can be accounted, at least in part, by alterations in apoAI gene transcription rates (ref. 15 and refs. therein), neither the precise nature of signals regulating transcription nor relevant signaling mechanisms are clearly understood.

The studies summarized in this communication strongly suggest that at least one mechanism by which apoAI gene is regulated involves signal tranduction pathways similar to those involved in regulation of genes responsive to steroid hormones. Specifically, the observation that one of the cis-acting elements in the apoAI gene liver specific enhancer (ie: site A) can be occupied by at least two members of the steroid/thyroid receptor superfamily of ligand dependent transcription factors (ie: ARP-1 and RXRα) taken together with the established role of this family of transcription factors in modulation of gene transcription in response to small hydrophobic extracellular signaling molecules, for example steroid and thyroid hormones (reviewed in refs. 7-9), raise the possibility that the apoAI gene is also regulated by such small hydrophobic signaling molecules. It is, therefore, tempting to speculate that since apoAI plays a major role in plasma lipid metabolism the identification of such signaling molecules may help to establish the existence of communication networks between intravascular lipid metabolism and apoAI gene regulation.

Although for the sake of simplicity, the binding of only ARP-1 and RXRα to site A was emphasized in the current communication, other published and unpublished observations indicate that many different members of the steroid/thyroid receptor superfamily also bind to site A with high affinity. The functional consequences of binding of these proteins on the expression of the apoAI gene basal promoter from site A vary, from constitutive activation by the hepatocyte nuclear factor 4 (HNF4, unpublished observations) and inducible activation by RXRα and RXRα/retinoic acid receptor α (RARα) heterodimers in the presence of RA (ref. 15 and unpublished observations) to repression of either constitutive or inducible activation by ARP-1, ear3-COUP-TF and ARP-1/ear3-COUP-TF and ARP-1/RXRα heterodimers (ref. 15 and unpublished observations). These observations, together with the recent finding that the ligand responsiveness of RXRα can be redirected by formation of heterodimers with the thyroid hormone receptor (TR), vitamin D3 receptor (VDR) and RARα that respond to thyroid hormone, Vitamin D3 and RA respectively (18-21), strongly suggest that site A is the receiving end of signals from diverse signaling pathways. Furthermore, the remarkable recent finding that the activity of various members of the steroid/thyroid receptor superfamily is regulated by the Jun and Fos protooncogenes which transmit transcriptional signals generated by a completely different signal tranduction pathways involving cell surface receptors and various intracellular second messengers (reviewed in refs 22-24) argues that apoAI gene expression is connected, through site A, to an extensive signaling network that monitors and integrates a large number of signals influencing cell behavior.

Assuming that this astonishing diversity of signals channeled directly or indirectly to site A is operational in vivo, it may not be surprising that occupation of site A by a given trans-acting factor is tightly controlled by both positive and negative mechanisms. Although the possibility has not been excluded that ARP-1 in the presence of an appropriate ligand may function as an activator, it is clear that in the absence of such a ligand ARP-1, when in high enough intracellular concentrations, displaces endogenous or exogenously added activators thus repressing transcription from site A (see also ref. 16 for similar findings with the apolipoprotein CIII gene). Thus the observation that RXRα and RA, although incapable of activating apoAI gene expression, are effective in alleviation of ARP-1 mediated repression of the apoAI gene in liver cells raises the intriguing possibility that repression by ARP-1 is a prerequisite step for replacement of endogenous activators bound to site A by RXRα. Whether ARP-1 repression represents a general mechanism for switching occupation of site A from one transactivator to another and thus facilitating responsiveness of the apoAI gene to diverse signaling pathways is a very interesting possibility and it is currently under investigation.

In conclusion, although the recently established mechanisms for eukaryotic gene regulation provide the guiding concepts for the unraveling of signal transduction pathways and for the identification of relevant signaling molecules influencing apoAI gene expression using the reverse (ie: from the nucleus to the extracellular environment) physiology approach outlined in this communication, the existence and utilization of these pathways must also be substantiated by forward physiology. In this context it is interesting that we have recently observed that RA feeding to rabbits increases their apoAI plasma levels. We are currently investigating whether this is due to the RXRα signaling pathway described in this communication.

## ACKNOWLEDGEMENTS

I would like to thank Drs. Alan R. Tall and Aldons J. Lusis for critically reading the manuscript, Liisa Warren for typing and editing the manuscript, and Dawn Dykstra for the art work. I would also like to thank Drs. Yisheng Wang, Myungchull Rhee, Patricia Costa-Giomi, Andrew Katocs and Elwood Largis for permitting referencing of some of their unpublished results.

# REFERENCES

1. **Karathanasis, S.K.** In: Lusis AJ, Rotter JI, Sparkes RS, eds. Molecular Genetics of Coronary Artery Disease. Candidate Gnes and Processes In Atherosclerosis. Monogr Hum Genet. Basel: Karger, 1992; vol 14, 140-171.

2. **Sorci-Thomas, M., M. M. Prack, N. Dashti, F. Johnson, L. L. Rudel, and D.L. Williams.** J. Lipid Res. 1989; 30:1397-1402.

3. **Apostolopoulos, J.J., M.J. La Sala, and G.J. Howlett.** Biochem Biophys. Res. Commun. 1988;154:997-1002.

4. **Wilcox, H.G., R.A. Frank, and M. Heimberg.** J. Lipid Res. 1991; 32:395-405.

5. **Karin, M.** Curr. Opin. Cell Biol. 1991; 3:467-473.

6. **Roeder, R.G.** Trends Biochem. Sci. 1991; 16:402-408

7. **Evans, R.M.** Science. 1988; 240:889

8. **Green, S., and P. Chambon.** Trends Genet. 1988; 4:309

9. **Beato, M.** Cell. 1989; 56:335

10. **Zannis, V.I., F.S. Cole, C.L. Jackson, D.M. Kurnit, and S.K. Karathanasis.** Biochemistry. 1985; 24:4450-4455.

11. **Haddad, I.A., J.M. Ordovas, T. Fitzpatrick, and S.K. Karathanasis.** J. Biol. Chem. 1986; 261:13268-13274.

12. **Sastry, K.N., U. Seedorf, and S.K. Karathanasis.** Mol. Cell. Biol. 1988; 8: 605-614.

13. **Widom, R.L., J.A.A. Ladias, S. Kouidou, and S.K. Karathanasis.** Mol. Cell. Biol. 1991; 11:677-687.

14. **Ladias, J.A.A., and S.K. Karathanasis.** Science. 1991; 251:561-564.

15. **Widom, R.L., M. Rhee, S.K. Karathanasis.** Mol. Cell. Biol. 1992; (in press)

16. **Mietus-Snyder, M., F.M. Sladek, G.S. Ginsburg, C.F. Kuo, J.A.A. Ladias, J.E. Darnell, Jr., and S.K. Karathanasis.** Mol. Cell. Biol. 1992; 12:1708-1718.

17. **Rottman, J.N., R.L. Widom, B. Nadal-Ginard, V.Mahdavi, and S.K. Karathanasis.** Mol. Cell. Biol. 1991; 11: 3814-3820.

18. **Kliewer, S.A., K. Umesono, D.J. Mangelsdorf, and R.M. Evans.** Nature. 1992; 355:446-449.

19. **Leid, M., P. Kastner, R. Lyons, H. Nakshatri, M. Saunders, T. Zacharewski, J-Y. Chen, A. Staub, J-M. Garnier, S. Mader, and P. Chambon.** Cell. 1992; 68:377-395.

20. **Yu, V.C., C. Delsert, B. Andersen, J.M. Holloway, O. Devary, A.M.Naar, S.Y. Kim, J-M. Boutin, C.K. Glass, and M.G. Rosenfeld.** Cell. 1991; 67:1251-1266.

21. **Zhang, X-K., B. Hoffman, P.V-V. Tran, G. Graupner and M. Pfahl.** Nature. 1992; 355: 441-446.

22. **Miner, J.N. and K.R. Yamamoto.** Trends Biochem. Sci. 1991; 16:423-426.

23. **Miner, J.N., M.I. Diamond, and K.R. Yamamoto.** Trends Biochem. Sci. 1991; 2:525:530.

24. **Schule, R., and R.M. Evans.** Trends Genet. 1991; 7:377-381.

High density lipoproteins and atherosclerosis III.
N.E. Miller and A.R. Tall, editors.

# Genetic Variation in Mouse Apolipoprotein A-IV Expression

Karen Reue, Deborah A. Purcell-Huynh, Thomas H. Leete, Mark H. Doolittle, Andres Durstenfeld, and Aldons J. Lusis

Department of Medicine, University of California, Los Angeles, and Wadsworth VA Medical Center, Los Angeles, California.

## INTRODUCTION

Inbred mouse strains exhibit genetic differences in susceptibility to diet-induced atherosclerosis, as well as in levels and structures of lipoproteins. Analysis of these variations has lead to the identification of genetic factors controlling lipoprotein structure, concentration, and atherosclerosis susceptibility. For example, studies with inbred mice have provided evidence for a strong relationship between high density lipoprotein (HDL) levels and atherosclerosis, and allowed the identification of a genetic locus on chromosome 1 that determines HDL levels and atherosclerosis susceptibility (1). Among the genes which likely contribute to genetic variation in lipoprotein levels are those encoding the apolipoproteins. A striking example of such genetic variation occurs among mouse strains in apolipoprotein A-IV structure and expression. To better understand the factors that regulate apolipoprotein expression, we have begun to characterize naturally occuring genetic variations in apolipoprotein A-IV expression in mouse strains.

Apo A-IV is synthesized in liver and intestine, and is a protein constituent of triglyceride-rich and high density lipoproteins. Although the physiological role of apo A-IV is not well understood, some evidence suggests that it may have a role in the intravascular metabolism of HDL, and in reverse cholesterol transport. For example, apo A-IV is known to activate lecithin:cholesterol acyltransferase (LCAT), a key enzyme in the esterification of HDL cholesterol (2); it appears to potentiate the activity of an "HDL conversion factor" isolated from human plasma (3); it has been shown to modulate the activation of lipoprotein lipase in the presence of apo C-II (4); it can act as a ligand for binding of HDL to rat hepatocytes (5); and apo A-IV containing particles promote cholesterol efflux from fibroblasts and adipose cells (6).

Extreme genetic variation occurs in apo A-IV gene expression among inbred mouse strains. In a survey of 13 strains, we found that the basal levels of apo A-IV mRNA in liver vary significantly, with the largest difference (20-fold) occuring between strains C57BL/6J and 129/J (7). Apo A-IV levels in intestine, however, vary less than 2-fold between these two strains. Genetic variation in apo A-IV mRNA levels in the liver also occurs in response to eating a high fat diet, with some strains exhibiting an increase and others a decrease in apo A-IV mRNA. In addition to variations in apo A-IV expression, genetic differences occur among mouse strains in apo A-IV mRNA and protein structure. Apo A-IV mRNA from strain 129 differs from

C57BL/6 and several other *Mus musculus* inbred strains in having a 12 nucleotide deletion near the 3' end of the protein coding region (8). Genetic polymorphisms are known to occur in the analogous region of human apo A-IV (9), and population studies have provided evidence for a correlation between apo A-IV polymorphism and HDL cholesterol levels (10).

## MOLECULAR BASIS FOR GENETIC VARIATION IN APO A-IV EXPRESSION

*Genetic variation in apo A-IV mRNA and protein expression* To identify molecular mechanisms that determine genetic variation in apo A-IV mRNA levels, we characterized further the apo A-IV expression phenotype in strains C57BL/6 and 129. To determine whether the difference in C57BL/6 and 129 mRNA levels is reflected in apo A-IV protein synthetic rate, the relative rates of apolipoprotein synthesis were measured in the two strains. Freshly isolated hepatocytes from C57BL/6 and 129 were pulse-labeled with $^{35}$S-methionine for timed intervals, and apolipoproteins A-IV, A-I, and A-II were immunoprecipitated and analyzed on SDS-polyacrylamide gels (figure 1). The incorporation of label into immunoprecipitable counts was linear with time, and the two strains exhibited equivalent rates of apolipoproteins A-I and A-II synthesis. However, the rate of [$^{35}$S]methionine incorporation into apo A-IV was 10-fold lower in hepatocytes isolated from C57BL/6 compared to 129. reflecting the variation in apo A-IV mRNA levels between the two strains.

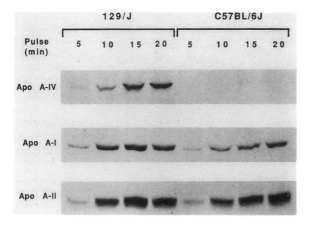

**Figure 1**. *Genetic variation in hepatic apo A-IV mRNA levels is reflected in apo A-IV protein synthetic rates.* Hepatocytes from 129/J and C57BL/6J mice were pulse-labeled with [$^{35}$S]methionine for 5, 10, 15, and 20 minutes. Apolipoproteins A-IV, A-I, and A-II were immunoprecipitated from equivalent amounts of total protein and analyzed on SDS-polyacrylamide gels.

Apo A-IV in the blood is derived from both hepatic and intestinal synthesis (11). As demonstrated previously, however, intestinal apo A-IV mRNA levels do not vary significantly between strains C57BL/6 and 129 (7). We were therefore interested to determine whether the genetic variation in hepatic apo A-IV synthesis alone could have an effect on the level of circulating apo A-IV. Using immunoblot analysis, we found that the levels of apo A-IV in plasma from 129 mice is approximately 3-fold higher than in C57BL/6. Thus, the genetic variation in liver apo A-IV expression appears to influence the steady state concentration of apo A-IV in the blood, although it remains to be determined whether a difference in apo A-IV catabolism could also contribute to higher plasma levels in strain 129.

**Genetic variation in apo A-IV expression occurs at both transcriptional and post-transcriptional levels.** Steady state mRNA levels represent a balance between rates of transcription, transport, and turnover. We performed nuclear run-off assays to directly compare rates of apo A-IV transcription in liver nuclei from C57BL/6 and 129. When normalized to actin, the rate of apo A-IV transcription in liver nuclei from 129 was 2.7-fold higher than in C57BL/6 nuclei. This difference does not reflect the 20-fold difference between C57BL/6 and 129 steady state mRNA levels, and indicates that post-transcriptional events, such as mRNA turnover, may also contribute to the genetic variation.

A standard approach to measure mRNA turnover is to treat cells with drugs that inhibit transcription, and determine the amount of the specific mRNA remaining at timed intervals. Freshly isolated hepatocytes were incubated with actinomycin D to inhibit transcription, and RNA was isolated at timed intervals up to 24 hours. In hepatocytes from both strains, apo A-I mRNA decreased gradually over 24 hours of treatment, to 50% of the original concentration. However, the levels of apo A-IV mRNA decreased only for the first 6 hours of actinomycin treatment (in C57BL/6 hepatocytes), or not at all (in 129 hepatocytes). These results suggest that the normal turnover of apo A-IV mRNA requires continued synthesis of a protein that becomes rapidly depleted in transcription-inhibited cells. Interestingly, when hepatocytes were cultured for 24 hours without actinomycin, mRNA levels for apo A-I and for albumin diminished considerably, to 5% (apo A-I) and 20% (albumin) of the levels in freshly isolated hepatocytes. In contrast, apo A-IV mRNA in hepatocytes from both mouse strains were not altered after 24 hours in culture. Taken together, these results suggest that apo A-IV is a long-lived mRNA, and that the mechanism for its decay may differ from other liver expressed mRNAs.

The results described above indicated that the traditional methodology is not adequate for apo A-IV mRNA half-life determination. We therefore employed an alternative method that allows an estimation of mRNA turnover rates based on the simultaneous measurement of mRNA synthesis and steady state concentration within the same sample. With this approach, newly synthesized mRNA is tagged by incorporation of thiolated nucleoside triphosphates, and separated from pre-existing RNA by affinity chromatography (12). The concentration of mRNAs of interest are determined in both the newly synthesized fraction and in an analogous amount of total RNA. From this mRNA synthesis data, a rate constant for mRNA degra-

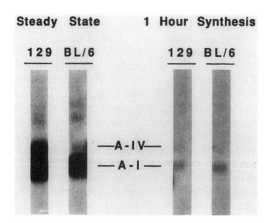

**Figure 2**. *Apo A-IV mRNA concentration in C57BL/6J and 129/J hepatocytes after one hour of synthesis and at steady state.* Hepatocytes from C57BL/6 and 129 were incubated with 4-thiouridine for one hour, and harvested for total RNA extraction. Newly synthesized RNA, which had incorporated the thiol label, was isolated from a portion of total RNA by mercurated agarose affinity chromatography (12). Total RNA and thiol-labeled RNA prepared from an equivalent amount of total mRNA were electrophoresed, transferred to nylon menbrane, and hybridized with cDNAs for apo A-IV and apo A-I.

dation can be calculated, assuming that steady-state conditions exist. Results of a representative experiment using freshly isolated hepatocytes from C57BL/6 and 129 are shown in figure 2. As shown at the left, the two strains have similar steady state levels of apo A-I mRNA, whereas strain 129 has an approximately 20-fold higher concentration of apo A-IV mRNA. The levels of these mRNAs synthesized during a one hour period and isolated from an equivalent amount of total RNA are shown at the right in figure 2. Whereas the amount apo A-I mRNA is indistinguishable for the two strains, the concentration of thiolated apo A-IV mRNA is approximately 2-fold higher in strain 129. Thus, although 129 has a much higher steady state concentration of apo A-IV mRNA, the rate of synthesis is only 2-fold higher, in agreement with the nuclear run-off data. The results indicate that the decay constant for apo A-IV mRNA is 10-fold higher in hepatocytes from C57BL/6 compared to 129. Thus, a genetic variation in the rate of apo A-IV mRNA turnover contributes to the difference in hepatic apo A-IV mRNA levels in strains C57BL/6 and 129.

*Apo A-IV mRNA 3' portion specifically binds liver cytosol proteins.* In the case of many eucaryotic mRNAs, turnover involves the interaction of cytosolic proteins with sequences or secondary structures present in the 3' portion of the mRNA (reviewed in 13). We prepared *in vitro* RNA transcripts corresponding to the 3' end of C57BL/6 and 129 apo A-IV mRNAs, and incubated them with protein extracts from mouse liver. The synthetic transcripts contain the final 132 nucleotides of coding sequence and 80 nucleotides of 3' untranslated sequence, but exclude the poly A addition signal. As shown by electrophoretic mobility shift assay, protein extracts prepared from liver cytosol contain proteins which form a specific complex with the 3' apo A-IV transcripts derived from C57BL/6 and 129. Protein binding to the labeled transcript is successfully competed by the addition of increasing amounts of unlabeled apo A-IV transcript. In contrast, transcript derived from the 3' portion of actin mRNA does not compete effectively, demonstrating the specificity of the protein-RNA interaction. Since both C57BL/6 and 129 transcripts bind the protein it appears that the 12 nucleotide sequence polymorphism does not have an effect on this interaction.

We have further characterized the proteins that interact with the apo A-IV transcripts by ultraviolet crosslinking. With this method, proteins acquire radioactive label by virtue of their interaction with, and crosslinking to, the labeled RNA transcript. In experiments with equal amounts of protein extract from liver of C57BL/6 and 129 mice, proteins of approximately 74 kDa and 52-60 KDa become crosslinked to the apo A-IV transcripts (figure 3). A comparison of proteins in C57BL/6 and 129 liver extracts reveals a quantitative difference in RNA binding to the 74 KDa protein. Interestingly, no binding activity is detected in intestinal protein extracts. Thus, the RNA binding protein appears to be expressed in a tissue specific manner, and exhibits

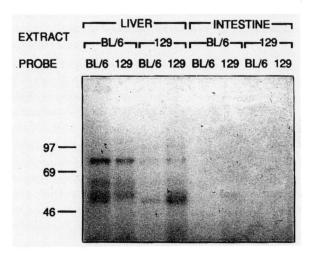

**Figure 3**. *Specific proteins in mouse liver interact with apo A-IV 3' RNA transcripts*. Radiolabeled synthetic RNA transcripts corresponding to the 3' end of C57BL/6 and 129 mRNA were incubated with cytosolic protein extracts (50 µg) from C57BL/6 liver and intestine. Reactions were irradiated with ultraviolet light, and proteins specifically complexed to RNA were detected by SDS-polyacrylamide gel electrophoresis and autoradiography. Combinations of probes and extracts are indicated above the lanes.

genetic variation in binding activity between strains C57BL/6 and 129. The function of this RNA-binding protein and its ability to interact with additional mRNA species remains to be determined.

## GENETIC CONTROL OF APO A-IV EXPRESSION

*Cis- and trans-acting genetic factors control apo A-IV mRNA levels.* Genetic variation in apo A-IV mRNA levels may be controlled by *cis*-acting elements linked to the structural gene, and/or by genetically distinct *trans*-acting factors. To identify genetic elements that control apo A-IV mRNA levels, we produced (C57BL/6 X 129)$F_1$ mice, and measured the relative concentration of apo A-IV mRNA derived from each parent, using the 12 nucleotide sequence variation to distinguish transcripts derived from the two alleles. Whereas strain 129 has a 20-fold higher level of apo A-IV mRNA than C57Bl/6, the ratio of 129 to C57BL/6 transcripts in $F_1$ mice is 3:1, and the total apo A-IV mRNA concentration is intermediate between the two parental strains. This *cis/trans* test indicates that *trans*-acting genetic loci influence apo A-IV expression. The apo A-IV mRNA-binding protein is a candidate for a *trans*-acting factor that controls apo A-IV mRNA levels. Nevertheless, since 129 mRNA is present at a 3-fold higher concentration than C57BL/6 mRNA, *cis*-acting elements must also play a role.

*Genetic mapping of trans-acting loci that influence apo A-IV mRNA levels.* The level of apo A-IV mRNA in mouse liver is a quantitative trait that exhibits continuous variation among different mouse strains and appears to be controlled by multiple genes. Recently, it has become possible to identify genetic loci, known as quantitative trait loci (QTL), that contribute to complex phenotypes using experimental crosses in plants or animals (14). We have begun to utilize QTL mapping to identify genetic loci that control apolipoprotein expression. This method relies on the production of a genetic linkage map based on DNA polymorphisms, and uses interval mapping to assess the effect of each genomic segment in determining a particular trait. To identify *trans*-acting loci that control apo A-IV mRNA expression, we quantitated mRNA levels in a backcross produced between strain C57BL/6 and the wild-derived species *Mus spretus*. *Mus spretus* was chosen because it is the most evolutionarily divergent mouse species that interbreeds with laboratory strains, and therefore most likely to exhibit genetic polymorphism. In an initial set of 67 backcross mice that were fed a high fat diet, we have detected a genetic locus on chromosome 11 that appears to control apo A-IV mRNA levels in response to fat feeding. In contrast, apo A-I mRNA levels are not influenced by this locus. Since the structural gene for mouse apo A-IV is on chromosome 9, the chromosome 11 locus represents a *trans*-acting gene that specifically influences apo A-IV expression. In the future, we will apply this technique to identify genetic loci that control expression of other apolipoproteins, and to determine whether common *trans*-acting factors regulate their expression.

# REFERENCES

1. Paigen B, Mitchell D, Reue K, Morrow A, Lusis AJ, LeBoeuf RC. (1987) *Proc. Natl. Acad. Sci. USA* 84:3763-3767.
2. Steinmetz A and Utermann G. (1985) *J. Biol. Chem.* 260:2258-2264.
3. Barter PJ, Rajaram OV, Chang LBF, Rye KA, Gambert P, Lagrost L, Enholm C, and Fidge NH. (1988) *Biochem. J.* 254:179-184.
4. Goldberg IJ, Scheraldi CA, Yacoub LK, Saxena U, and Bisgaier C. (1990) *J. Biol. Chem.* 265:15714-15718.
5. Dvorin E, Gorder NL, Benson DM, and Gotto AM, Jr. (1986) *J. Biol. Chem.* 261:15714-15718.
6. Steinmetz A, Barbaras R, Ghalim N, Clarey V, Fruchart J-C, and Ailhaud G. (1990) *J. Biol. Chem.* 265:7859-7863.
7. Williams SC, Grant SG, Reue K, Carrasquillo B, Lusis AJ, and Kinniburgh AJ. (1989) *J. Biol. Chem.* 264:19009-19016.
8. Reue K, and Leete TH. (1991) *J. Biol. Chem.* 266:12715-12721.
9. Lohse P, and Brewer HB, Jr. (1991) *Curr. Opin. Lipidol.* 2:90-95.
10. Menzel H-J, Sigurdsson G, Boerwinkle E, Schrangl-Will S, Dieplinger H, and Utermann G. (1990) *Hum. Genet.* 84:344-346.
11. Elshourbagy NA, Boguski MS, Liao WSL, Jefferson LS, Gordon JI, and Taylor JM. (1985) *Proc. Natl Acad. Sci. USA* 82:8242-8246.
12. Johnson TR, Rudin SD, Blossey BK, Ilan J, Ilan J. (1991) *Proc. Natl. Acad. Sci. USA* 88:5287-5291.
13. Peltz SW, Brewer G, Bernstein P, Hart PA, and Ross J. (1991) *Crit. Rev. Eucar. Gene Expr.* 1:99-126.
14. Lander ES and Botstein D. (1989) *Genetics* 121:185-199.

# ENZYMES AFFECTING HIGH DENSITY LIPOPROTEINS

© 1992 Elsevier Science Publishers B.V. All rights reserved.
High density lipoproteins and atherosclerosis III.
N.E. Miller and A.R. Tall, editors.

# Lipase structural domains involved in HDL generation and processing

Richard C. Davis and Howard Wong.

Lipid Research, VA Wadsworth Medical Center and the Department of Medicine, University of California, Los Angeles, California, USA

## INTRODUCTION

HDL generation and processing are intimately involved with the metabolism of triglyceride-rich lipoproteins. Early studies showed that lipolysis of triglycerides from chylomicra and VLDL by lipoprotein lipase (LPL) is accompanied by the release of excess surface coat (1). The remodeled surface coat, consisting of phospholipids, unesterified cholesterol, and apolipoproteins, is then isolated in a fraction with HDL-like density, and having a discoidal structure appropriate for nascent HDL (2). These HDL precursors quickly acquire the characteristic apoproteins and lipid constituents of mature HDL by interactions with other circulating lipoproteins or with cells (3). Through the action of lecithin cholesterol acyltransferase (LCAT) (1) and cholesteryl ester transfer protien (CETP) (4), HDL play a major role in the transfer of excess cholesterol from cellular membranes. Ultimately, this cholesterol is transported to the liver, either by direct HDL uptake, or indirectly, by transfer to IDL, LDL, or chylomicron remnants (5). However, during the HDL lifetime, excess HDL triglycerides and, to some extent, phospholipids are hydrolyzed by hepatic lipase (HL) (6). Thus, both lipoprotein lipase and hepatic lipase play major roles in the generation and processing of HDL, a major factor in cholesterol homeostasis.

What then is the structural basis for lipase function in lipid metabolism? Although our understanding of lipase structure/function is far from complete, a variety of experimental approaches have yielded significant insights. This chapter outlines some of these insights.

## GENE HOMOLOGIES

LPL and HL are closely related genes. Together with pancreatic lipase, they constitute a dispersed gene family (7,8) with LPL mapped to chromosome 8 (9), HL located on chromosome 15 (9) and pancreatic lipase on chromosome 10 (10). The genes for LPL (7,11) and HL (12) are also very similar, each about 30 Kb and consisting of 10 exons and 9 introns with a strong preservation of exon size and of intron/exon boundary locations. The gene for pancreatic lipase is slightly more distant evolutionarily, containing introns at sites homologous with those in LPL and HL, as well as 3 additional introns not present in those two lipases (7). Thus, it has been suggested that the genes for LPL and HL evolved from the pancreatic lipase gene, with an accompanying loss of introns (7).

## AMINO ACID HOMOLOGIES

There is also high conservation of amino acid sequence within the gene family. For instance, the positions of most cysteine residues are conserved (13), suggesting a conserved set of disulfide bonds and implying a similar overall three dimensional structure. Between LPL and HL, there is a conserved pair of N-linked glycosylation sites, both of which are utilized (14,15). This strong structural homology has led to the conclusion that LPL, HL and pancreatic lipase perform triglyceride and phospholipid hydrolysis by basically identical mechanisms. Interestingly, the other lipases with known sequence, including hormone sensitive lipase (16) and cholesterol ester lipase (17), share very little sequence homology with the pancreatic lipase gene family.

## A CONSERVED GLY-XAA-SER-XAA-SER MOTIF

In an initial search for lipase functional domains, it was noted that all known species of LPL, HL, or pancreatic lipase showed conservation of the sequence motif: Gly-Xaa-Ser-Xaa-Gly, where Xaa can be any amino acid (18). Historically, there has been some ambiguity about the significance of the conserved serine. The Gly-Xaa-Ser-Xaa-Gly motif has been found as a conserved element at the catalytic site of almost all serine esterases and thioesterases (19-21). There it functions as the acylatable catalytic center of the enzyme. This strongly suggested that the conserved serine in the lipase family served a similar function. However studies with porcine pancreatic lipase suggested a different role. Pancreatic lipase was stably acylated on the conserved serine 152 (22,23). This acylated enzyme lost the ability to hydrolyze longchain (lipase) substrates presented as emulsified droplets, but reportedly retained its weak ability to hydrolyze short chain (esterase) substrates present in monodisperse solution (24). This suggested that acylation of pancreatic lipase serine 152 blocked enzyme binding to lipid interfaces of substrate emulsions, but that the catalytic center, located elsewhere on the molecule, was capable of hydrolyzing substrate molecules that reached it by diffusion. Thus, two possible roles were suggested for the conserved Gly-Xaa-Ser-Xaa-Gly motif in lipases: (a) catalytic site residues, or (b) lipid interfacial binding.

## SITE DIRECTED MUTAGENESIS OF THE CENTRAL SERINE

The role of the conserved serine in the Gly-Xaa-Ser-Xaa-Gly motif was further examined by altering its amino acids using site directed mutagenesis. Clones for cDNAs of both human LPL (25) and rat HL (26) have been isolated and used with expression systems to produce active lipase enzyme. For both enzymes, it has been possible to express a mutant clones modified to encode a conservative amino acid substitution for the conserved serine (27,28). In each case, mutations to the serine in the Gly-Xaa-Ser-Xaa-Gly motif (Ser 147 of rat HL and Ser 132 of human LPL) caused complete loss of hydrolase activity for both lipase and esterase substrates, but apparently did not significantly affect the ability of the mutant lipase to bind lipid emulsions. Five other serines are also absolutely conserved in the lipase gene family. However, for each of these other serines in LPL, some amino acid substitutions allowed at least partial activity (28). These data strongly support the idea that the Gly-Xaa-Ser-Xaa-Gly motif is part of the catalytic site, and that LPL contains no secondary catalytic center with an acylatable serine.

## PANCREATIC LIPASE CRYSTAL STRUCTURE

The catalytic role of the central serine is further supported by X-ray crystallography data. While no crystal structures have been obtained for HL or LPL, crystals of human pancreatic lipase have been successfully analyzed (29). The putative catalytic serine (Ser 153) is positioned in a triad with Asp176 and His263 with a geometry that closely matches the geometry of the Ser-Asp-His catalytic triad of other serine esterases. In addition, all known examples of LPL, HL, and pancreatic lipase have absolutely conserved the analogous serine, aspartate and histidine residues.

Thus, the crystal structure for pancreatic lipase has established the structural environment of the catalytic serine and has identified histidine and aspartate residues likely to participate in catalysis. In fact, subsequent site directed mutagenesis experiments and work with naturally occurring LPL mutants (30) supports the assignment of the catalytic Asp residue. More importantly, the domain structure of pancreatic lipase establishes a framework for identifying general functional structures for the entire lipase family, even though LPL and HL will differ from pancreatic lipase in many fine details.

The most obvious structural feature of the pancreatic lipase molecule is a subdivision into two well resolved domains. The N-terminal domain consists of the first 338 residues of the mature protein and contains a large beta sheet of five strands. The catalytic serine extends from the tip of the central beta strand into a hydrophobic groove that is covered by a lid or flap. The last 111 pancreatic lipase residues constitute the C-terminal domain containing two four-stranded beta sheets that form a pocket or clamshell-like structure reminiscent of fatty acid binding protein.

## ASSIGNING FUNCTION TO THE LIPASE STRUCTURE

The structure of the N-terminal domain is very similar to the three dimensional structures observed for the lipases of Rhizomucor (31) and Geotrichum (32). These fungal lipases also have a large beta sheet with the catalytic serine mounted on the tip of the central beta strand. All the lipases have a lid structure that blocks access to the catalytic groove. However, in response to the presence of substrate, the lid of the Rhizomucor lipase has been shown to fold back and expose the catalytic triad (33). This motion also exposes a large hydrophobic surface surrounding the catalytic groove and including the underside of the lid structure itself. Presumably, the hydrophobic surface acts to bind the lipase to lipid interfaces, and the motion of the lid is the mechanism responsible for the classical activation of lipases in the presence of emulsified substrates (33). Thus, the N-terminal domain possesses all the necessary features for a general lipase: a catalytic triad in a hydrophobic groove, a domain for binding lipid interfaces, and a mechanism for interfacial activation. The C-terminal domain of pancreatic lipase has no currently obvious function. Indeed, the fungal lipases have no corresponding domain, suggesting that the C-terminal domain of the pancreatic lipase family carries out a function or modulates a property specific to the family.

## HEPARIN BINDING AND N-LINKED GLYCOSYLATION

While pancreatic lipase functions in the duodenum, both LPL and HL bind the intimal surfaces of the vascular endothelium (34,35), presumably via an interaction with heparan-sulfate proteoglycans (34). Injected heparin displaces this endothelially bound LPL and HL into the plasma. A set heparin binding consensus sequences has been identified in other proteins and homologous sequences have been identified in both LPL and HL (36) in the last twenty to thirty amino acids of their N-terminal domains. That these residues actually serve to bind the lipases to heparan sulfates *in vivo*, or to heparin *in vitro* has never been directly demonstrated.

LPL, HL and pancreatic lipase sequences from different species contain varying numbers of potential sites for N-linked glycosylation. Since pancreatic lipase from some species lack potential sites, N-linked glycans are unlikely to be generally important to pancreatic lipase function. However, there is a conserved pair of potential sites present in all known sequences for HL and LPL. Both these sites are apparently used and site directed mutagenesis experiments to measure the importance of these glycans have been performed (14,15).

Interestingly, the N-terminal domain and the C-terminal domain each contain one of the conserved sites. The C-terminal site (Asn359 in human LPL and Asn376 in rat HL) seems to be entirely dispensable so that mutations eliminating this site have no effect on lipase activity or secretion (14,15). The N-terminal site is more puzzling. Mutations in the human LPL N-terminal site (Asn43) completely block activity or secretion of the mutant lipase in COS cell based expression systems (15). It appears that this glycan must be present and must undergo processing by glucosidase I in order to produce active LPL (37). By contrast, mutation of the rat HL N-terminal site (Asn57) had minimal effect on lipase activity expressed in Xenopus oocytes (14), although the same mutation may cause a several fold reduction in activity secreted from COS cells (unpublished data). The reason for this difference is unclear.

## MAPPING DIFFERENCES BETWEEN LPL AND HL

Although LPL and HL are very similar in their structures and properties, several important biochemical characteristics distinguish these two enzymes. Most obviously, LPL activity is strongly stimulated by the presence the protein cofactor apolipoprotein C-II (apoC-II) (34) whereas there is no strong cofactor requirement for HL. Also, there are important differences in substrate preferences for the two enzymes. For instance, HL has much higher phospholipase activity than LPL (38), whereas the preferred substrates for LPL, chylomicra and VLDL, are only poorly hydrolyzed by HL. Finally, *in vitro* assays of HL activity are essentially unaffected by the presence of 1 M NaCl, whereas high salt strongly inhibits LPL activity (39).

It is now possible to localize the structural bases of these differences by taking advantage of the high degree of homology between HL and LPL. The basic strategy is to construct chimeric lipases by joining appropriate segments of HL and LPL cDNA sequences. These chimeric lipases are then expressed in tissue culture systems and monitored to determine if their properties are HL-like or LPL-like. The initial construct (HL/LPL chimera) joined the N-terminal domain of rat HL (codons 1-329) to the C-terminal domain of human LPL (codons 313-STOP) (40). This construct was compared with the LPL/HL chimera (LPL codons 1-312 joined to rat HL, codons 330-STOP) and to unmodified LPL and HL.

## CHIMERIC LIPASE CONSTRUCTION AND EXPRESSION

Chimera construction was carried out using the polymerase chain reaction (PCR) (41) with the strategy of splicing overlapping ends (42). Appropriate segments of the cDNAs for human LPL (25) and rat HL (26) were amplified using primers that created overlapping sequences on the ends of the two pieces to be joined. In a secondary PCR reaction, each amplified fragment then serves both as primer and as template for the other when making the spliced cDNA. VENT polymerase with proofreading capability was used in these reactions to avoid errors in the amplified lipase sequence. The chimeric and parental lipase cDNA clones were cloned in the expression vector pSVL and the structures of the chimeras were confirmed by nucleotide sequencing. These lipases were then transiently expressed in COS-7 (43) cells, using electroporation for transfection of the plasmid DNAs and their lipase activity was monitored in the cell medium and cellular homogenates.

## CHARACTERISTICS OF THE CHIMERIC LIPASES

The LPL/HL and HL/LPL chimeric lipases both show strong catalytic activity with emulsified triolein and with dissolved tributyrin substrates (40). As expected, both chimeric lipases were inhibited by the appropriate antisera to either HL or LPL. Otherwise, these antisera showed no crossreactivity. Thus the chimeric lipases carried epitopes from both parental lipases.

More importantly, the chimeric lipases made it possible to map specific properties of HL and LPL on the domain structure of the lipase family. The LPL/HL chimera was stimulated by apoC-II and inhibited by 1 M NaCl. Conversely, the HL/LPL chimera was unstimulated by apoC-II and uninhibited by 1 M NaCl. This shows that the apoC-II interaction site of LPL occurs in its N-terminal domain. It also suggests that certain critical N-terminal structures of LPL are destabilized by 1 M NaCl and that HL either has no corresponding structure or that the analogous structure in HL has a more stable bonding structure or resides in a more protected environment.

Interestingly, the triolein hydrolase activity of the HL/LPL chimera is inhibited by monoclonal antibody to LPL as well as by $F_{ab}$ fragments derived from that monoclonal, demonstrating that the monoclonal epitope lies in the LPL C-terminal domain. However, hydrolysis of the esterase substrate (monodisperse tributyrin) was unaffected by this monoclonal (40) suggesting that the LPL C-terminal domain, while important to lipase activity, is not essential for esterase activity or to general function of the catalytic site. This is the first indication that the lipase C-terminal domain is specifically important in the hydrolysis of longchain emulsified substrates. Thus far, all other lipase properties map to the N-terminal domain. This includes common features of the lipases including the catalytic triad, the lid structure conferring lipid binding and interfacial activation, and the putative heparin binding region. Also, the lipase-specific cofactor requirement and salt sensitivity are N-terminal.

## FURTHER OBJECTIVES

As demonstrated above, chimeric constructs are powerful tools for further structure/function studies of the lipase gene family. One immediate possibility is to investigate the importance of the C-terminal domain to lipase substrate specificity. Initial experiments suggest that the LPL/HL chimera is a more efficient phospholipase than LPL. Does the HL C-terminal domain confer this increased activity? Perhaps it is the altered interaction of domains rather than innate specificity of the domains themselves. Ultimately, these kinds experiments will be used to examine the structural basis for lipase interactions with circulating lipoproteins and their apoprotein components. This will be an important step in understanding the complex HDL processing cascade.

## ACKNOWLEDGEMENTS

This study was supported by funds from the Veterans Administration and the National Institutes of Health (HL28481).

## REFERENCES

1. Eisenberg, S. Metabolism of apolipoproteins and lipoproteins. *Current Opinion in Lipidology* 1:205-215, 1990.

2. Hamilton, R.L., Williams, M.C., Fielding, C.J. and Havel, R.J. Discoidal bilayer structure of nascent high density lipoproteins from perfused rat liver. *J.Clin.Invest.* 58:667-680, 1976.

3. Albers, J.J. Lipid transfer proteins. In: *Disorders of HDL*, edited by Carlson, L.A. London: Smith-Gordon/Nishimura, 1990, p. 25-30.

4. Tall, A.R. Plasma lipid transfer proteins. *J.Lipid Res.* 27:361-367, 1986.

5. Grundy, S.M. *Cholesterol and Atherosclerosis*, Philadelphia:J.B. Lippincott Co., 1990.

6. Patsch, J.R. High density lipoproteins and alimentary lipaemia. In: *Disorders of HDL*, edited by Carlson, L.A. London: Smith-Gordon/Nishimura, 1990, p. 133-136.

7. Kirchgessner, T.G., Chuat, J-C., Heinzmann, C., Etienne, J., Guilhot, S., Svenson, K., Ameis, D., Pilon, C., D'Auriol, L., Andalibi, A., Schotz, M.C., Galibert, F. and Lusis, A.J. Organization of the human lipoprotein lipase gene and evolution of the lipase gene family. *Proc.Natl.Acad.Sci.USA* 86:9647-9651, 1989.

8. Ben-Zeev, O., Ben-Avram, C.M., Wong, H., Nikazy, J., Shively, J.E. and Schotz, M.C. Hepatic lipase: a member of a family of structurally related lipases. *Biochim.Biophys.Acta* 919:13-20, 1987.

9. Sparkes, R.S., Zollman, S., Klisak, I., Kirchgessner, T.G., Komaromy, M.C., Mohandas, T., Schotz, M.C. and Lusis, A.J. Human genes involved in lipolysis of plasma lipoproteins: Mapping of loci for lipoprotein lipase to 8p22 and hepatic lipase to 15q21. *Genomics*. 1:138-144, 1987.

10. Davis, R.C., Diep, A., Hunziker, W., Klisak, I., Mohandas, T., Schotz, M.C., Sparkes, R.S. and Lusis, A.J. Assignment of human pancreatic lipase gene (PNLIP) to chromosome 10q24-q26. *Genomics* 11:1164-1166, 1991.

11. Deeb, S.S. and Peng, R. Structure of the human lipoprotein lipase gene. *Biochemistry* 28:4131-4135, 1989.

12. Ameis, D., Stahnke, G., Kobayashi, J., McLean, J., Lee, G., Büscher, M., Schotz, M.C. and Will, H. Isolation and characterization of the human hepatic lipase gene. *J.Biol.Chem.* 265:6552-6555, 1990.

13. Kirchgessner, T.G., Svenson, K.L., Lusis, A.J. and Schotz, M.C. The sequence of cDNA encoding lipoprotein lipase: A member of a lipase gene family. *J.Biol.Chem.* 262:8463-8466, 1987.

14. Stahnke, G., Davis, R.C., Doolittle, M.H., Wong, H., Schotz, M.C. and Will, H. Effect of N-linked glycosylation on hepatic lipase activity. *J.Lipid Res.* 32:477-484, 1991.

15. Semenkovich, C.F., Luo, C-C., Nakanishi, M.K., Chen, S-H., Smith, L.C. and Chan, L. In vitro expression and site-specific mutagenesis of the cloned human lipoprotein lipase gene. *J.Biol.Chem.* 265:5429-5433, 1990.

16. Holm, C., Kirchgessner, T.G., Svenson, K.L., Fredrikson, G., Nilsson, S., Miller, C.G., Shively, J.E., Heinzmann, C., Sparkes, R.S., Mohandas, T., Lusis, A.J., Belfrage, P. and Schotz, M.C. Hormone-sensitive lipase: Sequence, expression, and chromosomal localization to 19cent-q13.3. *Science* 241:1503-1506, 1988.

17. Reue, K., Zambaux, J., Wong, H., Lee, G., Leete, T.H., Ronk, M., Shively, J.E., Sternby, B., Borgström, B., Ameis, D. and Schotz, M.C. cDNA cloning of carboxyl ester lipase from human pancreas reveals a unique proline-rich repeat unit. *J.Lipid Res.* 32:267-276, 1991.

18. Ameis, D., Kobayashi, J., Davis, R.C., Ben-Zeev, O., Lee, G., Wong, H. and Schotz, M.C. Lipases: a molecular view. In: *Disorders of HDL*, edited by Carlson, L.A. London: Smith-Gordon/Nishimura, 1990, p. 13-18.

19. Brenner, S. The molecular evolution of genes and proteins: A tale of two proteins. *Nature* 334:528-530, 1988.

20. Kraut, J. Serine proteases: Structure and mechanism of catalysis. *Ann.Rev.Biochem.* 46:331-358, 1977.

21. Randhawa, Z.I., Naggert, J., Blacher, R.W. and Smith, S. Amino acid sequence of the serine active-site region of the medium-chain S-acyl fatty acid synthetase thioester hydrolase from rat mammary gland. *Eur.J.Biochem.* 162:577-581, 1987.

22. Maylie, M.F., Charles, M. and Desnuelle, P.A. Action of organophosphates and sulfonyl halides on porcine pancreatic lipase. *Biochim.Biophys.Acta* 276:162-175, 1972.

23. Guidoni, A.A., Bendouka, F., De Caro, J.D. and Rovery, M. Characterization of the serine reacting with diethyl p-nitrophenyl phosphate in porcine pancreatic lipase. *Biochim.Biophys.Acta* 660:148-150, 1981.

24. Chapus, C. and Sémériva, M. Mechanism of pancreatic lipase action. 2. Catalytic properties of modified lipases. *Biochemistry* 15:4988-4991, 1976.

25. Wion, K.L., Kirchgessner, T.G., Lusis, A.J., Schotz, M.C. and Lawn, R.M. Human lipoprotein lipase complementary DNA sequence. *Science* 235:1638-1641, 1987.

26. Komaromy, M.C. and Schotz, M.C. Cloning of rat hepatic lipase cDNA: Evidence for a lipase gene family. *Proc.Natl.Acad.Sci.USA* 84:1526-1530, 1987.

27. Davis, R.C., Stahnke, G., Wong, H., Doolittle, M.H., Ameis, D., Will, H. and Schotz, M.C. Hepatic lipase: Site-directed mutagenesis of a serine residue important for catalytic activity. *J.Biol.Chem.* 265:6291-6295, 1990.

28. Faustinella, F., Smith, L.C., Semenkovich, C.F. and Chan, L. Structural and functional roles of highly conserved serines in human lipoprotein lipase: Evidence that serine 132 is esential for enzyme catalysis. *J.Biol.Chem.* 266:9481-9485, 1991.

29. Winkler, F.K., D'Arcy, A. and Hunziker, W. Structure of human pancreatic lipase. *Nature* 343:771-774, 1990.

30. Faustinella, F., Chang, A., Van Biervliet, J.P., Rosseneu, M., Vinaimong, N., Smith, L.C., Chen, S-W. and Chan, L. Catalytic triad residue mutation (Asp 156-Gly) causing familial lipoprotein lipase deficiency: Co-inheritance with a nonsense mutation (Ser 447-Ter) in a Turkish family. *J.Biol.Chem.* 266:14418-14424, 1991.

31. Brady, L., Brzozowski, A.M., Derewenda, Z.S., Dodson, E., Dodson, G., Tolley, S., Turkenburg, J.P., Christiansen, L., Huge-Jensen, B., Norskov, L., Thim, L. and Menge, U. A serine protease triad forms the catalytic centre of a triacylglycerol lipase. *Nature* 343:767-770, 1990.

32. Schrag, J.D., Li, Y., Wu, S. and Cygler, M. Ser-His-Glu triad forms the catalytic site of the lipase from *Geotrichum candidum*. *Nature* 351:761-764, 1991.

33. Brzozowski, A.M., Derewenda, U., Derewenda, Z.S., Dodson, G.G., Lawson, D.M., Turkenburg, J.P., Bjorkling, F., Huge-Jensen, B., Patkar, S.A. and Thim, L. A model for interfacial activation in lipases from the structure of a fungal lipase-inhibitor complex. *Nature* 351:491-494, 1991.

34. Smith, L.C. and Pownall, H.J. Lipoprotein Lipase. In: *Lipases*, edited by Borgström, B. and Brockman, H.L. Amsterdam, New York, Oxford: Elsevier, 1984, p. 263-305.

35. Persoon, N.L.M., Hülsmann, W.C. and Jansen, H. Localization of the salt-resistant heparin-releasable lipase in the rat liver, adrenal and ovary. *J Cell Biol* 41:134-137, 1986.

36. Cardin, A.D. and Weintraub, H.J.R. Molecular modeling of protein-glycosaminoglycan interactions. *Arteriosclerosis* 9:21-32, 1989.

37. Ben-Zeev, O., Doolittle, M.H., Davis, R.C., Elovson, J. and Schotz, M.C. Maturation of lipoprotein lipase. *J.Biol.Chem.* 1992.(In Press)

38. Nilsson, A., Landin, B. and Schotz, M.C. Hydrolysis of chylomicron arachidonate and linoleate ester bonds by lipoprotein lipase and hepatic lipase. *J.Lipid Res.* 28:510-517, 1987.

39. Kinnunen, P.K.J. Hepatic endothelial lipase: Isolation, some characteristics and physiological role. In: *Lipases*, edited by Borgström, B. and Brockman, H.L. Amsterdam: Elsevier, 1984, p. 307-328.

40. Wong, H., Davis, R.C., Nikazy, J., Seebart, K.E. and Schotz, M.C. Domain exchange: Characterization of a chimeric lipase of hepatic lipase and lipoprotein lipase. *Proc.Natl.Acad.Sci.USA* 88:11290-11294, 1991.

41. Saiki, R.K., Gelfand, D.H., Stoffel, S., Scharf, S.J., Higuchi, R., Horn, G.T., Mullis, K.B. and Erlich, H.A. Primer-directed enzymatic amplification of DNA with a thermostable DNA polymerase. *Science* 239:487-491, 1988.

42. Horton, R.M., Cai, Z., Ho, S.N. and Pease, L.R. Gene splicing by overlap extension: Tailor-made genes using the polymerase chain reaction. *BioTechniques* 8:528-535, 1990.

43. Gluzman, Y. SV40-transformed simian cells support the replication of early SV40 mutants. *Cell* 23:175-182, 1981.

CHOLESTERYL ESTER TRANSFER PROTEIN (CETP) TRANSGENIC MICE: LIPOPROTEIN METABOLISM AND REGULATION OF CETP GENE EXPRESSION

Authors: Alan R. Tall, Luis B. Agellon, Tony Hayek, Annemarie Walsh, Xian Cheng Jiang, Tova Chajek-Shaul, and Jan L. Breslow.

Institutions: Division of Molecular Medicine, Department of Medicine, Columbia University, New York, NY 10032 and Laboratory of Biochemical Genetics, and Metabolism, Rockefeller University, New York, NY, 10021

## INTRODUCTION

The cholesteryl ester transfer protein (CETP) is a hydrophobic plasma glycoprotein of Mr approximately 70,000, which mediates the exchange and transfer of neutral lipids and phospholipids between the plasma lipoproteins (1). By mediating the net transfer of cholesteryl esters (CE) from HDL to triglyceride-rich lipoproteins, the CETP appears to play an important role in the catabolism of HDL CE. Recent studies of human genetic CETP deficiency indicate that CETP plays a major role in HDL catabolism, and also influences the CE content of apoB-containing lipoproteins (2). Studies of CETP metabolism in animal models suggest that CETP may act as a pro-atherogenic factor (3), although this issue is controversial since CETP is also thought to be involved in reverse cholesterol transport (4). The mRNA for CETP is found in a variety of tissues, including liver, spleen and adipose tissue (5). The CETP mRNA is induced in both liver and in peripheral tissues in animals placed on a high cholesterol diet (6,6a).

Recently, human CETP transgenic mice have been developed in order to investigate the impact of CETP expression on lipoprotein metabolism and atherosclerosis (7) and to study the regulation of CETP gene expression (8). The mouse is an ideal model in which to study the effects of CETP expression, since mice are normally deficient in plasma cholesteryl ester transfer activity. The specific goals of the studies in transgenic mice are 1) to investigate the effects of CETP expression on lipoprotein levels; 2) to study the interaction of CETP with other genes influencing lipoproteins metabolism such as apoA-I (9) and apoC-III (10); 3) to determine the effects of CETP expression on the development of atherosclerosis in mice; 4) to define the DNA elements in or around the CETP gene which mediate tissue-specific expression, and to elucidate the molecular mechanisms of the induction of the CETP mRNA in response to a high cholesterol, high fat diet. This paper will summarize progress to date in some of these goals.

## RESULTS AND DISCUSSION

CETP transgenic mice were developed employing a minigene, including several native exons and introns of the CETP gene, as well as a portion of the CETP cDNA (Fig 1). This minigene was placed under the control of the mouse metallothionein promoter (mT-CETP), which permits induction of expression in response to increased dietary Zn. In later studies the minigene was used in conjunction with the natural flanking sequences of the CETP gene (NFR-CETP transgene) in order to investigate the regulation of expression of the CETP gene (see below).

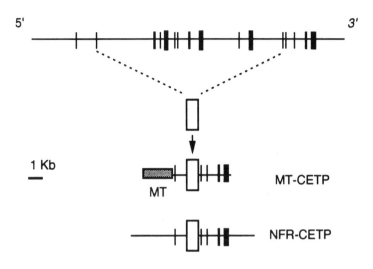

Figure 1. Structure of CETP transgenes. The organization of human CETP gene is shown (top). The vertical bars represent exons. A minigene was constructed by combining genomic fragments with a portion of the cDNA, representing exons 2 to 12, and placed under control of the metallothionein (MT) promoter, or assembled with the natural flanking sequences of the CETP gene (NFR-CETP).

Using the MT-CETP gene construction a line of CETP transgenic mice was developed, which expresses human CETP of normal Mr and specific activity (7). In the basal state the levels of plasma CETP in these mice are similar to that in normolipidemic humans (about 2 ug/ml). With Zn induction the levels are approximately doubled (to about 4 ug/ml), producing CETP levels similar to those observed in certain human dyslipidemic states [dysbetalipoproteinemia (Type III), probucol therapy and nephrotic syndrome]. Analysis of plasma lipoproteins in these MT-CETP transgenic animals indicated that the Zn induction resulted in a modest decrease in HDL cholesterol. The reduction in HDL cholesterol was approximately 20 to 30% compared to non-transgenic animals. CETP expression resulted in reductions of HDL cholesterol of similar magnitude in mice of both sexes, and on diets consisting of chow, high fat and cholesterol or high fat and cholesterol supplemented with bile salts (7). Analysis of VLDL and LDL lipids revealed no significant differences between transgenic and non-transgenic mice (7. These results support a role of CETP in HDL cholesteryl ester catabolism and suggest that increased levels of CETP observed in certain human dyslipidemias may be causally related to reductions in HDL cholesterol levels.

Compared to the dramatic increase in HDL cholesterol observed in human genetic CETP deficiency, the magnitude of the change in HDL cholesterol comparing Tg and nonTg mice was relatively modest. Recent studies of human apoA-I transgenic mice indicate that apoA-I expression leads to increased HDL levels and produces speciation of HDL (i.e. formation of distinct $HDL_2$ and $HDL_3$ subclasses) similar to that observed in humans (11,12). In order to investigate the possibility of a specific interaction between CETP and HDL containing human apoA-I, CETP transgenic mice were crossed with human apoA-I transgenic mice and the effects of CETP expression on plasma lipoproteins were evaluated (13). The crossing of heterozygous CETP transgenic mice with heterozygous apoA-I transgenic mice produced offspring with four different genotypes: non-transgenic, (nonTg), apoA-I transgenic (AI Tg), CETP transgenic (CETP Tg) or apoA-I and CETP transgenic (A-I CETP Tg). Plasma lipoproteins were analyzed before and after Zn induction. Comparing CETP Tg and non-Tg mice, the reduction in HDL cholesterol was similar to that observed previously (i.e. about 25%). However, comparing A-I Tg with CETP AI Tg mice, the reduction in HDL cholesterol was much more pronounced (about 70% in the Zn induced state). The expression of both transgenes also resulted in a much more profound reduction in HDL cholesterol when the results were expressed in absolute terms. Lipoprotein turnover studies indicated an approximate 20% increase in the FCR of HDL cholesteryl ethers, comparing CETP Tg and non TG mice. By contrast, in A-I CETP Tg mice the FCR of HDL cholesteryl ethers was increased 100% compared to A-I Tg mice. Analysis of HDL particles by native gradient gel electrophoresis showed a marked reduction in HDL particle size in AI CETP Tg mice, compared to AI Tg mice. These results suggest that the HDL particles formed by human apoA-I are much better substrates for CETP than mouse HDL particles. The results would also be consistent with a specific interaction between human CETP and human apoA-I, leading to enhanced CETP activity. Although plasma CETP levels were similar in AI CETP Tg and CETP Tg mice, an analysis of CETP distribution, using the CETP mAb TP2 to probe Western blots of native gels of plasma lipoproteins, revealed a marked difference in CETP distribution. In AI CETP Tg mice more than 90% of CETP was associated with HDL particles, as occurs in normal human plasma. This was true in both basal and Zn induced plasma samples. However, in CETP Tg mice a minority of the CETP was HDL associated, and about 80% of CETP was lipoprotein-free following Zn induction. Previous biochemical studies have shown that the ability of CETP to employ HDL as a substrate parallels its binding to the HDL (14). Thus, the low binding of CETP by mouse HDL in vivo provides an explanation for its relatively poor ability to act as a substrate for CETP. Interestingly, the difference in binding of human CETP to mouse versus human HDL cannot be reproduced by in vitro incubations of human CETP with isolated mouse or human HDL fractions, suggesting that an additional factor (such as incorporation during lipoprotein biosynthesis) is acting in vivo to produce the specific binding of CETP to HDL particles formed by human apoA-I.

In order to investigate the in vivo regulation of CETP gene expression, transgenic mice were prepared using the CETP minigene linked to its natural flanking sequences (NFR-CETP Transgene), rather than to the metallothionein promoter (Fig 1) (8). The NFR CETP transgene contained about 3.4 Kbp of 5′ flanking sequence and 2 Kbp of 3′ flanking sequence. Using the NFR CETP transgene, several lines of transgenic mice were obtained, with plasma CETP activities, varying from about 30% to 200% of human plasma CETP activity.

In four lines of NFR CETP Tg mice the abundance of the CETP mRNA was determined in various tissues by RNAse protection assay (8). In two of the NFR CETP Tg lines, the pattern of expression was similar to that of the human gene, with highest levels of CETP mRNA in liver, spleen, small intestine, kidney, and adipose tissue. In two other lines the tissue distribution was more restricted with major expression in liver and spleen, or liver and small intestine. In response to a high cholesterol, high fat diet, there was a marked induction of CETP in mRNA in liver and a variable induction in several peripheral tissues. The induction of the CETP mRNA was most pronounced in liver where the abundance of CETP mRNA was increased from 4 to 10-fold by the high cholesterol diet in different lines of transgenic mice. In marked contrast to these findings, the mT-CETP transgene was expressed in a wide variety of tissues, including the liver, but gave rise to no increase in CETP mRNA in response to a high cholesterol diet. In parallel with the mRNA results, plasma CETP activity and mass was increased about 2.5-fold in NFR CETP Tg mice in response to the high cholesterol diet, but was not changed in the mT CETP Tg mice in response to the same diet. Nuclear run-on assays in the NFR CETP Tg mice showed an approximate five-fold increase in transcriptional rate of the CETP transgene in response to the high cholesterol diet.

A time course study in one line of NFR CETP Tg mice indicated that the increase in CETP mRNA occurred within 48 h of beginning the high cholesterol diet (8). A comparison of different diets revealed that the increase in CETP mRNA was largely due to dietary cholesterol. Increased dietary fat alone caused only a slight increase in CETP-mRNA, but increased dietary fat amplified the increase in CETP mRNA when added to a high cholesterol diet.

The studies in NFR CETP Tg mice suggest that relatively limited portions of the flanking sequences of the gene (or the minigene itself) contain the elements mediating tissue-specific patterns of human CETP mRNA expression. The variable expression in different lines of mice probably arises from positional effects due to different sites of integration of the transgene in the chromosome in the different lines of mice. The marked induction of liver CETP mRNA in response to increased dietary cholesterol in the NFR CETP Tg mice resembles the increase in tissue CETP mRNA observed in rabbits, hamsters, monkeys, and humans in response to a high cholesterol diet (3,6,7). A comparison of results in mT CETP and NFR CETP Tg mice indicates that the increase in plasma CETP activity and mass in response to a high cholesterol diet is entirely due to an increase in CETP-mRNA, and is not the passive consequence of increased plasma lipoprotein mass resulting from increased dietary cholesterol, as had been suggested (15). In NFR CETP Tg mice the increase in liver CETP mRNA produced by a high cholesterol diet can be attributed entirely to increased transgene transcription. The contrasting responses of the NFR CETP and mT-CETP transgenes suggests that the natural flanking sequences of the human CETP gene contain one or more cholesterol response elements, responsible for increased transcription in response to increased dietary cholesterol. Studies of CETP mRNA in isolated parenchymal or non-parenchymal cell fractions prepared from perfused livers of cholesterol fed NFR CETP Tg mice or Zn induced mT CETP Tg mice show that the CETP mRNA is expressed primarily in the hepatocyte fraction (16). Since both induced transgenes are expressed in the same cell type, the different cholesterol response of the NFR CETP transgene is not simply the result of expression in a different cell type.

A limited number of genes are known to be regulated in response to changes in dietary or cellular cholesterol content. The best characterized of these are the LDL receptor and HMG CoA reductase genes which are down-regulated by cholesterol (17). This effect is mediated by a highly conserved, proximal promoter sequence called the sterol regulatory element (SRE) (17). It is notable that the proximal promoter sequences of the CETP gene do not contain an SRE (18), suggesting that there may be a distinctive mechanism for the cholesterol-induced increased CETP gene transcription. The marked increase in CETP gene transcription response to a high cholesterol diet probably provides a mechanism to enhance reverse cholesterol transport to the liver. Since this occurs by decreasing the cholesterol content of HDL, and increasing the cholesterol content of VLDL, this may nonetheless produce a pro-atherogenic effect. In the future it should be possible to test the hypothesis that CETP expression enhances the atherogenicity of the plasma lipoproteins (14) in mice expressing the CETP transgene.

## REFERENCES

1   Hesler, CB, Swenson TL, Tall AR. J Biol Chem 1987; 262: 2275-2282.
2   Inazu A, Brown ML, Hesler CB, Agellon LB, Koizumi J, Takata K, Maruhama Y, Mabuchi H, Tall AR. N Eng J Med 1990; 323: 1234-1238.
3   Quinet EM, Rudel LL, Tall AR. J Clin Invest 1991; 87: 1559-1566.
4   Tall AR. J Clin Invest 1990; 86: 379-384.
5   Drayna D, Jarnagin AS, Mclean J, Henzel W, Kohr W, Fielding C, Lawn R. Nature 1987; 327: 632-634.
6   Quinet EM, Agellon LB, Kroon PA, Marcel YL, Lee Y-C, Whitlock ME, Tall AR. J Clin Invest 1990; 85: 357-363.
6a  Jiang XC, Moulin P, Quinet EM, Goldberg IJ, Yacoub LK, Agellon LB, Compton D, Schnitzer-Polokoff R, Tall AR. J Biol Chem 1991; 266: 4631-4639.
7   Agellon LB, Walsh A, Hayek T, Moulin P, Jiang XC, Shelanski SA, Tall AR. J Biol Chem 1991; 266: 10796-10801.
8   Jiang XC, Agellon LB, Walsh, A, Breslow JL, Tall AR. (Submitted for publication).
9   Walsh A, Ito Y, Breslow JL. J Biol Chem 1989; 264: 6488-6494.

10   Ito Y, Azrolan N, O'Connell A, Walsh A, Breslow JL. Science 1990;
     249: 790-793.
11   Chajek-Shaul T, Hayek T, Walsh A, Breslow JL. Proc Natl Acad Sci
     USA 1991; 88: 6731-6735
12   Rubin EM, Ishida BY, Clift SM, Krauss RM. Proc Natl Acad Sci USA
     1991; 88: 434-438.
13   Hayek T, Chajek-Shaul T, Walsh A, Agellon LB, Moulin P, Tall AR,
     Breslow JL. (Submitted for publication).
14   Tall AR. J Lipid Res 1986; 27: 359-365.
15   Quig DW, Zilversmit DB. Annu Rev Nutr 1990; 10: 169-193.
16   Unpublished.
17   Goldstein JL, Brown MS. Nature 1990; 343: 425-430.
18   Agellon LB, Quinet EM, Gillette TG, Drayna DT, Brown ML, Tall AR.
     Biochemistry 1990; 29: 1372-1376.

High density lipoproteins and atherosclerosis III.
N.E. Miller and A.R. Tall, editors.

# Molecular Defects in the Lecithin:Cholesterol Acyltransferase Gene

John W. McLean

Department of Cell Biology, Genentech Inc.
460 Point San Bruno Boulevard
South San Francisco, CA 94080
USA

## INTRODUCTION

Lecithin:Cholesterol Acyltransferase (LCAT, EC 2.3.1.43) is the enzyme that catalyzes the formation of cholesteryl esters by the transesterification of the unsaturated $sn$-2 fatty acids from phosphatidylcholine (lecithin) to the $3\beta$ hydroxyl group of cholesterol. LCAT is synthesized in the liver and circulates in the plasma predominantly as a complex with high density lipoprotein (HDL). LCAT is a key component in the process of reverse cholesterol transport, whereby cholesterol of peripheral origin is transported through the plasma for catabolism in the liver. The esterification of difussible cholesterol to its insoluble ester form in plasma is important in maintaining a concentration gradient between cell membranes and plasma. Virtually all the cholesteryl ester formation in plasma can be accounted for by the action of this enzyme.

Much of our understanding of the role of LCAT has come from examining patients genetically defective in LCAT activity. Two different disorders, familial LCAT deficiency and fish-eye disease have been found to originate from defects in the LCAT gene. Both these disorders are autosomal recessive, with obligate heterozygotes showing none of the symptoms of enzyme deficiency. The biochemical and clinical manifestations of these diseases are highly variable and most probably represent different impaired activities of the enzyme.

Familial LCAT deficiency has been identified in more than 50 patients in approximately 30 families. It is most often seen in populations with a limited gene pool, or in consanguineous marriages. The most distinctive clinical finding is massive corneal opacities. Other clinical symptoms are variable, but include renal insufficiency, proteinuria, hemolytic anemia and early atherosclerosis of aorta, coronary and renal arteries. Tissue abnormalities are caused by lipid deposition, especially in the cornea, renal parenchyma, and aorta. Patients often die in their fourth or fifth decade due to kidney failure. There are marked changes in all plasma lipoproteins in both composition and physical properties. Total plasma concentrations of unesterified cholesterol, lecithin and triglycerides are elevated, whereas cholesteryl ester and lysolecithin are decreased.

In contrast, fish-eye disease has only been described in five families to date. As in familial LCAT deficiency, there are massive corneal opacities, but patients only appear defective in the esterification of cholesterol in HDL particles. Cholesterol esterification in apoB-containing particles appears normal, giving rise to a near normal cholesteryl ester/unesterified cholesterol ratio in plasma, but decreased in HDL. No renal involvement is seen in these patients.

Of particular interest is the severely reduced HDL levels in patients with familial LCAT deficiency and fish-eye disease. Although epidemiological studies have shown an inverse correlation between plasma HDL levels and the risk of myocardial infarction, these patients do not seem to show an increased prevalence of coronary heart disease. For the most recent review of the clinical and biochemical manifestations resulting from LCAT gene defects see Assmann *et al.* [1]

## FAMILIAL LCAT DEFICIENCY MUTATION STUDIES

This report details five new families with defects in the LCAT gene that lead to familial LCAT deficiency.

The LCAT gene residues on the long arm of chromosome 16, and the 440 amino acids of the protein are encoded on 6 exons that span about 4.2 kb of genomic DNA [2]. The cDNA sequences for human, rat, and mouse LCAT, as well as partial protein sequence of the porcine enzyme are known.

The strategy for determining the mutation sites in LCAT genes was as follows: Patient genomic DNA was cloned into bacteriophage λ vectors, and recombinant clones containing the entire gene were selected. Gene fragments were subcloned, and all exons, and intron/exon boundaries were subject to DNA sequencing. Any differences from the wild type DNA sequence were evaluated by several methods to confirm whether the mutation was the basis of altered enzyme function. Mutations were confirmed by amplifying genomic DNA from patients and family members by the polymerase chain reaction (PCR). Amplified DNA fragments were subjected to direct DNA sequencing, and if a change in restriction site was predicted from the wild type sequence, this was also checked. When this analysis revealed that the patient phenotype was caused by two different mutations giving a compound heterozygote, a second strategy was employed. LCAT gene fragments were amplified from patient DNA by PCR {exons 1-5 and exon 6 were amplified to give two fragments}. PCR fragments were analyzed directly by DNA sequencing, and also subcloned into plasmid vectors. Plasmid clones that did not contain the initial mutation were also subjected to DNA sequence analysis. Putative mutations that were found by this approach were also analyzed as described above.

## FAMILY 1

For a clinical and biochemical report on this extensive family see Vrabec *et al.*[3].

This is a family of North American Indians of the Laccourte Oreilles, resident in Northern Wisconsin. Four members of the family were found to be homozygotes for familial LCAT deficiency. The parents of the proband are unrelated, but members of the same tribe. DNA was available from the proband and his son. The proband was assessed to have 13% of normal LCAT activity and 26% of normal LCAT mass.

The proband (Subject 1) was found to be homozygous for the mutation R244G caused by a single base change in exon 6. His son, an obligate heterozygote, was found to carry one copy of the mutant gene.

```
      HinPI
...CAGCGCATA...        ->        ...CAGGGCATA...
    Q   R   T                      Q   G   T
        244                            244
```

## FAMILY 2

An unpublished family of Drs John Kane and Mary Malloy, UCSF San Francisco.

The proband JC is one of three siblings who are all afflicted with familial LCAT deficiency. The parents are heterozygotes, unrelated, and are of German and Irish extraction. DNA was available from the proband and both parents. LCAT activity was assessed at <10% in all three siblings. No data is available regarding LCAT mass.

The first mutation was found to be L32P, caused by a single base change in exon 2. This mutation was inherited from the mother HC.

```
                                    AvaI
                                    SmaI
...TGCCTGGGG...        ->        ...TGCCCGGGG...
    C   L   G                      C   P   G
        32                             32
```

The second mutation was found to be T321M, caused by a single base change in exon 6. This mutation was inherited from the father RC.

```
                                    NlaIII
...CCCACGCCC...        ->        ...CCCATGCCC...
    P   T   P                      P   M   P
        321                            321
```

## FAMILY 3

For a discussion of this family see Bethell *et al.* [4].

The proband BH is one of three siblings, his brother also being affected with familial LCAT deficiency. DNA was only available from the proband. The parents are unrelated and of Swiss Mennonite - English extraction. The proband was assessed to have 2% of normal LCAT activity, and 4% of normal mass.

The first mutation was found to be a deletion/change at the beginning of exon 4, giving rise to a frameshift.

```
     KpnI
...ccacagGGTACCTGCAC...      ->      ...ccacagGGTTCTGCACA...
        G  Y  L  H                             G  F  C  T
        119                                    119   terminates at
                                                     residue 238
```

The second mutation was found to be single base change in exon five to give G183S.

```
                                                PvuII
...GGCCACAGCCTCGGCTGT...      ->      ...GGCCACAGCCTCAGCTGT...
   G  H  S  L  G  C                      G  H  S  L  S  C
               183                                    183
```

This mutation alters one of the residues close to the active site serine (at position 181 in LCAT). The sequence G-X-S-X-G is a motif that appears conserved in many lipases and transacylases [5]. The replacement of the glycine residue downstream of the serine would be expected have a major effect on enzyme activity.


FAMILY 4

For a discussion of this family see Ohta *et al.*, and Murano *et al.* [6,7].

This is a Japanese family in which both the parents and paternal grandparents of the proband were in consanguineous marriages between first cousins. DNA was available from the proband S5 and both parents. The proband was assessed to have between 0 and 9% normal LCAT activity and 4% normal mass.

The proband was homozygous for the insertion of a single C residue in exon 1 at the position of proline 10, which gave rise to a frameshift that would cause termination downstream after 16 amino acid residues. Analysis of both parents by DNA sequencing of PCR products encompassing this mutation confirmed that they were heterozygous at this position.

```
...CCGCACACC...      ->      ...CCCGCACACCACGCCCAAGGCTGAG...
   P  H  T                      P  A  H  H  A  Q  A  •
   10                           10
```

It might be expected that such a short peptide lacking any functionality might not even be secreted from the hepatocyte, rather, being rapidly degraded intracellularly.

## FAMILY 5

For a discussion of this family see Albers *et al.* [8,9].

This is a Japanese family in which the parents of the probands (brother and sister) are first cousins. The probands had 8-9% normal LCAT activity and 40-46% normal LCAT mass. DNA was only available from the probands.

The probands were found to be homozygous for a single base mutation in exon 6, giving rise to M293I.

```
                                       NdeI
   ...TACATGTGG...      ->       ...TACATATGG...
       Y  M  W                       Y  I  W
         293                           293
```

## DISCUSSION

The heterogeneity of the clinical and immunological presentation of both familial LCAT deficiency and fish-eye disease originally suggested that this might be accounted for by many different defects in the LCAT gene. The widespread geographical and ethnic distribution of familial LCAT deficiency, and the differences in immunologically-detectable LCAT mass also lent credence to this notion. This heterogeneity has been borne out by recent studies identifying the mutations in the LCAT gene that give rise to these disorders (see 1 for review). The emerging picture is that this highly-conserved enzyme has undergone mutation many different times at different locations to give rise to these disorders. However it is difficult to equate particular mutations with specific phenotypes at present due to several considerations. Because of the severity of the disease in the patients diagnosed so far, it as yet unknown whether mutations causing less severe phenotypes have gone undetected.

The figures reported for mass measurements, should be viewed with caution, since sequence changes might easily destroy epitopes. This would most likely occur if gross misfolding of the protein were to take place, or in frameshift mutations.

Although some attempts have been made to elucidate the functional domains of LCAT, there have been conflicting reports in this regard. Expression of recombinant LCAT with site-directed mutations should provide important new insights [10].

This report brings that number of reported mutations in the LCAT gene to 18, including 3 frameshifts, 1 amino acid insertion, and the rest single base substitutions giving rise to missense mutations. The fish eye mutations have all so far been missense [1, 11, Hans Prydz, *pers. comm.*].

As yet no obvious reason as to why a particular mutation should give rise to the fish-eye phenotype rather than the classical familial LCAT deficiency phenotype has emerged. Many questions are raised by these observations. Why does familial LCAT deficiency but not fish-eye disease lead to renal dysfunction, but both lead to corneal opacification? Are the renal changes seen the result of lipid deposition (perhaps from abnormal lipoprotein particles), or are they the result of an impairment in reverse cholesterol transport? What is the basis of the differential ability of fish-eye patients to esterify cholesterol in apoB-containing particles, but not in HDL? Another major conundrum is the lack of evidence that patients have any major increased risk for CHD, even though HDL levels are very low.

## ACKNOWLEDGMENTS

The author would like to acknowledge Drs John Albers, John Kane, Mary Malloy, Christopher Fielding, Shinichi Murano, Elizabeth Koller, Donald Wiebe, Jiri Frohlich and Aubie Angel for their generous contribution of patient DNA, as well as clinical and biochemical data.

## REFERENCES

1    Assman, G., von Eckardstein, A., and Funke, H. (1991) *Curr. Opin. Lipid.* **2** 110-117.

2    McLean, J., Wion, K., Drayna, D., Fielding, C., and Lawn, R. (1986) *Nucleic Acids Res.* **14** 9387-9406.

3    Vrabec, M.P., Shapiro, M.B., Koller, E., Wiebe, D.A., Henricks, J., and Albers J.J. (1988) *Arch. Opthal.* **106** 225-229.

4    Bethell, W., McCulloch, C., and Ghosh, M. (1975) *Canad. J. Ophthal.* **10** 494-501.

5    Yang, C.-H., Gu, Z.-W., Yang, H.-X., Rohde, M.F., Gotto, A.M., and Pownall, H.J. (1989) *J. Biol. Chem.* **264** 16822-16827.

6    Ohta Y., Yamamoto, S., Tsuchida, H., Murano, S., Saitoh, Y., Tohjo, S., and Okada, M. (1986) *Am. J. Kidney Dis.* **7** 41-46.

7    Murano, S., Shirai, K., Saito, Y., Yoshida, S., Ohta, Y., Tsuchida, H., Yamamotot, S., Asano, G., Chen, C.-H., and Albers, J.J. (1987) *Scand. J. Lab. Invest.* **47** 775-783.

8    Albers, J.J., Chen, C.-H., Adolphson, J., Sakuma, M., Kodama, T., and Akanuma, Y. (1982) *Hum. Genet.* **62** 82-85.

9    Albers, J.J., Adolphson, J., Chen, C.-H., Murayama, N., Honma, S., and Akanuma, Y. (1985) *Biochim. Biophys. Acta* **835** 253-257.

10   Francone, O., and Fielding, C.J. (1991) *Proc. Natl. Acad. Sci. USA* **88** 1716-1720.

11   Klein, H.G., Lohse, P., Pritchard, P.H., Bojanovski, D., Schmidt, H., and Brewer, H.B. Jr. (1991) *Arterio. Thromb.* **11** 1415a.

# Regulation of the reaction of high density lipoproteins with lecithin cholesterol acyltransferase

A. Jonas, D. J. Bolin, and F. S. Bonelli

Department of Biochemistry, College of Medicine at Urbana-Champaign, University of Illinois, 506 South Mathews Avenue, Urbana, IL 61801, USA

## INTRODUCTION

The role of lecithin cholesterol acyltransferase (LCAT) in lipoprotein metabolism is determined not only by the chemical reaction it catalyzes but also by the sites where this reaction occurs. LCAT carries out the transfer of an acyl chain from a phospholipid, most commonly a phosphatidylcholine (PC), to cholesterol, on the surface of nascent high density lipoproteins (HDL) and smaller spherical HDL subclasses. As depicted in Figure 1, the esterification of cholesterol on HDL promotes the flow of cholesterol from cell membranes and other lipoproteins into HDL, and results in the storage of cholesterol esters in the core of HDL particles. In the process, the HDL particles are converted from nascent discoidal subspecies to mature spherical $HDL_3$ and to larger $HDL_2$ subspecies. The cholesterol esters in the core of HDL can be redistributed to less dense lipoproteins via the cholesterol ester transfer protein and then delivered to the liver, thus completing the "reverse cholesterol transport" pathway from the peripheral tissues [1].

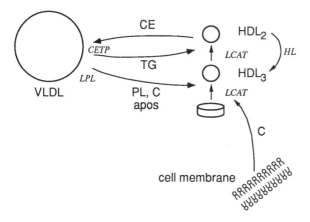

Figure 1. The role of LCAT in HDL metabolism. Aside from LCAT, lipoprotein lipase (LPL), the cholesterol ester transfer protein (CETP), and hepatic lipase (HL) participate in the metabolism of HDL and of other lipoproteins (VLDL). During these processes, lipids (CE, TG, PL, C) and apoproteins (apos) are transferred between the lipoproteins.

The preferential reaction of LCAT on the surface of HDL is determined, to a large extent, by its activation by apolipoprotein A-I (apo A-I); however, other factors also control the reaction since other apolipoproteins also activate LCAT, and diverse lipoprotein subclasses containing apo A-I are not equally reactive with this enzyme. Our laboratory has been engaged for the past ten years in the investigation of the various steps of the interaction of LCAT with HDL and their regulation. Figure 2 shows the reaction steps that occur on the surface of HDL. The first step is the reversible binding of the enzyme to the lipoprotein surface, probably involving interaction of the enzyme with surface lipids. Next, the optimal activation of the reaction requires the participation of apo A-I bound to the particle surface. Following the activation step, phospholipid binds to the active site of the enzyme, and the first catalytic step releases lyso-phospholipid and forms an acyl-enzyme intermediate. Finally, binding of cholesterol to the acyl-enzyme intermediate leads to the formation of the cholesterol ester product and its release from the enzyme into the core of HDL. The enzyme may then participate again in the catalytic cycle or may be released into solution.

The objective of this paper is to review some of our recently published work and to describe current, unpublished work on these individual steps of the LCAT reaction.

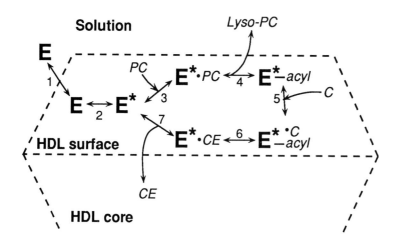

Figure 2. Steps of the LCAT reaction on the surface of HDL. **E** represents LCAT in solution and bound to the surface; **E\*** is the activated form of the enzyme; *PC* and *C* are the lipid substrates of LCAT; and *Lyso-PC* and *CE* are the products.

## BINDING OF LCAT TO HDL

Measurements of the enzymatic activity of LCAT or binding of specific antibodies for LCAT on fractionated plasma has shown that LCAT may exist free in plasma, or bound to various fractions of HDL [2,3], and even associated with LDL in small amounts [2]. Until our current work [unpublished work, Bolin and Jonas, 1991], direct quantitative binding measurements of the affinity and stoichiometry of LCAT for lipoproteins had not been performed. We developed two high-sensitivity methods for this purpose: one of the methods is based on the inhibition of the enzymatic activity by competing HDL particles included in the reaction mixture, and the other is a solid phase binding assay that uses microtiter wells coated with HDL in conjunction with [125]I-labeled LCAT. The *activity inhibition* method relies on a standard kinetic assay where the reconstituted HDL (rHDL) substrate is labeled with [3]H-PC, which produces radiolabeled cholesterol ester upon reaction with the enzyme. The apparent Michaelis-Menten kinetics of the reaction are measured and analyzed for the rHDL substrate in the absence and in the presence of increasing concentrations of the unlabeled test HDL particle. Enzyme dissociation from the substrate and binding to the test particle results in an apparent inhibition of activity with a competitive pattern, as shown in Figure 3.

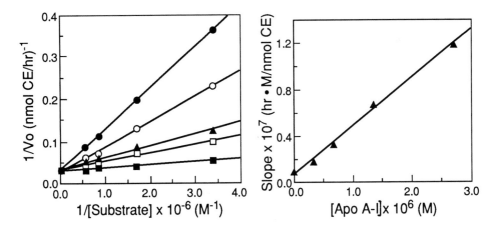

Figure 3. Inhibition kinetics of LCAT reacting with a substrate rHDL in the presence of increasing concentrations of an unlabeled rHDL containing apo A-I.

Analysis of the inhibition results yields an inhibition constant, $K_I$, that can be equated with the dissociation constant, $K_d$, of LCAT from the "inhibitor" particle. The $K_d$ values determined by this method are summarized in Table 1 for rHDL particles containing apo A-I or apo A-II, having similar average particle sizes (96 and 100 Å, respectively), and identical lipid compositions. The preliminary results for two series of apo A-I particles of different diameters prepared with either POPC or DPPC are also included. It is evident from these results that differences in apolipoprotein composition, PC composition, and particle size result, at most, in 5-fold differences in $K_d$ values, whereas reactivity of these particles with LCAT, when the rHDL are radiolabeled and assayed directly, can vary by as much as 200-fold as indicated by the apparent $V_{max}$/apparent $K_m$ values in Table 1 [4-6; unpublished results, Jonas and Kézdy, 1990]. Thus, the main control of the reaction rate for these systems must occur at a step beyond the initial binding step of the enzyme to the interface.

Table 1
Binding affinities ($K_d$) and reactivities (apparent $V_{max}$/apparent $K_m$) of rHDL with LCAT

| rHDL Particles [a] | | | $K_d$ [b] (M) | App. $V_{max}$/App. $K_m$ [d] (nmol CE/hr·M) |
|---|---|---|---|---|
| Apo | PC | Diam.(Å) | | |
| A-I | egg-PC | 96 | $2.1 \times 10^{-7}$ | $96.5 \times 10^4$ |
| A-II | egg-PC | 100 | $1.1 \times 10^{-6}$, $3.7 \times 10^{-7}$ [c] | $1.9 \times 10^4$ |
| A-I | POPC | 78 | $8.5 \times 10^{-7}$ | $6.1 \times 10^4$ |
| | | 96 | $3.2 \times 10^{-7}$ | $97.6 \times 10^4$ |
| | | 109 | $8.3 \times 10^{-7}$ | $8.5 \times 10^4$ |
| A-I | DPPC | 97 | $9.5 \times 10^{-7}$ | $10.9 \times 10^4$ |
| | | 136 | -- | $1.6 \times 10^4$ |
| | | 186 | $9.9 \times 10^{-7}$ | $0.5 \times 10^4$ |

[a]Discoidal rHDL were prepared by the Na cholate method using the PC listed and 5-10 mol % cholesterol. The diameters were measured by nondenaturing gradient gel electrophoresis.
[b]The $K_d$ values are the inhibition constants measured by the activity-inhibition method.
[c]This value of $K_d$ was obtained by the solid phase method which also gave a stoichiometry of one LCAT per rHDL particle (4 apo A-II/particle).
[d]From Lineweaver-Burk analysis of initial velocity versus apolipoprotein concentration, using rHDL particles containing $^{14}$C-cholesterol.

In order to confirm the results for the binding of LCAT to rHDL particles containing apo A-I and apo A-II, we carried out parallel experiments using $^{125}$I-LCAT binding to microtiter plates coated with the same rHDL particles, in the *solid-phase assay*. After correction for nonspecific binding, the usual saturation curves were observed with increasing LCAT concentrations (Figure 4). The $K_d$ value for LCAT binding to rHDL particles containing apo A-II calculated from these experiments and given in Table 1, is of the same order of magnitude as that obtained by the activity-inhibition method. A stoichiometry of approximately 1 LCAT bound per rHDL particle is derived from the same data [unpublished results, Bolin and Jonas, 1991].

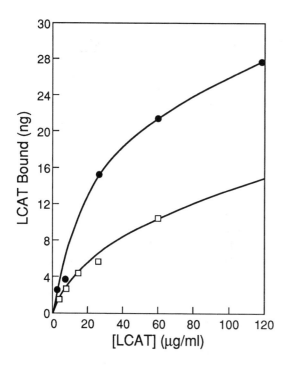

Figure 4.  Binding of $^{125}$I-LCAT to microtiter plates coated with rHDL containing apo A-II(●); binding of $^{125}$I-LCAT to plates without rHDL (□).

## ACTIVATION BY APOLIPOPROTEINS

It was first reported by Fielding et al. [7] that apo A-I added to PC/cholesterol vesicles dramatically activates the LCAT reaction.   Subsequent studies by Soutar et al. [8], Albers et al. [9], and our laboratory [10,11] showed unequivocally that other water soluble apolipoproteins also activate.  Table 2 gives the relative specificity constants (apparent $V_{max}$/apparent $K_m$) for several rHDL particles of equivalent morphology (discs), comparable sizes (96-145 Å), and identical lipid composition [unpublished results, Jonas and Steinmetz, 1991].  Other apolipoproteins are, at best, 25% as effective as apo A-I in activating the LCAT reaction; however, apo A-I can vary dramatically in its activating ability depending on the composition and morphology of the substrate particle.

Table 2
Reactivities of rHDL, containing different apolipoproteins, with LCAT

| rHDL Particles [a] | | App. $V_{max}$/App. $K_m$ [b] (nmol CE/hr·M) |
|---|---|---|
| Apo | Diameter (Å) | |
| A-II | 100 | $0.7 \times 10^5$ |
| A-I | 96 | $37.0 \times 10^5$ |
| E | 109 | $7.4 \times 10^5$ |
| A-IV | 145 | $8.5 \times 10^5$ |

[a]Discoidal particles prepared with POPC and 5 mol % cholesterol; the diameters are those of the major particles ($\sim$ 50% of total protein) in a heterogeneous mixture.
[b]These parameters vary from experiment to experiment depending on the concentration of LCAT used [unpublished results, Jonas and Steinmetz, 1991].

We recently found that the structure of apo A-I, in homogeneous rHDL discs made with POPC, changes depending on the diameter of the particles and the number of apo A-I molecules per particle [4]: 78 Å and 109 Å discs with 2 and 3 apo A-I per particle, respectively, have equivalent apo A-I structures as determined by spectroscopic measurements, whereas 96 Å discs with 2 apo A-I per particle have a distinct apo A-I structure. The reactivity with LCAT correlates with the apo A-I structure as can be seen in Table 1: the 96 Å particles are 12- to 16-fold more reactive than the 78 and 109 Å species. The most plausible explanation for this phenomenon is that the structure of apo A-I required for LCAT activation is well defined and is expressed in the 96 Å discs but not in the other two particles. In other studies [12,13] we found that these particles can be interconverted as a result of changes in the phospholipid content. Since this interconversion involves the region of apo A-I including the $Lys_{107}$ residue [14], it is also likely that the same region is implicated in the LCAT activation process. Other investigators, using monoclonal antibodies for different sequences of apo A-I [15] or synthetic peptide analogs of apo A-I sequences [16], have also suggested that this central region of apo A-I is involved in activation. In contrast, point mutations in this region of apo A-I, $Lys_{107} \rightarrow$ deletion [14], $Glu_{110} \rightarrow$ Lys [17], and $Glu_{111} \rightarrow$ Gln [18] do not affect significantly the activation. Therefore, a structural motif rather than a precise sequence are probably responsible for the activation of the LCAT reaction by apo A-I.

The mechanism of the activation is still unknown, but our observation that LCAT is active in solution with water soluble substrates in the absence of apo A-I, and is not activated further by excess apolipoprotein [19], indicates that the active site and the catalytic steps are not influenced by apo A-I, rather that binding of the water insoluble lipid substrates to the active site or removal of the products are facilitated by apo A-I. Whether the activation mechanism involves an interaction of the enzyme and apolipoprotein on the particle surface and modification of LCAT structure, or an activation of lipid substrates by apo A-I, is an open question.

## EVENTS AT THE ACTIVE SITE

The reaction of LCAT with different molecular lipid substrates can be studied independently from steps 1 and 2 in the overall reaction scheme (Figure 2) only when the interfaces presented to LCAT are equivalent. This was achieved by Pownall et al. [20] and by our laboratory [21] by using rHDL particles containing apo A-I and an unreactive ether PC matrix with small amounts of added PC substrates. Using this system Pownall et al. [20] have shown that phosphatidylethanolamines and phosphatidylcholines are the best phospholipid substrates for LCAT, and that PCs with saturated acyl chains shorter than C-18 are better substrates than PCs with longer, and more unsaturated chains. Presumably, the active site is not big enough to accommodate the longest and bulkiest acyl chains.

Another approach to the investigation of the catalytic steps of the LCAT reaction is to use water soluble substrates. We have developed continuous spectroscopic assays for the reaction of LCAT with p-nitrophenyl (PNP) esters of fatty acids [19] and dipyrene PC [unpublished results, Bonelli and Jonas, 1990] in solution, and have demonstrated that the phospholipase reaction of LCAT with these substrates has turnover numbers (16 nmol PNPB hydrolyzed/hr/$\mu$g) comparable to those of the cholesterol acyltransferase reaction on the best rHDL substrates (34 nmol cholesterol ester formed/hr/$\mu$g). The enzyme is active in solution and is not activated further by apo A-I or other apolipoproteins [19]. Clearly, the catalytic events are not influenced by apolipoproteins, and the activation of the LCAT reaction by apolipoproteins is an interfacial event.

Analysis of the reaction kinetics with PNP fatty acid esters (C-3 to C-6) indicated that binding affinity at the active site increases with chain length, but the catalytic efficiency decreases somewhat, probably because tighter binding decreases the probability that the ester bond will be in the proper location and orientation for enzymatic cleavage.

Using the PNP-butyrate (PNPB) and dipyrene PC substrates, we demonstrated that various amphiphiles, including lyso-PC and long chain fatty acids, at concentrations below their critical micellar concentration, inhibit the LCAT reaction in solution [unpublished results, Bonelli and Jonas, 1990]. The inhibition is competitive in the case of lyso-PC and simple noncompetitive in the case of fatty acids, indicating binding to the active site, and to specific negative effector sites, respectively. Therefore, the products of the LCAT reaction can potentially inhibit the enzymatic reaction by direct effects on the enzyme in addition to any interfacial effects they may have.

## PRODUCT RELEASE AND ENZYME RECYCLING

The first product of the LCAT reaction, lyso-PC (step 4 of the scheme in Figure 2), is quite soluble in water; it diffuses through plasma and binds to serum albumin [22]. Whether the enzyme must desorb from the interface to allow lyso-PC to leave the active site is unknown. The second product of the LCAT reaction, the cholesterol ester (step 7), diffuses out of the active site into the nonpolar core of the HDL. There is some evidence that cholesterol ester may bind reversibly to the enzyme since Sorci-Thomas et al. [23] have demonstrated a partial reversal of the LCAT reaction with a radiolabeled cholesterol ester.

Regarding the recycling of the enzyme on the same particle, or its desorption from the interface, our activity-inhibition experiments modified so that the competing rHDL was added after the reaction was initiated with substrate rHDL, provide evidence that LCAT desorbs from particles and equilibrates rapidly with other particles present in the solution [unpublished results, Jonas and Kézdy, 1990]. However, so far, we have no information on the numbers of reaction cycles the enzyme completes before its release.

## CONCLUSIONS

Much remains to be learned about the molecular and kinetic details of each step of the LCAT reaction, but it is evident that the chemical composition of the HDL substrate particle, as well as its physical properties will influence critically the kinetics of the overall reaction. Thus, the apolipoprotein and lipid composition and content of the particles, the structure of the apolipoproteins (especially apo A-I), and the size and shape of the particles will affect the reaction rates with LCAT. Furthermore, it must be noted that these chemical and physical properties of HDL are not independent parameters. The surface and core lipid composition, and the proportion of lipid to apolipoprotein affect the particle size and shape. In turn, size and shape of the particles influence the structure of the apolipoproteins. Therefore, a clear understanding of the preference of LCAT for different HDL particles as substrates will require a better understanding of the structure and dynamics of HDL, its interaction with LCAT, and the subsequent steps of the reaction at the surface of HDL.

## REFERENCES

1    Glomset J. In: Nelson G, ed. *Blood Lipids and Lipoproteins*. New York: Wiley, 1972; 745-787.
2    Chen CH, Albers JJ. *Biochem Biophys Res Commun* 1982; 107: 1091-1096.
3    Francone OL, Gurakar A, Fielding C. *J Biol Chem* 1989; 264: 7066-7072.
4    Jonas A, Kézdy KE, Wald JH. *J Biol Chem* 1989; 264: 4818-4824.
5    Wald JH, Krul ES, Jonas A. *J Biol Chem* 1990; 265: 20037-20043.
6    Jonas A, Wald JH, Harms KLT, Krul ES, Kézdy KE. *J Biol Chem* 1990; 265: 22123-22129.
7    Fielding CJ, Shore VG, Fielding PE. *Biochem Biophys Res Commun* 1972; 46: 1493-1498.
8    Soutar AK, Garner CW, Baker HN, Sparrow JT, Jackson RL, Gotto AM Jr., Smith LC. *Biochemistry* 1975; 14: 3057-3064.
9    Albers JJ, Lin J, Pretorius Roberts G. *Artery* 1979; 5: 61-75.
10   Jonas A, Sweeny SA, Herbert PN. *J Biol Chem* 1984; 259: 6369-6375.
11   Zorich N, Jonas A, Pownall HJ. *J Biol Chem* 1985; 260: 8831-8837.
12   Jonas A, Kézdy KE, Williams MI, Rye K-A. *J Lipid Res* 1988; 29: 1349-1357.

13    Jonas A, Bottum K, Kézdy KE. *Biochim Biophys Acta* 1991; 1085: 71-76.
14    Jonas A, von Eckardstein A, Kézdy KE, Steinmetz A, Assmann G. *J Lipid Res* 1991; 32: 97-106.
15    Banka CL, Bonnet DJ, Black AS, Smith RS, Curtiss LK. *J Biol Chem* 1991; 266: 23886-23892.
16    Anantharamaiah GM, Vankatachalapathi YV, Bruillette CG, Segrest JP. *Arteriosclerosis* 1990; 10: 95-105.
17    Takada Y, Sasaki J, Ogata S, Nakanishi T, Ikehara Y, Arakawa K. *Biochim Biophys Acta* 1990; 1043: 169-176.
18    Bruhn H, Stoffel W. *Biol Chem Hoppe-Seyler* 1991; 372: 225-234.
19    Bonelli FS, Jonas A. *J Biol Chem* 1989; 264: 14723-14728.
20    Pownall HJ, Pao Q, Massey JB. *J Biol Chem* 1985; 260: 2146-2152.
21    Jonas A, Zorich NL, Kézdy KE, Trick WE. *J Biol Chem* 1987; 262: 3969-3974.
22    Nakagawa M, Nishida T. *J Biochem* 1973; 74: 1263-1266.
23    Sorci-Thomas M, Babiak J, Rudel LL. *J Biol Chem* 1990; 265: 2665-2670.

**ACKNOWLEDGEMENTS**

The work from the A. Jonas' laboratory cited in this paper was supported by NIH Grants HL-16059 and HL-29939. We wish to thank the Champaign County Blood Bank, Health Resource Center, for the gift of human plasma, and Dr. A. Steinmetz for the apo E and apo AIV samples.

# HIGH DENSITY LIPOPROTEIN STRUCTURE

© 1992 Elsevier Science Publishers B.V. All rights reserved.
High density lipoproteins and atherosclerosis III.
N.E. Miller and A.R. Tall, editors.

# Modulation of HDL Precursor Structure and Metabolism

A.V. Nichols [a], E.L. Gong [a] and A. R. Tall [b]

[a]Lawrence Berkeley Laboratory, University of California, Berkeley, California 94720, USA

[b]Columbia University College of Physicians and Surgeons, 630 168th Street, New York, New York 10032, USA

## INTRODUCTION

Numerous epidemiologic studies have established a strong inverse relationship between plasma HDL levels and coronary heart disease (CHD) (1). Recent studies suggest that factors influencing levels and metabolism of HDL include both the composition and size of HDL and the fractional catabolic rates of apoAI or apoAII (2). Factors modulating HDL composition and size include lipid transfer proteins (cholesteryl ester transfer protein {CETP} and phospholipid transfer protein {PLTP}) as well as enzymes, such as lecithin:cholesterol acyltransferase {LCAT} and lipases, hepatic triglyceride lipase {HTGL} and lipoprotein lipase {LPL}. Like mature HDL in human plasma, HDL precursors (designated as nascent HDL or nHDL) are also potentially subject to the above modulating agents. However, except for LCAT little is known what effect these factors may have on the structural and metabolic properties of the precursor particles or how such remodeling may influence the channeling of precursors towards specific HDL subpopulations in human plasma. LCAT-mediated transformation of discoidal analogs of precursor nHDL to HDL-like products is characterized by a strong positive correlation between the size of the precursor particles and the size of their core-containing transformation products (3). Thus, modulation-induced change in size of nHDL particles by transfer proteins or enzymes would be expected to correspondingly shift the size of their LCAT-transformation products. In view of the association between HDL level and HDL particle size and composition, reduction in nHDL size may contribute to lower HDL levels and increased risk of CHD. Since nHDL lack core lipids and consist almost exclusively of phospholipid, unesterified cholesterol and apolipoproteins, their remodeling mainly involves phospholipid depletion as facilitated by CETP and PLTP and phospholipid lipolysis as facilitated by HTGL.

nHDL from various sources exhibit discrete species of discoidal and small (77Å) particles with unique apolipoprotein stoichiometry (4). Like plasma HDL, nHDL exhibit apolipoprotein-specific populations including, nHDL(AIw/oAII) {nascent HDL containing apoAI without apoAII} and nHDL(AIwAII) {nascent HDL containing apoAI with apoAII} that are comprised, to a greater or lesser extent, of discoidal and small particles (5). Discoidal nHDL(AIw/oAII) species can be modeled in vitro by reassembly of apoAI with phosphatidylcholine (PC) into complexes with and without unesterified cholesterol (UC) using detergent-dialysis procedures (6,7). The present study is concerned with three classes of complexes identified by their number of apoAI per complex: 2AI-class, 3AI-class and 4AI-class. Subclasses within each class exhibit unique sizes, molar ratios of PC:apoAI and, based on a recently proposed model of discoidal complexes (8), may contain a specific number of helices per apoAI in their structure . The discoidal model hypothesis proposes that the unique size and phospholipid content of a specific subclass is largely determined by its number of apoAI molecules and by the number of helices per apoAI assumed by apoAI upon interaction with the phospholipid bilayer. We have examined the fit of the model to major subclasses we have identified during reassembly of complexes within the 2AI-, 3AI-and 4AI-classes. In addition, we have used the model to predict properties of hypothetical discoidal complexes, having a specific number of apoAI and helices per apoAI, but which appear either to be unstable or to occur as minor or trace components under the reassembly conditions used. Table 1 presents properties of both experimentally-defined and predicted minor subclasses within each of the three classes. Based on the discoidal complex model, addition or depletion of phospholipid from a subclass, within a specific class of complexes, would be expected to increase or reduce, respectively, the number of helices per apoAI within the structure of the product complexes. At the present time, it is not clear whether phospholipid depletion of 4AI-subclasses or 3AI-subclasses produces intraclass or interclass conversions or both. Interclass conversions may involve particle destabilization leading to production of subclasses with lower number of apoAI per particle.

Table 1

Phosphatidlycholine-Apolipoprotein AI Discoidal Complex Classes[a]

| | 4AI-Class | | | 3AI-Class | | | 2AI-Class | | |
|---|---|---|---|---|---|---|---|---|---|
| Subclass size (Å) | 170±3[b] | (149)[c] | (130) | 130±3 | (118) | (101) | 95±2 | 86 | 77 |
| Molar ratio PC/AI | 155/1 | (124/1) | (87/1) | 119/1 | (90/1) | (59/1) | 83/1 | (55/1) | 40/1 |
| Helices/AI | (8) | (7) | (6) | (8) | (7) | (6) | (8) | (7) | (6) |
| Nomenclature: | | | | | | | | | |
| Nichols et al. | 4AI-170Å | (4AI-149Å) | (4AI-130Å) | 3AI-130Å | (3AI-118Å) | (3AI-101Å) | 2AI-95Å | (2AI-86Å) | 2AI-77Å |
| Jonas et al. (8)[d] | | | | | | | rHDL3 | rHDL2 | rHDL1 |

[a] Experimental procedures: Preparation and characterization of complexes (6,7); gradient gel electrophoresis (GGE) (9); number of apoAI/complex (10); PC content/AI in predicted complexes and estimated number of helices/AI in all complexes (8)

[b] ± Standard deviation

[c] Values in parentheses derived from discoidal model (8)

[d] Complexes contain unesterified cholesterol

In the present study, we investigated phospholipid depletion using the largest subclass experimentally identified within each of the classes, specifically the 2AI-95Å, 3AI-130Å and 4AI-170Å subclasses. Depletion was effected by spontaneous and CETP-mediated transfer of phospholipid to human plasma HDL3 (11). HDL3 was used as PC acceptor in view of its avidity for vesicle and chylomicron phospholipid. Specific questions addressed in the present study were: [1] does CETP facilitate phospholipid depletion of discoidal complexes, [2] do intraclass conversions occur and are the products consistent with the discoidal complex model, and [3] do interclass conversions occur and what products are formed?

## Spontaneous and CETP-Mediated Conversion of 2AI-Class Complexes

According to Table 1, the 2AI-class of PC-apoAI complexes includes 3 subclasses: 2AI-95Å; 2AI-86Å and, 2AI-77Å, with a predicted number of helices per apoAI of 8, 7 and 6, respectively. All of these subclasses are formed in reassembly mixtures with 75:1 PC:apoAI molar ratio. Spontaneous transfer of PC from the 2AI-95Å to HDL$_3$ over a period of 24 hr results in its progressive conversion to a smaller product with size corresponding to the 2AI-77Å subclass (Fig. 1A,B). The size and

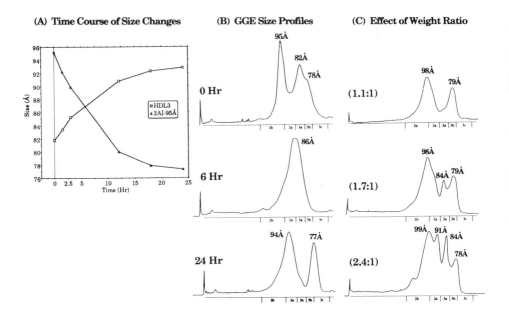

Figure 1. Spontaneous PC transfer between 2AI-95Å subclass and HDL$_3$. Weight ratio of PC (subclass): protein (HDL$_3$) in interaction mixture (37°C) was 1.1:1 and was used in all subsequent studies unless otherwise noted. Subclass complexes were prepared as in Table 1; HDL$_3$ were isolated ultracentrifugally (12). Analyses were performed as in Table 1. (A) Time course of size changes; (B) size profiles at 0, 6 and 24 hr; (C) size profiles at 18 hr when weight ratio of PC (subclass):protein (HDL$_3$) in mixture is increased as indicated.

composition of this product (2AI; 77Å; 33:9:1, PC:UC:AI) are comparable to those of small (77Å) particles identified in native nHDL (4). The UC observed in the conversion product was picked up from the HDL$_3$ during PC depletion. Based on area measurements from protein-stained profiles (from gradient gel electrophoresis), there appears to be little dissociation of apoAI during this conversion, indicating that the process is primarily one of PC depletion from the complexes. Reflecting its uptake of PC, HDL$_3$ size increases and approaches a plateau when conversion of the complexes nears completion. Higher levels of 2AI-95Å in the interaction mixture result in saturation of HDL$_3$ by PC and the appearance of conversion products now including not only the 2AI-77Å but also 2AI-84Å particles (Fig. 1C), both of which are predicted by the discoidal model based on number and conformation of apoAI molecules. These observations suggest that PC transfer can drive sequential conversion of the 2AI-95Å to the other stable subclasses of the 2AI-class (2AI-84Å and 2AI-77Å, with predicted helices/AI of 7 and 6, respectively). The above observations also suggest that small 2 apoAI-particles as observed in native nHDL may arise in part from conversion of discoidal particles driven by PC transfer.

Addition of CETP markedly accelerated PC transfer to HDL$_3$ and conversion of the 2AI-95Å (Fig. 2A,B). Under the same conditions shown in Figure 1, at 3 hr the CETP-mediated decrease in size of the 2AI-95Å was approximately fourfold greater than the decrease from spontaneous transfer. Similar to the conversion observed during spontaneous transfer, CETP-mediated conversion was associated with minimal change in apoAI content of the complexes.

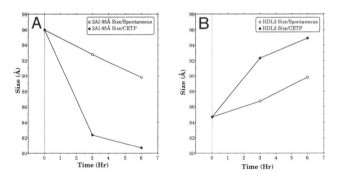

Figure 2. CETP-mediated PC transfer between 2AI-95Å subclass and HDL$_3$. Experimental conditions were as described in Table 1 and Fig. 1. CETP, prepared by Dr. Alan Tall, was recombinant CETP expressed by CHO cell line; partially purified CETP was prepared from human plasma (13). Time course of size changes in (A) 2AI-95Å subclass; (B) HDL$_3$.

## Spontaneous and CETP-Mediated Conversion of 3AI-Class Complexes

According to Table 1, the 3AI-class of PC-apoAI complexes includes 3 subclasses: 3AI-130Å; 3AI-118Å and, 3AI-101Å, with predicted number of helices of 8, 7 and 6 per apoAI, respectively. The 3AI-131Å is formed in PC-AI reassembly mixtures prepared at a PC:AI molar ratio of 200:1. On the other hand, the 3AI-118Å and 3AI-101Å are not detected under the conditions used. Reasssembly of a stable 3AI-109Å complex requires incorporation of a significant amount of unesterified cholesterol and yields a discoidal complex with molar composition of approx. 78:22:1 (PC:UC:AI) (8,14). Thus, except for the 3AI-130Å, the 3AI-subclasses predicted by the discoidal model for PC-apoAI complexes appear unstable under the reassembly conditions used. Smaller 3AI-complexes can be formed under these conditions but their formation requires incorporation of UC.

Spontaneous and CETP-mediated PC transfer from the 3AI-130Å to HDL3 was evaluated in mixtures with the same level of complex PC as in experiments with the 2AI-95Å. Unlike our observations with the 2AI-subclass, the rate of size decrease of the 3AI-subclass was similar both in the presence and absence of CETP (Fig. 3a). In the course of a 6 hr incubation with or without CETP, the size of the 3AI-130Å was reduced to 122Å which may correspond to that of the predicted 3AI-118Å (7 helices/AI) complex. No peaks were observed corresponding to a 3AI-101Å (6 helices/AI) complex, although its peak may have merged with that of the PC-enriched HDL3. Compared to spontaneous transfer, the increase in HDL3 size was markedly greater in the presence of CETP (Fig. 3b), indicating that considerable transfer to the HDL3 was facilitated by CETP.

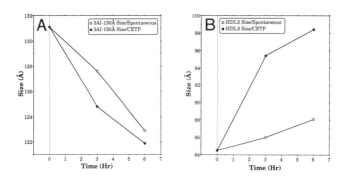

Figure 3. CETP-mediated PC transfer between 3AI-130Å subclass and HDL3. Conditions and analyses as in Table 1 and Fig. 2. Time course of size changes in (A) 3AI-130Å subclass; (B) HDL3.

However, this transfer occurred without facilitating size reduction of the 3AI-130Å. Interestingly, the increased transfer to HDL3 was correlated with a dramatic decrease in peak area of the 3AI-130Å (Fig. 4a). Thus, in the presence of CETP, the 3AI-130Å peak area decreased 77% at 6 hr

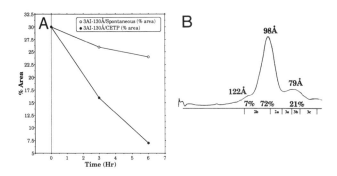

Figure 4. CETP-mediated PC transfer between 3AI-130Å subclass and HDL₃. Conditions and analyses as in Fig. 3. (A) Time course of change in subclass peak area expressed as % of total size profile area; (B) total size profile of interaction mixture at 6 hr, with % distribution of peak areas indicated.

compared to a 20% decrease without CETP. The redistribution of subclass mass appeared mainly as PC enrichment of the $HDL_3$ and appearance of additional peaks (approx. 21% of total profile area) primarily in the size interval ($HDL_{3b/c}$) containing the smaller 2AI-subclasses (Fig.4b). CETP-mediated interclass conversion of the 3AI-subclass complexes is indicated, since product particles in the $HDL_{3b/c}$ size interval would be expected to have 2 apoAI per particle. Thus, in the case of the 3AI-130Å, CETP appears to directly facilitate interclass conversion of the subclass with minimal influence on intraclass conversion. This suggests that the transfer mechanism may include CETP-mediated fusion of the 3AI-131Å with HDL3 resulting in extensive PC transfer and interclass conversion.

### Spontaneous and CETP-Mediated Conversion of 4AI-Class Complexes

According to Table 1, the 4AI-class of PC-apoAI complexes includes 3 subclasses: 4AI-170Å; 4AI-149Å; and 4AI-130Å, with a predicted number of helices per apoAI of 8, 7 and 6, respectively. The 4AI-170Å is formed in PC-AI reassembly mixtures prepared at molar ratio of 200:1. The other two 4AI-subclasses are not detected in these mixtures under the reassembly conditions used and their properties in Table 1 were derived using the discoidal model. Possibly, as with 3AI-complexes, incorporation of UC may be required to stabilize smaller 4AI-complexes.

Spontaneous and CETP-mediated transfer of PC from the 4AI-170Å to HDL3 was investigated in interaction mixtures providing complex PC at the same level as in experiments with the 2AI-95Å. As with the 2AI-subclass, CETP markedly increased the rate of size change in both the 4AI-170Å and

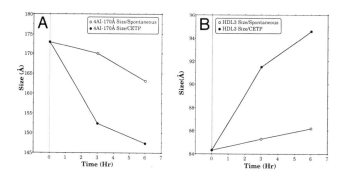

Figure 5. CETP-mediated PC transfer between 4AI-170Å subclass and HDL3. Conditions and analyses as in Fig. 3. Time course of size changes in (A) 4AI-170Å subclass; (B) HDL3.

the HDL3 (Fig. 5A,B). CETP-mediated PC transfer promoted intraclass conversion of the 4AI-170Å to the 4AI-147Å. whose size corresponds closely to that of the predicted 4AI-149Å (7 helices/AI) (Table 1). During spontaneous transfer, a 149Å conversion product is attained only after 18 hr incubation. At much higher levels of HDL3 relative to that of the 4AI-170Å in the interaction mixture, a product with size of 135Å is formed after 18 hr of spontaneous transfer. This particle may correspond to the predicted 4AI-130Å (6 helices/AI) shown in Table 1. In the presence of CETP, the size increase in HDL3 approximates that observed with 2AI-95Å indicating comparable PC transfer. At 3 hr, the CETP-mediated decrease in size of the 4AI-170Å, relative to the spontaneous decrease, is approximately five-to-sevenfold greater and at 6 hr approaches a limiting size of 147Å. A major feature of the CETP-mediated intraclass conversion of the 4AI-170Å is a concurrent and marked reduction in its peak area of approx. 60% at 6 hr (Fig. 6A). During spontaneous transfer, the decrease in this subclass' size is considerably less and is associated with a minimal decrease in peak area. In summary, these results suggest that the 4AI-170Å subclass undergoes intraclass conversions which are associated with PC transfer and with changes in AI conformation. However, in addition to promoting intraclass conversion, CETP also promoted extensive interclass redistribution of its protein and phospholipid mass. The size distribution of products formed during CETP-mediated conversion of the 4AI-170Å was evaluated from protein-stained gradient gels after electrophoresis of the interaction mixture (Fig. 6B). The reductions in peak area correlate with area increases within the size interval of the PC-enriched HDL3 and within the size interval of smaller HDL particles, namely the HDL3b/c. Since complexes in the HDL3b/c interval are primarily the smaller 2AI-subclasses, these results would be consistent with CETP-induced interclass conversion. The size interval containing the PC-enriched HDL$_3$ also may include 2AI-subclass products, such as the larger 2AI-95Å.

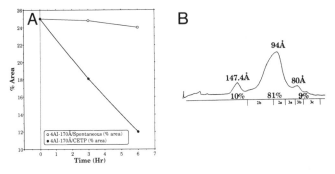

Figure 6. CETP-mediated PC transfer between 4AI-170Å subclass and HDL$_3$. Conditions and analyses as in Fig. 3. (A) Time course of change in subclass peak area expressed as % of total size profile area; (B) total size profile of interaction mixture at 6 hr, with % distribution of peak areas indicated.

## SUMMARY

The present study utilized model discoidal complexes 2AI-95Å, 3AI-130Å, and 4AI-170Å to evaluate structural remodeling (intraclass and interclass conversion) in response to spontaneous and CETP-mediated PC transfer to HDL$_3$ (Table 2). Compositional and structural properties of the

Table 2
Intraclass Conversions During PC Depletion

| Size of conversion products (Å) | 4AI-Class | | | 3AI-Class | | | 2AI-Class | | |
|---|---|---|---|---|---|---|---|---|---|
| | 170 → 147 → 135 | | | 130 → 122 → ? | | | 95 → 84 → 77 | | |
| Predicted # of helices/AI | 8 | 7 | 6 | 8 | 7 | 6 | 8 | 7 | 6 |
| Complex sizes (Å) predicted from # of apoAI & helices/AI | 168 | 149 | 130 | 130 | 115 | 101 | 91 | 82 | 72 |
| Complex sizes (Å) in reassembly mixtures | 170 | --- | --- | 130 | --- | --- | 95 | 86 | 77 |

substrate complexes were consistent with those predicted by the discoidal complex model (8). Properties of product complexes generated by PC depletion were also generally consistent with those predicted by the model.

Under the experimental conditions used, CETP markedly facilitated transfer of PC from all of the above complexes to $HDL_3$. With the 2AI-95Å subclass, CETP facilitated intraclass conversion associated with the PC transfer. With the larger 3AI-130Å and 4AI-170Å subclasses, PC transfer was associated with interclass conversions apparently involving fission with formation of smaller products having a lower number of apoAI per particle. Our studies suggest that CETP-mediated and, most likely, PLTP-mediated remodeling of nHDL can have significant impact on precursor size, number of apoAI and apoAI conformation. By affecting precursor size, remodeling can significantly influence the size of HDL particles (whether $HDL_2$ or $HDL_3$) resulting from LCAT-mediated transformation of the remodeled precursor particles.

## ACKNOWLEDGEMENTS

This work was supported by National Institutes of Health Grants HL 46281-02 (A.V.N.) and HL 22682 (A.R.T.), and was conducted at the Lawrence Berkeley Laboratory (Department of Energy Contract DE-AC03-76SF00098 to the University of California).

## REFERENCES

1.  Miller NE. Am Heart J 1987; 113: 589-597.
2.  Brinton EA, Eisenberg S, Breslow JL. J Clin Invest 1991; 87: 536-544.
3.  Nichols AV. In: Esfahani M, Swaney J, eds. Advances in Cholesterol Research. Caldwell: Telford Press, 1990; 315-365.
4.  Nichols AV, Gong EL, Blanche PJ, Forte TM, Shore VG. In: Lippel K, ed. Proceedings of the Workshop on Lipoprotein Heterogeneity. NIH Publication No. 87-2646, 1987; 331-340.
5.  Nichols AV, Gong EL, Blanche PJ, Forte TM. In: Miller NE, ed. Proceedings of the 2nd International Workshop on HDL and Atherosclerosis. Amsterdam: Elsevier, 1989; 159-171.
6.  Matz CE, Jonas A. J Biol Chem 1982; 257: 4535-4540.
7.  Nichols AV, Gong EL, Blanche, Forte TM. Biochim Biophys Acta 1983; 750: 353-364.
8.  Jonas A, Kezdy KE, Wald JH. J Biol Chem 1989; 264: 4818-4824.
9.  Nichols AV, Blanche PJ, Gong EL. In: Lewis L, Opplt J, eds. CRC Handbook of Electrophoresis Vol III. Boca Raton: CRC Press, 1983; 29-47.
10. Swaney JB. J Biol Chem 1980; 255: 877-881.
11. Tall A, Swenson T, Hesler C, Granot E. In: Gotto AM Jr., ed. Plasma Lipoproteins. Amsterdam: Elsevier, 1987; 277-297.
12. Anderson DW, Nichols AV, Forte TM, Lindgren FT. Biochim Biophys Acta 1977; 493: 55-68.
13. Ohnishi T, Yokoyama S, Yamamoto A. J Lipid Res 1990; 31: 397-406.
14. Nichols AV, Gong EL, Blanche PJ, Forte TM. J Lipid Res 1987; 28: 719-732.

© 1992 Elsevier Science Publishers B.V. All rights reserved.
High density lipoproteins and atherosclerosis III.
N.E. Miller and A.R. Tall, editors.

# APOLIPOPROTEIN A-IV AND HIGH DENSITY LIPOPROTEINS: A TENUOUS INTERACTION

Richard B. Weinberg[a]

[a]Department of Medicine, The Bowman Gray School of Medicine, Medical Center Boulevard, Winston-Salem, North Carolina, 27157, USA

## INTRODUCTION

Human apolipoprotein A-IV (apo A-IV) is a 46,000 dalton plasma glycoprotein (1-3) of intestinal origin (4,5,6). Originally described in 1978 (1), apo A-IV was initially regarded as an unimportant curiosity, for it appeared to circulates primarily as a lipid-free apolipoprotein (2,4,5,7-9). Although the specific function of apo A-IV in human lipid metabolism has yet to be determined, recent studies have demonstrated that apo A-IV can activate lecithin cholesterol acyltransferase (10,11), catalyze the interconversion of high density lipoprotein (HDL) subfractions by lipid transfer proteins (12,13), and effect the efflux of cholesterol from peripheral cells (14-16). These observations constitute a growing body of evidence which suggests that apo A-IV plays an important role in the intravascular metabolism of high density lipoproteins and the process of reverse cholesterol transport.

## STRUCTURE OF APO A-IV

The biophysical properties of human apo A-IV are distinct from those of other human and mammalian apolipoproteins. Apo A-IV is an extremely hydrophilic apolipoprotein (17), and its affinity for lipid surfaces is considerably weaker than other apolipoproteins; consequently, it is easily displaced from native and model lipoproteins by other apolipoproteins (18,19). Like other apolipoproteins, apo A-IV contains a high content of amphiphilic alpha-helical structure (17,20), which is stabilized by association with lipid (21). However, the amphipathic helices in apo A-IV may not be capable of penetrating lipid monolayers to the same depth as those in other apolipoproteins (21); indeed, the hydrophobic faces of these helices may be oriented towards the interior of the protein where they are unavailable for binding to lipid surfaces (22). Moreover, in solution apo A-IV readily forms dimers with an unusually large association constant (23); this behavior may further limit its ability to bind to lipid.

## METABOLISM OF APO A-IV

In man, the gene for apo A-IV is expressed only in the small intestine (24). The synthesis of apo A-IV in the enterocytes of the small intestine is especially stimulated by fat absorption (5,25,26). Apo A-IV is initially incorporated onto the surface of nascent chylomicrons (5), but its subsequent intravascular metabolism is unique in that it rapidly dissociates from the chylomicron surface following their entry into the bloodstream (8,27) and thereafter circulates primarily unassociated with serum lipoproteins (5,7,8). The plasma residence time of apolipoprotein A-IV is less than 24 hours (8,27). Radiotracer studies in the rat have established that the liver and kidney are the major sites of apo A-IV catabolism (28).

Apo A-IV may play a physiologic role in the metabolism of high density lipoproteins. Apo A-IV activates lecithin-cholesterol acyl transferase (LCAT), the key enzyme in the metabolism of HDL (10,11). However, the catalytic efficiency of apo A-IV is only 20% of that of apo A-I, the physiologic activator of LCAT, and unlike apo A-I, is not affected by the saturation of the phospholipid fatty acyl chains (10,11). A common genetic variant, apo A-IV-2, demonstrates increased LCAT catalytic efficiency and phospholipid selectivity in comparison to the wild type apo A-IV, perhaps as a consequence of its ability to better penetrate lipid surfaces (29). Apo A-IV may also catalyze the interconversion of HDL subfractions by lipid transfer proteins (12,13), and may thereby modulate the speciation of HDL (13,30).

Apo A-IV may participate in the process of reverse cholesterol transport. Apo A-IV binds with high affinity to a variety of cells (15,16,31-33), and in cell culture promotes rapid efflux of cellular cholesterol (14-16). A distinctive discoidal HDL containing free cholesterol and apo A-IV appears in the peripheral nodal lymph of cholesterol-fed dogs (34); similar apo A-IV/lipid complexes have been observed in man (9,35). These observations further suggest that apo A-IV may participate in the earliest stages of peripheral HDL assembly.

## INTERACTION OF APO A-IV AND HDL

There is considerable disparity in the literature regarding the *in vivo* binding of apo A-IV to HDL. Following fractionation of serum by ultracentrifugation (5,7) or by electrophoretic techniques (2,23,36), essentially all apo A-IV is found in the lipoprotein-free fraction, unassociated with lipoproteins. When serum is fractionated by gel filtration chromatography, approximately 20% of the apo A-IV elutes with the HDL fraction (5,9). However, when serum is fractionated by FPLC on Superose 12 at 4 bar, almost all of the apo A-IV co-elutes with HDL (37). Although the true lipoprotein distribution of apo A-IV *in vivo* remains to be established, it is clear that the binding of apo A-IV to the HDL surface is a tenuous interaction, easily perturbed by physical forces.

In this regard, the *in vitro* binding and affinity of apo A-IV for the surface of HDL is transiently but dramatically increased by the action of LCAT; a second independent process thereafter effects the dissociation of apo A-IV from HDL (36,38,39). We have demonstrated that the association phenomenon is confined to the HDL$_3$ subfraction, requires cholesterol esterification, and is correlated with the amount of cholesterol ester formed (36). Recent findings suggest that the dissociation phenomenon may be mediated by cholesterol ester exchange protein (CETP) (40).

## A MONOLAYER MODEL OF APO A-IV/HDL INTERACTION

The most salient biophysical property of apo A-IV is its extremely labile interaction with the surface of serum lipoproteins, particularly high density lipoproteins. To date, the mechanisms which mediate the labile and reversible binding of apo A-IV to HDL have not been elucidated, nor has the relevance of these phenomena to the biologic function of apo A-IV been examined. The adsorption of protein solutions to lipid monolayers at equilibrium is a particularly appropriate model for the study of the interaction of apo A-IV and the surface of high density lipoproteins. Below we describe the use of a surface balance and surface radioactivity detector to investigate the biophysics of the adsorption of apo A-IV to phospholipid monolayers spread at the air/water interface.

## METHODS

Apo A-IV was prepared from lipoprotein-depleted serum (20) obtained from donors homozygous for the apo A-IV-1 allele (29). Apolipoprotein A-IV was labelled with $^{14}$C by reductive methylation (41); less than one lysine was labelled per molecule of protein. Egg yolk phosphatidylcholine (EPC) obtained from Sigma Chemical Company, St. Louis, MO was >99% pure by thin layer chromatography. A spreading solution of EPC was prepared by dissolving a known quantity of phospholipid in hexane/ethanol (9:1 v/v). EPC concentration was determined by analysis of phosphorus (42).

The adsorption of unlabeled and $^{14}$C-apo A-IV to the lipid/water interface was studied at 25°C using a 10.8 cm diameter Teflon dish which was mounted on a magnetic stirring plate, and enclosed in a humidified, temperature controlled cabinet. The surface pressure ($\pi$) of protein-lipid films was monitored with a mica Wilhelmy plate suspended from an electrobalance (43); the estimated error in $\pi$ was ± 1 mN/m. The surface concentration of $^{14}$C-apo A-IV ($\Gamma$) was monitored using a gas flow scintillation counter positioned 2 mm above the buffer surface (43). Calibration curves for converting cpm to mg/m$^2$ were generated by spreading known quantities of $^{14}$C-apolipoprotein at the air/buffer interface (44); the estimated error in $\Gamma$ was $\pm$ 5%.

EPC monolayers were spread at the air-water interface over phosphate-buffered saline to the desired initial pressure by dropwise addition of the phospholipid spreading solution from a Hamilton syringe. Thirty minutes were allowed to elapse to assure complete evaporation of all organic solvent. The desired amount of unlabeled or $^{14}$C-labelled apo A-IV was then injected beneath the monolayer, and the change in $\pi$ and $\Gamma$ were continuously recorded until they reached stable equilibrium values. The subphase was stirred with a magnetic flea throughout the course of each experiment to assure adequate mixing. Surface pressure-molecular area isotherms for apo A-IV were measured on a Langmuir-Adam surface balance, interfaced with a torsion balance (44). Surface pressure was recorded as a film of apo A-IV spread at the air/water interface was compressed in 1-3 Å$^2$/residue decrements.

## RESULTS

The adsorption of apo A-IV to EPC monolayers spread at an initial pressure of 10 mN/m was examined as a function of final subphase concentration, $C_P$ (FIGURE 1). At $C_P > 1 \cdot 10^{-6}$ gm/dl, $\pi$ and $\Gamma$ progressively increased, and reached maximum values of 19 mN/m and 0.31 mg/m$^2$, respectively, at $C_P > 1 \cdot 10^{-5}$ gm/dl. These values are similar to those previously reported for apo A-I (45). Subsequent lipid binding experiments were performed with $C_P = 3 \cdot 10^{-5}$ gm/dl, to assure surface saturation. It should be noted that at this concentration, greater than 99% of apo A-IV is in the monomeric form (23).

To assess the reversibility of binding, $^{14}$C-apo A-IV was injected beneath an EPC monolayer spread at a pressure of 10 mN/m, and allowed to equilibrate to constant $\pi$ and $\Gamma$. Following injection of an equal amount of unlabeled apo A-IV into the subphase, no change in $\pi$ was observed, but by 4 hours $\Gamma$ had decreased 57% to a new steady state value, indicating that the $^{14}$C-apo A-IV adsorbed to the monolayer had approached complete equilibrium with the unlabeled apo A-IV in the subphase. This established that the binding of apo A-IV to the EPC monolayer was reversible.

The effect of apo A-IV on the stability of the phospholipid monolayers was assessed by injecting unlabeled apo A-IV beneath monolayers of [$^{14}$C]-dipalmitoyl phosphatidyl choline spread at 10 mN/m. After 10 hours, $\Gamma$ had decreased by less than 8%, indicating that the adsorption of apo A-IV did not significantly disrupt or destabilize the phospholipid monolayer.

The monolayer exclusion pressure for apo A-IV was determined by injecting $^{14}$C-apo A-IV beneath EPC monolayers spread at increasing initial pressures ($\pi_i$), and monitoring the change in Γ and π. FIGURE 2 shows the resulting $\pi_i$-Δπ and $\pi_i$-Γ curves. The binding of apo A-IV to the lipid/water interface decreased in a linear manner with increasing πi; extrapolation of the $\pi_i$-Γ curve to zero indicated that apo A-IV could not penetrate the surface at $\pi_i$ > 28 mN/m. The change in surface pressure, which is more sensitive than the change in Γ to the presence of apo A-IV in the monolayer, also decreased linearly with increasing $\pi_i$; extrapolation of Δπ to zero indicated an exclusion pressure of $\pi_i$ > 29 mN/m. In comparison, exclusion pressures determined by extrapolation of $\pi_i$-Δπ curves for other human apolipoproteins are: apo A-I, 33 mN/m (46); apo A-II, 34 mN/m (43);apo C-III, 31 mN/m (47); apo C-II, 34 mN/m (47).

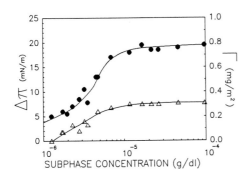

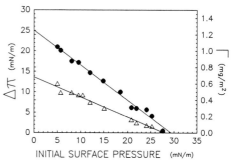

FIGURE 1. Adsorption of apo A-IV to EPC monolayers. (●) surface pressure; (Δ) surface concentration

FIGURE 2. Monolayer exclusion pressure for apo A-IV. (●) surface pressure; (Δ) surface concentration

To evaluate the relevance of the exclusion pressure data to the binding of apo A-IV to HDL$_3$, we estimated the surface pressure of native and LCAT-modified HDL$_3$ using the equation:

$$4\pi r_o^2 = (N_{aa} \times A_{aa}^{\pi=i}) + (N_{pl} \times A_{pl}^{\pi=i}) + (N_{fc} \times A_{fc}^{\pi=i})$$

where $N_x$ is the number of molecules of a given component present in the lipoprotein shell (aa, amino acid residues;pl, phospholipids;fc, free cholesterol) and $A_x^{\pi=i}$ is the area occupied by a molecule of that component at a surface pressure of i mN/m. This equation, when solved for i using the HDL$_3$ stochiometry calculated by Shen et al. (48) and the p-area curves for apo A-I (44), HDL phospholipids (49), and free cholesterol (49), predicted a surface pressure of 33 mN/m for native HDL$_3$. A similar analyses predicted that the surface pressure of HDL$_3$ is exquisitely sensitive to the action of

LCAT, and with only a 2% increase in the particle cholesterol ester content, the surface pressure falls below 29 mN/m, the predicted exclusion pressure of apo A-IV (FIGURE 3). This analysis also predicted that removal of newly synthesized cholesterol esters from the HDL$_3$ core by cholesterol ester transfer protein would return the HDL$_3$ surface pressure to 29 mN/m, assuming no replacement by triglyceride molecules.

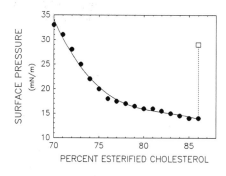 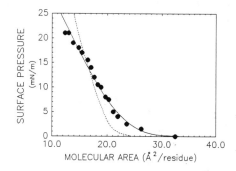

FIGURE 3. Calculated HDL$_3$ surface pressure vs %CE. (□) pressure after CETP removes CE molecules.

FIGURE 4. Surface pressure-molecular area isotherms. (—●—) apo A-IV; (···) apo A-I

## DISCUSSION

### The surface activity of apo A-IV

It is generally accepted that the binding of apolipoproteins to lipoproteins is mediated by the hydrophobic interaction of amphipathic alpha helical domains in the protein and lipid molecules on the lipoprotein surface (50-52). This necessitates both the physical penetration of the amphipathic helices into the lipid monolayer and the coordinate lateral compression of the lipid molecules (53). Hence the opposing forces which determine whether binding of an apolipoprotein is energetically favorable are the collective hydrophobicity of its alpha helical domains and the surface pressure of the monolayer. The alpha helical domains of human apo A-IV not only are extremely hydrophilic, but also have relatively low helical hydrophobic moments (17). On the basis of these properties we predicted that human apo A-IV would be at the bottom of apolipoprotein surface activity hierarchy. Our present observation that the monolayer exclusion pressure of apo A-IV is lower than other apolipoproteins, now directly confirms this prediction.

## The conformation of apo A-IV at the interface

A clue to the structural basis for the low surface activity of apo A-IV is provided by its unusual surface conformation. The $\pi$-area curve of an apo A-IV monolayer compressed at the air/water interface (FIGURE 4) reveals that at low surface pressures its mean residue molecular area is greater than apo A-I, consistent with a relatively expanded conformation. However, between 15-20 mN/m, the $\pi$-area curve for apo A-IV crosses the curve for apo A-I, and the mean residue area falls to 11.6 $\mathring{A}^2$, well below the predicted limiting area for closely packed amino acids, 15 $\mathring{A}^2$ (54). Similarly, the mean residue molecular area of apo A-IV adsorbed to EPC, calculated from the data in FIGURE 1, is 10.2 $\mathring{A}^2$/residue; this is consistent with exclusion of 33% of the amino acid residues in apo A-IV from the phospholipid/water interface. These data suggest that whereas at low surface pressure all of the amphipathic alpha helical domains in apo A-IV can penetrate the surface, at higher surface pressures weakly amphipathic domains no longer possess sufficient hydrophobicity to remain in the monolayer, are progressively forced out of the plane of the interface, and project in multiple loops or tails into the buffer subphase (53). Thus at surface saturation, a large part of the apo A-IV molecule is excluded from the interface by the pressure generated by its own adsorption.

## The labile association of apo A-IV with HDL

The partial exclusion of the apo A-IV molecule from the surface provides an explanation for its labile binding to HDL and the ease with which it is displaced from lipoproteins by other apolipoproteins. It also implies that the binding of apo A-IV to $HDL_3$ will be extremely sensitive to small changes in surface pressure, and that processes which modify the physical-chemical properties of the $HDL_3$ surface will have a dramatic effect on the association of apo A-IV and $HDL_3$. Therefore, a plausible mechanism of the effect of LCAT and CETP on the association of apo A-IV and $HDL_3$ is as follows: initially, the pressure of the $HDL_3$ surface monolayer is above the exclusion pressure of apo A-IV, and hence it cannot bind. However, when the action of LCAT lowers the $HDL_3$ surface pressure below 29 mN/m, apo A-IV may then penetrate the surface. Thereafter, when CETP depletes the $HDL_3$ core of newly synthesized cholesterol esters, the $HDL_3$ particle will shrink, its surface pressure will increase, and apo A-IV will again be excluded. Given the proximity of the exclusion pressure of apo A-IV to the predicted surface pressure of $HDL_3$, the changes in surface pressure would need not be great to effect the association/ dissociation phenomena in vivo; rather, the surface pressure of $HDL_3$ need only oscillate about a narrow range that spans the exclusion pressure of apo A-IV.

## The function of apo A-IV in the LCAT and CETP reactions

The labile and pressure sensitive binding of apo A-IV to the surface of HDL, rather than being an incidental curiosity, may in fact be of central importance to the molecular mechanisms of the LCAT and CETP reactions. Because both of these processes involve exchange or modification of lipids at the HDL surface, they can alter HDL surface pressure. If LCAT and CETP activity were sensitive to interfacial pressure - as is the case with two other surface active lipoprotein modifying enzymes, lipoprotein lipase (55) and hepatic lipase (56) - then reversible binding of apo A-IV to HDL from a "reservoir" of free protein could function as a barostatic mechanism to maintain HDL surface pressure in a critical range necessary for optimal LCAT and CETP activity. Two previous observations support this hypothesis: 1) although apo A-IV does not directly activate lipoprotein lipase in vitro, it accelerates the rate of triglyceride hydrolysis by lipoprotein lipase when it is activated by its co-factor, apo C-II (57); 2) although apo A-IV does not directly function as a lipid exchange protein, it accelerates the interconversion of HDL subfractions by CETP (13).

## SUMMARY

In summary, the surface activity and surface exclusion pressure of apo A-IV are lower than those of the other human apolipoproteins. Its binding and surface conformation are particularly sensitive to pressure, and at saturation, a significant portion of the molecule is excluded from the interface. The surface pressure of $HDL_3$ may be only slightly above the exclusion pressure of apo A-IV, and in vivo, the action of LCAT and CETP may cause the $HDL_3$ surface pressure to oscillate about a narrow range that spans the exclusion pressure of apo A-IV. The resultant labile association of apo A-IV and $HDL_3$ may be of central importance to its role in human lipoprotein metabolism.

## ACKNOWLEDGEMENT

The figures and portions of text have been adapted from an article currently in press in the Journal of Biological Chemistry, and are used with permission.

## REFERENCES

1. Weisgraber KH, Bersot TP, Mahley RW. Biochem Biophys Res Commun 1978;85:287-292.
2. Beisiegel U, Utermann G. Eur J Biochem 1979;93:601-608.
3. Weinberg RB, Scanu AM. J Lipid Res 1983;24:52-59.

4. Green PH, Glickman RM, Saudek CD, Blum CB, Tall AR. J Clin Invest 1979;64:233-242.
5. Green PH, Glickman RM, Riley JW, Quinet E. J Clin Invest 1980;5:911-919.
6. Elshourbagy NA, Walker DW, Paik YK, et al. J Biol Chem 1987;262:7973-7981.
7. Utermann G, Beisiegel U. Eur J Biochem 1979;99:333-343.
8. Ghiselli G, Krishnan S, Beigel Y, Gotto AM. J Lipid Res 1986;27:813-827.
9. Bisgaier CL, Sachdev OP, Megna L, Glickman RM. J Lipid Res 1985;26:11-25.
10. Steinmetz A, Utermann G. J Biol Chem 1985;260:2258-2264.
11. Chen CH, Albers JJ. Biochim Biophys Acta 1985;836:279-285.
12. Barter PJ, Rajaram OV, Chang LB, et al. Biochem J 1988;254:179-184.
13. Lagrost L, Gambert P, Dangremont V, et al. J Lipid Res 1990;31:1569-1575.
14. Stein O, Stein Y, Lefevre M, Roheim PS. Biochim Biophys Acta 1986;878:7-13.
15. Savion N, Gamliel A. Arteriosclerosis 1988;8:178-186.
16. Steinmetz A, Barbaras R, Ghalim N, et al. J Biol Chem 1990;265:7859-7863.
17. Weinberg RB. Biochem Biophys Acta 1987;918:299-303.
18. Weinberg RB, Spector MS. J Lipid Res 1985;26:26-37.
19. Rifici VA, Eder HA, Swaney JB. Biochim Biophys Acta 1985;834:205-214.
20. Weinberg RB, Spector MS. J Biol Chem 1985;60:4914-4921.
21. Weinberg RB, Jordan M. J Biol Chem 1990;265:8081-8086.
22. Weinberg RB. Biochemistry 1988;27:1515-1521.
23. Weinberg RB, Spector M. J Biol Chem 1985;260:14279-14286.
24. Elshourbagy NA, Walker DW, Bogusky MS, Gordon JI, et al. J Biol Chem 1986;261:1988-2002.
25. Apfelbaum TF, Davidson NO, and Glickman RM. Am J Physiol 1987;252:G662-666.
26. Go MF, Schonfeld G, Pfleger B, Cole TG, Sussman NL, Alpers DH. J Clin Invest 1988;81:1615-1620.
27. Ohta T, Fidge NH, Nestel PJ. J Clin Invest 1985;76:1252-1260.
28. Dallinga-Thie GM, Van't Hooft FM, Van Tol A. Arteriosclerosis 1986;6:277-284.
29. Weinberg RB, Jordan M, Steinmetz A. J Biol Chem 1990;265:18372-18378.
30. Nichols AV, Blanche PJ, Shore VG, Gong EL. Biochim Biophys Acta 1989;1001:2325-337.
31. Dvorin E, Gorder NL, Benson DM, Gotto, AM. J Biol Chem 1986;261:15714-15718.
32. Savion N, Gamliel A, Tauber JP, Gospodarowicz D. Eur J Biochem 1987;164:435-443.
33. Weinberg RB, Patton C. Biochem Biophys Acta 1990;1044:255-261.
34. Sloop CH, Dory L, Hamilton R, Krause B, Roheim PS. J Lipid Res 1983;24:1429-1440.

98

35. Ohta T, Fidge NH, Nestel PJ. J Biol Chem 1984;259:14888-14893.
36. Weinberg, R.B., and Spector, M.S. Biochem Biophys Res Commun 1986;135:756-763.
37. Lagrost L, Gambert P, Boquillon M, Lallemant C. J Lipid Res 1989;30:1525-1534.
38. DeLamatre JG, Hoffmeier CA, Lacko AG, Roheim PS. J Lipid Res 1983;24:1578-1585.
39. Bisgaier CL, Sachdev OP, Lee ES, et al. J Lipid Res 1987;28:693-703.
40. Bisgaier CL, Siebenkas MV, Hesler et al. J Lipid Res 1989;30:1025-1031.
41. Jentoff N, Dearborn DG. Methods Enzymol 1983;91:570-579.
42. Sokoloff L, Rothblat GH. Proc Soc Exp Biol Med 1974;146:1166-1172.
43. Phillips MC, Krebs KE. Methods Enzymol 1986;128:387-403.
44. Krebs KE, Ibdah JA, Phillips MC. Biochim Biophys Acta 1988:959:229-237.
45. Ibdah JA, Krebs KE, Phillips MC. Biochim Biophys Acta 1989;1004:300-308.
46. Ibdah JA, Phillips MC. Biochemistry 1988;27:7155-7162.
47. Krebs KE, Phillips MC, Sparks CE. Biochim Biophys Acta 1983;751:470-473.
48. Shen BW, Scanu AM, Kezdy FJ. Proc Natl Acad Sci USA 1977;74:837-841.
49. Ibdah JA, Lund-Katz S, Phillips MC. Biochemistry 1989;28:1126-1133.
50. Segrest JP, Jackson RL, Gotto AM. FEBS Lett 1974;38:247-253.
51. Morrisett JD, Jackson RL, Gotto AM. Biochim Biophys Acta 1977;472:93-133.
52. Atkinson D, Small DM. Ann Rev Biophys Biophys Chem 1986:15:403-456.
53. MaCritchie F. Adv Prot Chem 1978;32:283-320.
54. Jones MN. in Biological Interfaces, Chapter III, Elsevier, New York, 1975.
55. Vainio P, Virtanen JA, Kinnunen PKJ, et al. Biochemistry 1983:22:2270-2275.
56. Thuren T, Wilcox RW, Sisson P, Waite M. J Biol Chem 1991;266:4853-4861.
57. Goldberg IJ, Scheraldi CA, Yacoub LK, et al. J Biol Chem 1990;265:4266-4272.

High density lipoproteins and atherosclerosis III.
N.E. Miller and A.R. Tall, editors.

# Apolipoprotein A-I: structure, lipid interaction and activation of lecithin:cholesterol acyltransferase

Yves L. Marcel, Laura Calabresi and Qiang-Hua Meng

Laboratory of Lipoprotein Metabolism, Clinical Research Institute of Montreal, 110 Pine Avenue West, Montreal, Quebec, H2W 1R7, Canada

Progress in the characterization of HDL has demonstrated the great heterogeneity of particles, which characterize this lipoprotein density class, differing, not only in size, but in apolipoprotein composition and molar ratio of constitutive apolipoproteins (1). This complexity led several investigators to approach the study of HDL structure and metabolism through the definition of simpler precursor particles and through the *in vitro* preparation of such particles (2,3). Stable particles made of defined molar ratios of cholesterol, phosphatidylcholine and apoA-I have been now obtained which are believed to be analogous to biological intermediates in the genesis of HDL particles (4,5). These apoA-I-containing lipoproteins or LpA-I can be grouped in classes according to the number of apoA-I per particle, such as Lp2A-I, Lp3A-I and Lp4A-I, and within each class, in subclasses of defined and reproducible sizes depending on the apoA-I/lipid ratio. The existence in apoA-I gene of multiple repeats coding for 22-mers representing amphipathic α-helices has been the bases for the current model of apoA-I structure in discoïdal particles (6). In this model, apoA-I is bound to the edge of the disc with up to 8 repeats arranged as antiparallel amphipathic α-helices with their axis parallel to the axis of the disc. While the number of amphipathic α-helices in apoA-I is a matter of debate, Jonas and colleagues have observed that the Lp2A-I exist as particles of 7.8, 8.6 and 9.6 nm in which the α-helicity of apoA-I increases with the size of the particle. They could, in addition, calculate that the circumference of these particles can accommodate respectively 6, 7, and 8 α-helices for each molecule of apoA-I, thus providing an explanation for the increased α-helicity observed in the larger particles (5). Although largely based on indirect evidence, a logical model for apoA-I structure bound to discoïdal particles has been developed from these and other studies (6). Using this model as reference, we have undertaken to study the immunoreactivity of apoA-I epitopes to refine and validate the model with the aim of also defining the functional domains which mediate apoA-I interaction with lecithin: cholesterol acyltransferase (LCAT) and those which allow it to bind and interact specifically with cholesterol.

The first step in these studies has been the development and characterization of a large panel of monoclonal antibodies (mAbs) against apoA-I (7). A detailed mapping of the epitopes recognized by these mAbs has been carried out. On the N-terminal half of apoA-I, six overlapping epitopes have been identified which are complex discontinuous epitopes constituted by aminoacids or sequences dispersed throughout in the primary structure. The existence of such discontinuous epitopes implies that the N-terminal region has a complex tertiary structure although one cannot entirely rule out the possibility of intermolecular epitopes that may result from the presence of multiple copies of apoA-I on lipoproteins and the oligomeric nature of lipid-free apoA-I used in immunization and screening. In contrast, the epitopes present in the middle of apoA-I are shorter and usually constituted by residues forming a loop or ß-turn and the adjacent α-helix. We have proposed that these central epitopes, which are mostly limited to single helices, reflect the existence of a mobile domain (7), possibly constituted by a pair of adjacent helices which can be either free or bound to the lipid phase depending on the size of the lipoprotein, as suggested by others (8). On the C-terminal half of apoA-I, the epitopes identified consist of longer sequences which are thought to represent two adjacent antiparallel α-helices separated by a ß-turn. The nature and distribution of the epitopes, thus identified on apoA-I have been very informative. It is clear that the N-terminal region, which does not contain the regular amphipathic repeats characteristic of the rest of the molecule, has a distinct and complex folding which remains to be defined, while the central region, from residue 99 to 143, has multiple short epitopes compatible with the existence of a mobile domain.

Based on earlier evidence that the lipid composition of HDL influences its metabolism (9), we hypothesized that changes in lipid concentration of HDL should first alter apoA-I structure and that this would be reflected in specific modification of epitope immunoreactivity (10). Of particular interest in these studies was the observation that phospholipids and cholesterol had markedly different effects on epitopes and thus appeared to interact with distinct domains on apoA-I. While the extreme N-terminal sequence was specifically influenced by cholesterol, the immunoreactivity of a discontinuous epitope stretching from residue 1 to about 96 was inversely related to phospholipid concentration. This would indicate that the N-terminal domain, despite the absence of the amphipathic α-helical repeats, is in intimate contact with lipids. Adjacent to this region, the epitopes in the two antiparallel α-helices (residues 99 to 121) behaved differently, the expression being independent of phospholipids and decreased by cholesterol.

These studies have been pursued using well defined discoïdal LpA-I prepared by dialysis of mixtures of cholesterol, palmitoyl oleyl phosphatidylcholine, cholate and apoA-I followed by gel filtration separation of homogeneous populations of particles (5,11-12). Lp2A-I were obtained in the sizes of 7.8 and 9.6 nm, Lp3A-I in the sizes of 10.8 and 13.4 nm and Lp4A-I only as 17 nm particles. The immunoreactivity of all epitopes tested was significantly different in LpA-I compared to lipid-free apoA-I, which demonstrated that binding of apoA-I to lipids was accompanied by changes in structure affecting the entire molecule. In contrast, once associated with discoïdal particles the conformation of apoA-I was seen to vary little with the exception of the N-terminal region where the immunoreactivity of epitopes was significantly different in the small versus large particles in either of Lp2A-I or Lp3A-I. Elsewhere there was little difference in immunoreactivity of apoA-I epitopes in the Lp2A-I, LP3A-I and Lp4A-I regardless of sizes. This demonstrates that, with the exception of the N-terminal region, there is no major change in apoA-I conformation as a function of the number of apoA-I molecules in these particles and that no domain was found that could be masked as a function of lipid to protein ratio and particle size.

However when the relative position of epitopes was assessed by competition assay between pairs of mAbs, very significant differences were observed as a function of particle size but independently of the number of apoA-I molecules per particle. The most surprising observation was that competition between pairs of mAbs recognizing central epitopes was greater when they reacted with the large particles than with their small counterparts. If the structure of apoA-I was to remain the same in all discoïdal particles, one would expect more competition in small particles as a result of tighter packing of the polypeptide chain. Since this is not the case in either Lp2A-I or Lp3A-I, a different folding of the central portion of apoA-I must exist in the small compared to the large particles. This region coincides with the central helices which we proposed earlier may form a mobile domain based on the series of small epitopes found there that are constituted by one or part of one helix. Furthermore, the introduction of a hinged domain constituted by two adjacent antiparallel α-helices at either residues 99 to 143 or 121 to 165 in the model of apoA-I structure on these discoïdal particles improves the fit of the competition data with the model. This constitutes the first experimental data to support the existence of such a hinged domain on apoA-I (L. Calabresi, Q.-H. Meng and Y.L. Marcel, manuscript in preparation).

In our first attempt to characterize the functional domains of apoA-I, we tried to understand what particular structural feature, present in apoA-I, makes it the most efficient LCAT activator. All apolipoproteins, that share this property, also share a structural homology represented by series of amphipathic α-helical repeats. A priori this homology which is restricted to the secondary structure suggests that the capacity to activate LCAT may be related to the ability of these apolipoproteins to bind lipids and to generate a suitable structure, i.e. a discoïdal particle. Another hypothesis, to explain the higher rate of reaction observed with apoA-I, may also be a preferential interaction between LCAT and apoA-I perhaps due to the existence of an LCAT binding domain on apoA-I, as indeed plasma LCAT is for the most part associated with apoA-I-containing lipoproteins. We have evaluated this possibility by testing the capacity of mAbs reacting with various epitopes distributed along the apoA-I sequence to interfere in the reaction of LCAT with defined LpA-I. With these substrates, LCAT activity was highest with the largest particles and was a function of the ratio of phospholipid to apoA-I. The relative LCAT activity was correlated with the ratio of the particle circumference to the number of apoA-I molecules per particle, a parameter reflecting the space available per molecule of apoA-I and therefore the relative freedom or mobility of apoA-I on the particle's edge.

Out of 9 mAbs tested, only 3 inhibited the reaction of LCAT with LpA-I and the epitopes of these 3 mAbs were contained in the region of residues 96 to 186, a result in agreement with those of others (13). However, consideration of the exact position of epitopes for the inhibitory mAbs, shows that the process of antibody mediated inhibition is more complex than a simple process of steric hindrance. Indeed, other mAbs reacting with intervening epitopes, that is epitopes contained within residues 96 to 186, have been found which do not inhibit the LCAT reaction. Furthermore, some mAbs reacting in the same region have an enhancing effect on the reaction but only with specific particles, namely with the small particles, be they Lp2A-I or Lp3A-I. Antibodies can interfere in a reaction in a number of ways, such as by steric hindrance or by masking of a specific functional domain or by exerting a conformational change somewhere in the antigen. In the case of reaction enhancement, it is clear that certain mAbs may stimulate it by conformational change, i.e. by stabilization of an apoA-I conformation favorable to LCAT in the small particles or by prevention of the formation of an unfavorable conformation. The location of epitopes for inhibitory mAbs also suggests that they may act by interference with the hinged domain which we defined above (Q.-H. Meng, L. Calabresi, and Y.L. Marcel, manuscript in preparation).

In summary, our studies have contributed to define the structure of apoA-I, and to the understanding of its interaction with lipids. It is clear that the N-terminal region, which is characterized by a complex folding and a conformation different from that of the amphipathic repeats in the rest of the molecule, is also a lipid binding region. The differential effect of cholesterol and phospholipids on apoA-I epitopes has provided evidence for specific interaction of these lipids with distinct domains and suggests their possible segregation in HDL or LpA-I. Several lines of evidence demonstrate the existence, in apoA-I, of a flexible or mobile domain which is located between residues 99 and 143. The strongest evidence for this comes from the difference in apoA-I conformation in small and large LpA-I which can be explained by the introduction of hinged domains in the central region of apoA-I model structure.

Finally, the location of epitopes, recognized by mAbs inhibitory to the reaction of LCAT with LpA-I, demonstrates the importance of the central region of apoA-I in the activation of the reaction. The mechanism of activation itself may also depend upon the formation of these hinged domains or the existence of such domains which can be alternatively bound and unbound to lipids.

## REFERENCES

1    Eisenberg S. J Lipid Res 1984; 25: 1017-1057.
2    Matz CE, Jonas A. J Biol Chem 1982; 257: 4535-4540.
3    Nichols AV, Gong EL, Blanche PJ, Forte TM. Biochim Biophys Acta 1983; 750: 353-364.
4    Nichols AV, Gong EL, Blanche PJ, Forte TM, et al. J Lipid Res 1987; 28: 719-732.
5    Jonas A, Kezdy HE, Hefele Wald J. J Biol Chem 1989; 264: 4818-4824.
6    Brasseur R, De Meutter J, VanLoo B, Goormaghtigh, et al. Biochim Biophys Acta 1990; 1043: 245-252.
7    Marcel YL, Provost PR, Koa H, Raffai E, et al. J Biol Chem 1991; 266: 3644-3653.
8    Brouillette CG, Jone JL, Ng TC, Kercret H, et al. Biochemistry 1984; 23: 359-367.
9    Collet X, Perret B, Chollet F, Hullin F, et al. Biochim Biophys Acta 1988; 958: 81-92.
10   Collet X, Perret B, Simard G, Raffai E, et al. J Biol Chem 1991; 266: 9145-9152.
11   Jonas A, Hefele Wald J, Toohill KLH, Krul ES, et al. J Biol Chem 1990; 265: 22123-22129.
12   Hefele Wald J, Krul ES, Jonas A. J Biol Chem 1990; 265: 20037-20043.
13   Banka CL, Bonnet DJ, Black AS, Smith RS, et al. J Biol Chem 1991; 267: 23886-23892.

© *1992 Elsevier Science Publishers B.V. All rights reserved.*
*High density lipoproteins and atherosclerosis III.*
*N.E. Miller and A.R. Tall, editors.*

CONTRIBUTION OF HELIX-HELIX INTERACTIONS TO THE STABILITY
OF APOLIPOPROTEIN-LIPID COMPLEXES.

M. Rosseneu[a], B. Vanloo[a], L. Lins[b], J. Corijn[a], J-P. Van
Biervliet[a], J-M. Ruysschaert[b] and R. Brasseur[b]

[a]. Dept.Clinical Chemistry, A.Z. St-Jan, B-8000 Brugge
(Belgium)

[b]. Laboratoire de Chimie Physique des Macromolecules aux
interfaces, Fac. Sciences, Univ. Libre Bruxelles, B-1050,
Bruxelles, (Belgium).

INTRODUCTION.

Amphipathic helices in plasma apolipoproteins, were
first described by Segrest et al (1) in 1974. These
amphipathic helical regions are involved in the
interaction of apolipoproteins with lipids (2,3). An
important feature of the amphipathic helix is the
presence of two clearly defined faces, one hydrophobic
which interacts with the acyl chains of the phospholipid
and the other hydrophilic which is oriented towards the
aqueous phase. As most amphipathic helices do not have
exclusively polar or apolar residues on one face, the
localisation of the interface between hydrophobic and
hydrophilic sides, on the mere basis of this graphical
representation, might prove difficult. The hydrophobicity
potential concept, which provides a quantitative
definition of the relative magnitude of the two faces of
an amphipathic helice is quite informative in this
respect (4, 5).

Based both upon theoretical energy minimisation
calculations and upon infrared measurements by the ATR
technique, we proposed a general way of assembly for
apolipoproteins and phospholipid in a discoidal lipid-
protein complex (3, 6). In this model, the helices are
oriented parallel to the lipid acyl chains, around the
edge of the disc, with their hydrophobic face towards the
hydrophobic lipid core. The adjacent helices of apo AI,
A-IV and E, which are separated by beta-turns, are
oriented anti-parallel to each other. In this
configuration, the amino acid residues along the edges of
the helices are in close vicinity and can theoretically
form salt bridges. These ionic interactions can

contribute to the stability and cooperativity of the lipid-apolipoprotein complex structure.

In this paper we describe the identification of putative ion pairs in apo AI and A-IV, and the calculation of the energy of interaction between adjacent helices in apolipoprotein-phospholipid complexes. We also provide experimental evidence about the contribution of ionic inter-peptide interactions to the mode of association between apolipoprotein helical segments and synthetic phospholipids.


MATERIALS AND METHODS.


1. Reassembly of apolipoproteins with phospholipids.

Apolipoproteins A-I, CII and CIII were prepared from human plasma very low and high density lipoproteins by ultracentrifugation, delipidation and ion-exchange chromatography, according to well-established methodology (7). Apo A-IV was recovered from the ascites fluid of a patient with chylous lymphoma as previously described (8). The purity of the apolipoproteins was checked by SDS gel electrophorosis, isofocusing and amino acid analysis.

The apolipoproteins were reassembled with dimyristoylphosphatidylcholine (Sigma) vesicles, prepared by vortex mixing of the phospholipid in a 0.01 M Tris-HCl buffer, pH 8.1, 0.15 N NaCl. Complex formation with DMPC was followed by measurement of the absorbance of the protein-lipid mixture at 325 nm, as a function of temperature, between 16 and 30°C. Measurements were performed in the thermostated cells of a Kontron spectrophotometer equipped with a temperature programming device. These experiments were carried out in the presence of 0.15, 0.5 and 0.8 M NaCl, in order to investigate the effect of increasing salt concentrations on the properties of the lipid-apolipoprotein complexes.


2. Theoretical calculations.

The helical repeats in the apo A-I and A-IV sequences were identified using an autocorrelation matrix based upon similarities of hydrophobicity between amino acid residues (5). Molecular modelling of these segments, taken alone or as pairs of helices separated by a stretch of five residues, was carried out by a systematic calculation of the psi and phi angles of these five residues (9). The most stable structures obtained by this analysis were further optimized by energy minimisation techniques. For this purpose, an helical structure was imposed upon these segments and the three-dimensional structure was calculated using the classical values of the torsional angles psi and phi for alpha-helical residues. The lowest conformational energy was obtained by minimisation using the Simplex method (10) and considered as the most stable conformation for the peptides. The conformational energy was calculated as the sum of the Van der Waals, hydrophobic and electrostatic energies. The dielectric constant was taken as 16, corresponding to the value at a lipid/water interface (9). The hydrophobic and electrostatic potentials surrounding either a single helix or a pair of helical segments were calculated as previously described (11).

All calculations were performed on an Olivetti CP486 microcomputer equiped with an Intel 80486 arithmetic co-processor using the PC-Prot+ and PC-TAMMO programs. Graphs were drawn with the PC-PGM+ program.

RESULTS.

1. Characterisation of the helical repeats in apo AI and A-IV.

The 17-residue helical repeats identified in apo A-I and A-IV, using the auto-correlation matrix, are listed in Table I, together with the 5-residue segments separating these repeats. The homologous helical segments identified by this method coincide with those previously reported using either the Dayhoff matrix (12), or a matrix based on secondary structure homologies (13). The sequences of the five-residue segments separating the helices also share a strong homologoly, as most of them consist a Pro residue separating hydrophobic amino acids (Table I). The corresponding consensus sequences, respectively LXPYL for apo AI and LXPVA for apo A-IV, where X is mostly an hydrophobic residue, are homologous to those described for other proteins (14).

A systematic analysis of the angles phi and psi, followed by energy minimisation calculations for the pairs of helices of apo A-I, show that the helices are almost parallel in the lowest energy structure (Fig.1). The angle between the axes of the two helices varies between 10 and 25°. The Pro-containing segment separating the helices, consists of 5 residues in a beta-strand extended conformation.

Table I
Sequences of the helical and extended beta-strand segments
in apo A-I and apo A-IV.

| BETA-STRANDS | | |
|---|---|---|

| APO AI | | APO A-IV | |
|---|---|---|---|
| 64-68 | LGPVT | 60-64 | LVPFA |
| 97-101 | VQPYL | 93-97 | LLPHA |
| 119-123 | VEPLR | 115-119 | LEPYA |
| 141-145 | LSPLG | 137-151 | LDPLA |
| 163-167 | LAPYS | 159-163 | LRPHA |
| 185-189 | GGARL | 181-185 | LTPYA |
| 207-211 | AKPAL | 203-207 | LAPYA |
| | | 225-229 | MKKNA |
| | | 247-251 | LAPLA |
| | | 287-291 | VEPYG |
| | | 309-313 | LGPHA |

| HELICAL REPEATS: | | |
|---|---|---|

| APO AI | | APO A-IV | |
|---|---|---|---|
| 102-118 | DDFQKKWQEEMELYRQK | 98-114 | NEVSQKIGDNLRELQQR |
| 124-140 | AELQEGARQKLHELQEK | 120-136 | DQLRTQVNTQAEQLRRQ |
| 146-162 | EEMRDRARAHVDALRTH | 142-158 | QRMERVLRENADSLQAS |
| 168-184 | DELRQRLAARLEALKEN | 164-180 | DELKAKIDQNVEELKGR |
| 190-206 | AEYHAKATEHLSTLSEK | 186-202 | DEFKVKIDQTVEELRRS |
| 223-239 | ESFKVSFLSALEEYTKK | 208-224 | QDTQEKLNHQLEGLTFQ |
| | | 230-246 | EELKARISASAEELRQR |
| | | 252-258 | EDVRGNLKGNTEGLQKS |
| | | 292-308 | ENFNKALVQQMEQLRQK |
| | | 314-330 | GDVEGHLSFLEKDLRDK |

The length of this segment is sufficient to reverse the
orientation of the helices which lie anti-parallel
(Fig.1). In this configuration, the apolar helical faces
point towards the lipid phase, while the polar faces of
the two helices are oriented towards the aqueous phase
(Fig.2). The values of the different energies involved in
the stabilisation of such a pair of helices separated by
a beta-turn are listed in Table II. The lowest energy was
calculated for the peptides 128-162 and 168-206 followed
by peptide 146-184, while the 102-140 segment was less
stable. The greater stability of some of the helix pairs
was due to stronger electrostatic interactions between
charged residues (Fig.1).

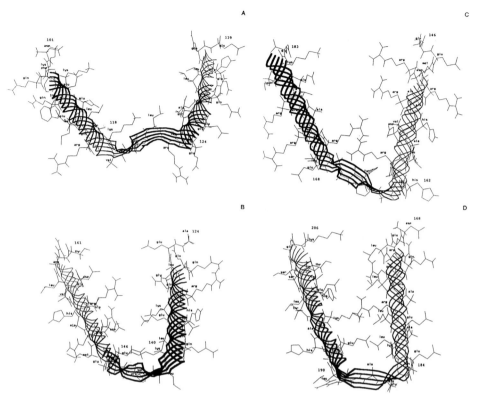

Fig.1. Computer modelling by energy minimisation of four pairs of helices separated by an extended beta-strand in apo A-I. The helical residues are: A:101-118; 124-139. B:124-140; 146-161. C:146-162; 168-183. D:168-184; 190-206. Beta-strand residues are: A:119-123; B;141-145; C:163-167; D:185-189.

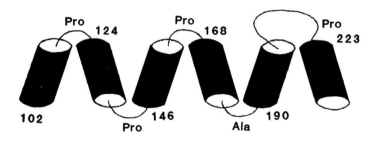

Fig.2. Schematic representation of the orientation of the helical repeats of apo A-I around the edge of a discoidal phospholipid-apoprotein complex.

110

Table II. Interaction energies (Kcal/mole peptide) between pairs of helices of apo A-I linked by an extended beta-strand.

| | helices | | | | | |
|---|---|---|---|---|---|---|
| 1st | Beta-strand | 2nd | $E_{tot}$ | $E_{V.d.W.}$ | $E_{pho}$ | $E_{electr.}$ |
| 102–118 | 119–123 | 124–140 | 0.1 | -0.3 | 0.2 | 0.2 |
| 124–140 | 141–145 | 146–162 | -9.2 | -2.5 | 0 | -6.7 |
| 146–162 | 163–167 | 168–184 | -7.1 | -0.8 | 0.04 | -6.4 |
| 168–184 | 185–189 | 190–206 | -9.2 | -0.9 | 0.3 | -8.7 |

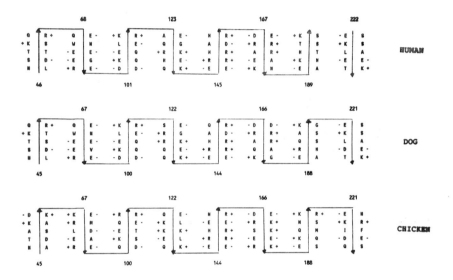

Fig.3. Charged residues located along the sides of the helical repeats in the sequences of human, dog and chicken apo A-I. These residues can be involved in intra-and inter-helical salt bridges.

Computer modelling of the anti-parallel pairs of helices separated by an extended beta-strand, showed that charged residues located along the edges of the helical segments are in close proximity. The formation of salt bridges becomes theoretically possible between the residues facing each other on both sides of the beta-strand. This particular configuration, shared also by apo A-IV and E, is due to the low hydrophobic angle of the helical segments, whose hydrophilic face covers 240° and to their ellipsoidal shape (5).

The residues susceptible to form salt bridges in the apo AI helices are shown on Fig.3. These residues are conserved in most apo AI species or replaced by residues with same charge, as shown for the sequences of human, dog and chicken apo A-I (Fig.3). The same holds also for the rat, rabbit and cow apo A-I (data not shown). The strongest polar interactions exist between residues of helices 120-145 and 148-163 in agreement with the energy minimisation data (Table II). Similar results were obtained for apo A-IV and E. The calculation of the electrostatic potential around the helices of apo A-I further showed that charged residues are uniformly distributed along most helical segments. Only helices 102-118 and 223-239 had a high density of positive charges around the N-terminal extremities.

## 2. Effect of the ionic strength on the cooperativity of the phospholipid-apoprotein complexes

The optical density decrease as a function of the temperature was used to monitor the extent of complex formation as it reflects the formation of small discoidal complexes compared to the original phospholipid liposomes (Fig.4). As previously observed (3), complex formation with the larger apoproteins A-I and A-IV, occurs close to the DMPC transition temperature. In contrast, the smaller apoproteins CII and CIII react at lower temperatures with the crystalline lipid, as the optical density decrease starts around 17°C. This behaviour is similar to that of synthetic peptides consisting of a single amphipathic helix such as the LAP-20 or 18A peptides (15). These data suggest that the peptide cooperativity is less pronounced in apo CII and CIII, each of which contains two helices separated a longer stretch of residues. Apo A-I and AI-IV consisting of respectively 6 and 8 repeats separated by 5-residue beta-strands, show greater cooperativity for lipid association (16).Increasing the salt concentration up to 0.5 and 0.8 M NaCl does not affect either the temperature or the amplitude of the association of phospholipids with apo A-I or A-IV. However with apo CII and CIII, the cooperativity of this process is reduced and the complex formation initiates at lower temperatures in the presence of high salt concentrations. This effect is similar to that observed with fusion-inducing peptides which form ionic inter-peptide interactions through their Lys and Glu residues (17). It is due to the shielding of the charged residues by NaCl and to a decrease of the ionic interactions.

112

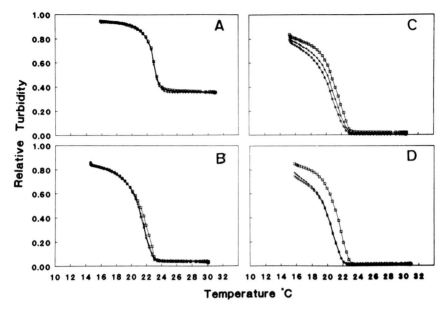

Fig.4. Influence of the ionic strength on the turbidity
decrease associated with the formation of discoidal
complexes between apoproteins and DMPC. The absorbance at
325 nm is measured as a function of temperature in the
presence of (□) .15 M; (+) .5 M and (◇) .8 M NaCl for :A:
apo A-I; B: apo A-IV; C: apo CII; D: apo CIII.


DISCUSSION.

    The results presented in this paper suggest that ionic
interactions and salt bridge formation between adjacent
residues in the helical repeats of the apoproteins can
significantly contribute to the stabilisation of the
apoprotein-phospholipid discoidal complexes. The concept
of pair complementarity between the helices of apo A-I is
further supported by recent data from Bruhn and Stoffel
(18), showing that the deletion of one pair of helices
does not affect either the lipid-binding or the LCAT
activation properties of apo A-I. The recent
crystallograpic data on apo E (19) have evidenced the
existence of specific interactions, both hydrophobic and
ionic between helical stretches in the protein crystals.
The cooperativity between helical segments of
apolipoproteins must therefore contribute to the
stability of these apolipoproteins and be involved in
their lipid-binding and enzyme co-factor properties.

The importance of the cooperativity between apolipoprotein helical repeats was also demonstrated from the experiments using synthetic peptides. Anantharamaiah et al (20) showed that the LCAT activation properties of the 18A-Pro-18A peptide were enhanced compared to those of the momomeric peptide. Fukushima et al (21) showed that the surface properties of the tetracontapeptide consisting of two 22-residue helical repeats of apo A-I separated by a Proline, mimicked more closely those of apo A-I than any single docosapeptide. The role of the beta strand stretch to ensure a proper match of the apolar faces of the helices seems therefore critical. A direct confirmation of the occurence of amphipathic helices in the structure of plasma apolipoproteins was provided by the crystallographic structure of apo E (19). The four helices found in the N-terminal fragment are arrranged to form a 2 by 2 bundle, a structure found in at least 18 other protein crystal structures. The charged residues in the apo E sequence include 24 acidic and 24 basic residues covering most of the surface of the bundle. Most participate in intramolecular salt bridges, 7 of which between pairs of helices.

We postulate that the same type of interaction is responsible for the cooperativity of the phospholipid transition in the apo AI and A-IV complexes. Such ionic interactions can also take place between residues of the helices of apo CII and CIII. As the distances between helices are larger, the ionic interactions are weaker and can be more easily disrupted by high salt concentrations.

REFERENCES.

1. Segrest JP, Jackson RL, Morrisett JD, Gotto AM, FEBS Lett.1974;3:247-250
2. Pownall HJ, Massey JB, Sparrow JT, Gotto AM. In: "Plasma lipoproteins". Gotto AM, ed. Amsterdam: Elsevier Sci, 1987;95-127
3. Brasseur R, De Meutter J, Vanloo B, Goormaghtigh E, Ruysschaert JM, Rosseneu M, Biochim. Biophys. Acta.1990;1043:245-252
4. Brasseur R, J. Biol. Chem.1991;266:16120-16127
5. Brasseur R, Lins L, Vanloo B, Ruysschaert JM, Rosseneu M, Proteins:.Structure, Function, and Genetics. (in press)
6. Vanloo B, Morrison J, Fidge N, Lorent G, Brasseur R, Ruysschaert JM, Baert G, Rosseneu M, J. Lipid Res.1991;32:1253-1264
7. Gotto AM, Pownall HJ, Havel RJ, Methods Enzymol.1986;128:3-40
8. Yang C-y, Gu Z-W, Chong I, Xiong W, Rosseneu M, Yang H-x, Lee B-r, Gotto AM, Chan L, Biochim. Biophys. Acta.1989;1002:231-237
9.Deleers M, Brasseur R, Proc. Natl. Acad. Sci. USA.1984;81:3370-3374

114

10. Nelder JA, Mead R, Comput. J.1965;7:308-313
11. Brasseur R, J. Biol. Chem.1988;263:12571-12575
12. Dayhoff MO, Barker WC, Hunt LT, Methods Enzymol.1983;91:524-544
13. Rosseneu M, Vanloo B, Lins L, Ruysschaert JM, Brasseur, R, in:"Structure and function of apolipoproteins", Rosseneu M, ed. Boca Raton FA: CRC Press. (in press)
14. Boguski MS,Freeman M, Elshourbagy NA, Taylor JM, Gordon JI, J. Lipid Res.1986;27:1011-1018
15. Anantharamaiah GM, Methods Enzymol. 1986;128:627-647
16. Lins L, Rosseneu M, Ruysschaert JM, Brasseur R, in:"Structure and function of apolipoproteins", Rosseneu M, ed. Boca Raton FA: CRC Press (in press)
17. Murata M, Kagiwada S, Takahashi S, Ohnishi S-i, J. Biol. Chem.1991;266:14353-14358
18. Bruhn H, Stoffel W, Biol. Chem. Hoppe-Seyler.1991;372:225-231
19. Wilson C, Wardell MR, Weisgraber KH, Mahley RW, Agard DA, Science.1991;252:1817-1822
20. Anantharamaiah GM, Venkatachalapathi YV, Brouillette CG, Segrest JP, Arteriosclerosis.1990;10:95-105
21. Fukushima D, Yokoyama S, Kroon DJ, Kezdy FJ, Kaiser ET, J. Biol. Chem.1980;255:10651-10657

# HIGH DENSITY LIPOPROTEIN-CELL INTERACTIONS

© 1992 Elsevier Science Publishers B.V. All rights reserved.
High density lipoproteins and atherosclerosis III.
N.E. Miller and A.R. Tall, editors.

Cholesterol transport between cells and high density lipo-proteins

Michael C. Phillips, William J. Johnson and George H. Rothblat

Department of Physiology and Biochemistry, Medical College of Pennsylvania, Philadelphia, PA 19129, USA

## INTRODUCTION

Cholesterol homeostasis in peripheral cells involves a balance between the influx and efflux processes. The acqui-sition of cholesterol by such cells is mediated by a variety of receptor and non-receptor processes involving both normal and modified lipoproteins (for reviews, see [1, 2]). The offsetting efflux process is believed to be mediated by high density lipoproteins (HDL) [3]. This clearance of cholester-ol from peripheral cells is the first step in the "reverse cholesterol transport" of excess cholesterol to the liver for excretion from the body [4].

A complete description of cholesterol transport between cells and HDL will require understanding of the following points. 1) The nature of the flux of cholesterol molecules from the cell surface (i.e. the plasma membrane). 2) The efflux of cholesterol from intracellular pools. 3) The effects of HDL structure and especially apolipoprotein con-formation on the transport process. This article addresses each of these issues in turn.

## RESULTS AND DISCUSSION

### Efflux of Plasma Membrane Cholesterol

It is well known that unesterified (free) cholesterol molecules can exchange between extracellular lipoproteins and cells. This exchange is a surface transfer process in the sense that internalization of the lipoprotein particles by the cell is not required. Free cholesterol exchange by surface transfer is a physical-chemical phenomenon that does not require metabolic energy (for reviews, see [3, 5]). A bidirectional flux of cholesterol occurs between extracellu-lar HDL particles and the cell plasma membrane (cf. Fig. 1). Efflux is defined as the rate of cholesterol movement from the cells to the medium (rate constant = $k_e$), and influx is the rate of movement in the opposite direction (rate constant = $k_i$). The kinetics of the cholesterol flux are consistent with a so-called "aqueous diffusion" mechanism.

In the aqueous diffusion process, cholesterol molecules desorb from the donor lipid-water interface and diffuse through the intervening aqueous layer until they collide with

118

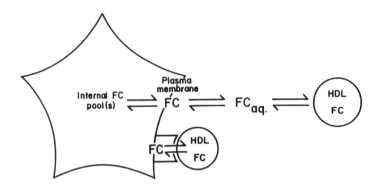

Figure 1. Schematic representation of the "aqueous diffusion" and receptor-mediated mechanisms of unesterified (free)
cholesterol (FC) flux between the cell plasma membrane and
extracellular HDL particles. $FC_{aq}$ in the aqueous diffusion
mechanism represents cholesterol molecules that have desorbed
into the aqueous phase and that are diffusing between the
cell surface and HDL. In the receptor-mediated process, the
high affinity binding of HDL apoprotein to the cell surface
receptor is postulated to facilitate the movement of cholesterol from the plasma membrane to the HDL particles.

and are absorbed by an acceptor particle; when excess acceptor particles are present, the rate-limiting step is the
desorption of cholesterol molecules from the donor particle.
The following kinetic criteria are characteristic of the
process [3, 5]: (1) the rate of free cholesterol exchange is
first order with respect to the concentration of free cholesterol in the given kinetic pool in the donor particles; (2)
the free cholesterol exchange process is strongly temperature
dependent and the activation energy is about 70 kJ/mol; and
(3) at high acceptor/donor particle ratios, the rate of
exchange is zero order with respect to the concentration of
acceptor particles. The transfer of cholesterol molecules to
the aqueous phase proceeds through a transition-state complex
where the cholesterol molecule is attached to the donor
lipid-water interface by the tip of its hydrophobic tail.
The height of the activation energy barrier for formation of
this transition state is affected by the interaction energy
of the cholesterol molecule with neighboring molecules in the
surface of the donor particle. Thus, if the Van der Waals
attraction between cholesterol and the host phospholipid is
relatively low, the rate of desorption of cholesterol molecules is enhanced. For this reason, decreases in: (1) the

degrees of saturation of the host phospholipid molecules; and (2) the sphingomyelin content of the lipid/water interface are accompanied by increases in the cholesterol exchange rate. Current understanding of the effects of proteins on the kinetics of cholesterol surface transfer by the aqueous diffusion mechanism are limited.

The influx and efflux of free cholesterol mass between cells and HDL can be expressed in terms of $k_i$ and $k_e$ and the concentrations of free cholesterol in the HDL and cell pools. Free cholesterol surface transfer processes drive the cell free cholesterol content towards a steady-state level defined by the external concentration of free cholesterol and the ratio of $k_i$ and $k_e$. The net movement of free cholesterol between cells and HDL seems to involve the diffusion of cholesterol molecules down their free energy gradient from regions with a high free cholesterol/phospholipid ratio to regions with a low ratio. Enrichment of the plasma membrane with cholesterol does not alter $k_e$ very much [6]; the flux of cholesterol out of the cell is increased because of the enlarged pool of plasma membrane cholesterol. HDL seems to participate in simple exchange (i.e., efflux = influx) with cells containing normal amounts of cholesterol, whereas HDL can cause the net release of cholesterol from cells enriched in cholesterol. Data demonstrating how the direction of net flux of cholesterol between HDL and fibroblasts is affected by the cholesterol content of HDL are summarized in Fig. 2. Influx is equal to efflux (i.e. exchange of cholesterol mass occurs) when the cholesterol content of $HDL_3$ is about 60 $\mu$g/mg protein which is similar to the normal free cholesterol content of this lipoprotein. It is apparent that net efflux of cellular cholesterol occurs when $HDL_3$ particles containing lesser amounts of free cholesterol are incubated with the cells. This effect arises because $k_e$ and $k_i$ are independent of HDL cholesterol content. Consequently the influx of cholesterol mass from HDL into cells is proportional to the cholesterol content of the HDL and is minimal with HDL that is very depleted of cholesterol [6].

As an alternative to the aqueous diffusion mechanism to explain HDL-mediated efflux of cellular cholesterol, it has been postulated that a cell surface receptor for HDL is in volved [7, 8]. As summarized in Fig. 1, the original hypothesis suggested that binding of HDL to the receptor facilitated movement of cholesterol molecules between the plasma membrane and the extracellular HDL particle. However, several lines of evidence show that the efflux of plasma membrane cholesterol is not coupled to the high affinity binding of HDL to the cell surface (for reviews, see [3, 5]). This lack of a role for HDL-receptor interactions is demonstrated by the data in Fig. 3. Treatment of HDL with dimethylsuberimidate crosslinks the apoprotein molecules and inhibits the specific interaction of HDL with the cell surface [9] but does not alter efflux of whole-cell [$^{14}$C] cholesterol (Fig. 3A). There is now general agreement that binding of HDL to

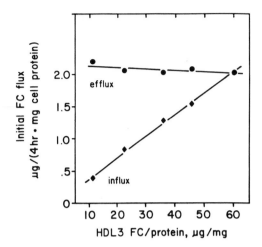

Figure 2. The dependence of cholesterol flux between HDL and fibroblasts growing in monolayer culture on the cholesterol content of HDL (from ref. [6]). The free cholesterol (FC) content of the HDL₃ was manipulated by reconstituting the lipoprotein particle. The cell and HDL FC pools were labeled with [$^{14}$C] and [$^{3}$H], respectively. The bidirectional flux of the two radiolabels was monitored to derive the FC efflux and influx. The influx (◆) and HDL-dependent efflux (●) of free cholesterol mass are depicted.

the cell surface does not affect the efflux of plasma membrane cholesterol [3, 5, 8]. However, as summarized in the next section, there are suggestions that binding of HDL to a receptor can stimulate efflux of intracellular cholesterol.

## Efflux of Intracellular Cholesterol

Intracellular pools of cholesterol that are particularly involved in the regulation of overall cell homeostasis are located in lysosomes (cholesterol delivered by endocytosis) the endoplasmic reticulum membranes (synthesized cholesterol), and in cytoplasmic cholesteryl ester inclusions (a storage form of cholesterol produced by acyl CoA:cholesterol acyltransferase (ACAT)) [1-3, 8]. Incubation of cells with HDL can lead to efflux of cholesterol from all of these intracellular sites. The current HDL-receptor hypothesis proposes that binding of HDL apoproteins to a cell surface receptor facilitates removal of excess intracellular cholesterol by stimulating translocation of cholesterol from internal sites to the plasma membrane [8]. Study of the efflux of newly synthesized cellular cholesterol formed from a radioactive precursor is problematic because of the occurrence of a series of sterol metabolites in addition to cholesterol [W.J. Johnson, M.C. Phillips and G.H. Rothblat, unpublished observations]. In this laboratory, we have focussed on the efflux of lysosomal cholesterol because, as described below, this pool can be selectively labeled quite readily [10]. The data summarized in Fig. 3B demonstrate that the efflux of lysosomally generated free cholesterol is unaffected by elimination of the specific binding of HDL to the cell surface.

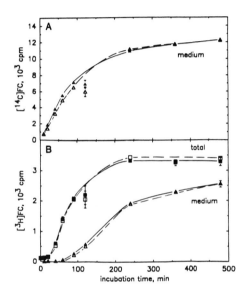

Figure 3. Effect of treating human HDL$_3$ with dimethylsuberimidate (DMS) on the efflux of whole-cell [$^{14}$C] and lysosomal [$^3$H] free cholesterol (FC) from Fu5AH rat hepatoma cells (from ref. [10]). Each efflux medium contained 0.2% bovine serum albumin and 1 mg protein/ml of either DMS-HDL$_3$ (open symbols) or unmodified HDL$_3$ (closed symbols) from the same donor. Panel A, whole-cell [$^{14}$C] FC. Panel B, lysosomal [$^3$H] FC.

The results depicted in Fig. 3B also give information about the rate of movement of cholesterol molecules from the lysosome to the plasma membrane. The lysosomal pool is labeled with [$^3$H] cholesterol by pulsing the cells with low density lipoprotein that has been reconstituted with [$^3$H] cholesteryl oleate and then incubating the cells at 37°C in the presence of HDL [10]. The hydrolysis of [$^3$H] cholesteryl oleate in lysosomes and the efflux of the resulting [$^3$H] cholesterol to the HDL are monitored after warming the cells to 37°C. Rapid hydrolysis of [$^3$H] cholesterol oleate to form [$^3$H] cholesterol begins after 10-20 min (Fig. 3B). This lysosomally generated [$^3$H] free cholesterol becomes available for efflux to HDL after an additional delay of 40-50 min (Fig. 3B).

The data in Fig. 3 show that in the Fu5AH cell 40-50 min elapses between the generation of free cholesterol in lysosomes and the availability of this sterol for desorption from the plasma membrane. This time is independent of the type of sterol acceptor in the medium, the concentration of the acceptor, the level of sterol in the cell, and the level of ACAT activity in the cell [10]. In the 40-50 min interval, several steps may need to occur in sequence for the delivery of lysosomal sterol to the cell surface. These are transfer of sterol from the surface of the partially degraded LDL to the lysosomal membrane, translocation across the lysosomal membrane, transport to the plasma membrane, and translocation across the plasma membrane. For this reason, the value of 40-50 min is an upper limit for the lysosome-to-plasma membrane transport time. The potential rate-limiting steps are movement of sterol from LDL to the lysosomal membrane and the transport of the sterol within the cytoplasm. Assuming rapid intracellular transport of lysosomal sterol in all cells, the slow desorption of plasma membrane cholesterol from most cells implies that typically this desorption step is absolutely rate limiting for the movement of cholesterol from lysosomes to HDL. Thus, in most cells, factors other than the rate of lysosome-to-plasma membrane sterol transport probably control the movement of lysosomal sterol out of cells to HDL. In general terms, the important controlling factors probably are those that determine the distribution of sterol between the plasma membrane and sites of esterification and that directly influence the rate of sterol desorption from the plasma membrane.

## Role of HDL Structure

Reflecting the fact that diverse pathways exist for formation and inter-conversion of HDL particles, circulating HDL in vivo comprises a heterogeneous population of lipid-protein complexes [3]. The major apolipoproteins of the HDL class of lipoproteins are A-I and A-II. A question of topical interest is the roles of the various subspecies of HDL particles in reverse cholesterol transport. We have been interested in understanding how HDL structure affects cholesterol efflux from cells.

Using immunoaffinity chromatography, human HDL can be separated into two subfractions: LP-AI, in which all particles contain apolipoprotein A-I (apoA-I) but no apoA-II, and LP-AI/AII, in which all particles contain both apoA-I and apoA-II [11]. To compare LP-AI and LP-AI/AII as acceptors of cell cholesterol, the isolated subfractions were diluted to

50 μg phospholipid/ml, and then incubated with monolayer
cultures of Fu5AH rat hepatoma cells in which whole-cell
cholesterol had been labeled with [14]C (Fig. 4). It is apparent that Lp-AI and Lp-AI/AII have similar capabilities to
remove cholesterol from the hepatoma cell. The [14]C] cholesterol essentially traces the efflux of plasma membrane cholesterol. The diffusion of cholesterol molecules from the
plasma membrane to the acceptor HDL particles and incorporation into the HDL seems to occur equally rapidly with Lp-AI
and Lp-AI/AII. Ultracentrifugally isolated HDL₃ particles
which contain both Lp-AI and Lp-AI/AII particles are more
efficient acceptors of cellular cholesterol in this system
(Fig. 4). The structural basis for this difference is not
clear at present. Similarly, the reasons for the particularly rapid delivery of cellular cholesterol to certain HDL
particles that exhibit pre-β mobility on electrophoresis in
agarose gels [12] are not understood. To better understand
the structure-function relationships of HDL particles it will
be necessary to define the conformation of the apoprotein
molecules at high resolution.

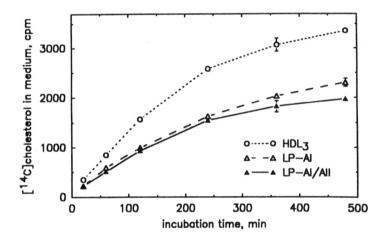

Figure 4. Efflux of whole cell [14]C] cholesterol from Fu5AH
rat hepatoma cells to human HDL₃, Lp-AI and Lp-AI/AII as a
function of time (from ref. [11]). The concentration of each
lipoprotein was 50 μg phospholipid/ml.

**ACKNOWLEDGMENTS**

We are indebted to our colleagues at the Medical College
of Pennsylvania who have contributed to various aspects of
the work from this laboratory described here. This research

was supported by NIH Program Project Grant HL22633 and Institutional Training Grant HL07443.

## REFERENCES

1   Brown MS, Goldstein JL.   Science 1986; 232: 34-47.
2   Rothblat GH, Phillips MC.   Current Opinion in Lipidology 1991; 2: 288-294.
3   Johnson WJ, Mahlberg FH, Rothblat GH, Phillips MC.   Biochim Biophys Acta 1991; 1085: 273-298.
4   Norum KR, Berg T, Helgerud P, Drevon CA.   Physiol Rev 1983; 63: 1343-1419.
5   Phillips MC, Johnson WJ, Rothblat GH.   Biochim Biophys Acta 1987; 906: 223-276.
6   Johnson WJ, Mahlberg FH, Chacko GK, Phillips MC, Rothblat GH.   J Biol Chem 1988; 263: 14099-14106.
7   Oram JF, Brinton EA, Bierman EL.   J Clin Invest 1983; 72: 1611-1621.
8   Oram JF.   Current Opinion in Lipidology 1990; 1: 416-421.
9   Chacko GK, Mahlberg FH, Johnson WJ.   J Lipid Res 1988; 29: 319-324
10  Johnson WJ, Chacko GK, Phillips MC, Rothblat GH.   J Biol Chem 1990; 265: 5546-5553.
11  Johnson WJ, Kilsdonk RPC, Van Tol A, Phillips MC, Rothblat GH.   J Lipid Res 1991; 32: 1993-2000.
12  Castro GR, Fielding CJ.   Biochemistry 1988; 27: 25-29.

# HDL receptor-mediated transport of cholesterol from cells

John F. Oram, Armando J. Mendez, and Edwin L. Bierman

University of Washington, Department of Medicine, Seattle, Washington 98195 USA

## INTRODUCTION

Numerous population studies have shown an inverse correlation between plasma HDL levels and the incidence and prevalence of atherosclerosis, suggesting that HDL protects against atherogenesis. This protection may be related to the role HDL plays in reverse cholesterol transport, a process by which cholesterol is transported from peripheral cells to the liver for excretion from the body. The first step of the reverse cholesterol transport pathway is the removal of cholesterol from cells. Studies from our laboratory have provided evidence that this step is mediated by binding of HDL to specific cell-surface receptors.

## HDL PROMOTES CHOLESTEROL EFFLUX FROM CELLS BY BOTH PASSIVE AND ACTIVE PROCESSES

HDL-mediated efflux of cellular cholesterol is complex and involves both passive and active processes. The interplay of these processes is influenced by the type of cell studied and its growth state and cholesterol status. Two examples of this are shown in Figure 1. When cells are in State A, they are either rapidly proliferating or cholesterol-depleted prior to radiolabeling with exogenous cholesterol. Under this condition, the demand for cholesterol as a structural component of membranes is relatively high, and the unesterified cholesterol (C) that enters the cells by uptake and lysosomal degradation of lipoproteins is transported rapidly and quantitatively to the plasma membrane [1,2]. The esterified cholesterol (CE) that accumulates in cells under this condition appears to be derived from plasma membrane C that recycles back into intracellular compartments that are accessible to the enzyme acyl CoA cholesterol acyltransferase (ACAT) [2,3]. When these cells are exposed to HDL or apolipoprotein-phospholipid vesicles, C efflux is promoted by a passive process that involves desorption of C from the plasma membrane and reabsorption to HDL particles [4]. This can also deplete CE content of cells by diverting C from the substrate pool for ACAT. This passive desorption/diffusion process is influenced largely by the physical properties of lipid domains in the plasma membrane and in HDL acceptor particles [4].

HDL-mediated cholesterol efflux becomes more complex when cells are growth-arrested, such as highly differentiated cells, and are overloaded with cholesterol prior to introduction of an exogenous source of radiosterol (State B, Fig. 1). Under these conditions, influx of exogenous C greatly exceeds the cell's requirements for C as a membrane structural component, and much of the excess C is diverted to intracellular pools where it can be converted to CE and stored as lipid droplets. When cells in this state are exposed to HDL, passive desorption processes may be too slow to remove the excess sterol, and active processes come into play. When cells are converted from State A to State B, the number of cell-surface binding sites for HDL increases [5,6], and the interaction of HDL with these sites actively stimulates translocation of excess C from intracellular sites to the plasma membrane (Fig. 1) [7,8]. The translocated C appears

126

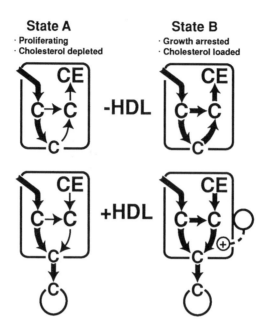

Figure 1. The effects of growth state and cholesterol status on cellular trafficking of lipoprotein-derived unesterified cholesterol (C) and on HDL-mediated cholesterol efflux.

to be packaged into plasma membrane domains that have a fast desorption rate, thus excess C is readily excreted from cells. These observations are consistent with the hypothesis that the stimulatory action of HDL on C translocation and efflux is mediated by a plasma membrane receptor.

## BINDING OF HDL APOLIPOPROTEINS TO CELLS STIMULATES EXCRETION OF INTRACELLULAR CHOLESTEROL

Early evidence for the existence of HDL receptors was obtained from studies showing that exposure of cultured cells to dense HDL particles caused a rapid depletion of an intracellular pool of C that regulates the synthesis of proteins involved in modulating cellular sterol metabolism [9,10]. Specifically, the interaction of HDL with cells rapidly induced the synthesis of sterol biosynthetic enzymes and LDL receptors by releasing feedback inhibition of these processes, and it decreased CE formation by depleting the cholesterol substrate pool for ACAT. These and other studies showed that one of the initial events that occurs when cells are exposed to HDL is the removal of cellular C that is in rapid equilibrium with the intracellular sterol regulatory pool.

To further test the possibility that HDL receptor interactions specifically stimulates removal of sterol from intracellular pools, it was necessary to devise a method to selec-

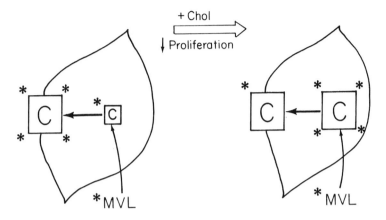

Figure 2. Model for translocation of newly-synthesized sterol from intracellular pools to the plasma membrane as influenced by the cholesterol status and growth state of cells. The model illustrates that most of the radiolabeled sterol tracer (asterisks) synthesized from radiolabeled mevalonolactone (*MVL) is incorporated into plasma membrane pools of cholesterol (C) in proliferating, cholesterol-depleted cells (left) but accumulates within intracellular cholesterol pools in cholesterol-loaded, growth-arrested cells (right).

tively introduce radiolabeled sterol tracer into these pools. One approach is to radiolabel cellular sterol by pulse-incubating cells with the sterol biosynthetic precursor $^3$H-mevalonolactone. When this protocol is used with proliferating cells that are cholesterol-depleted and exhibit high rates of sterol synthesis (State A), the newly synthesized sterol tracer is transported rapidly from the endoplasmic reticulum to the plasma membrane [7,8] (Fig. 2, left), presumably because a continual supply of C is required for membrane synthesis in replicating cells. However, a different transport pattern is observed when cells are first growth arrested and overloaded with cholesterol (State B, Fig. 2, right), conditions that lead to accumulation of cellular C in excess of that required for membrane synthesis. Instead of being rapidly transported to the plasma membrane, the sterol tracer enters an intracellular C pool that is accessible to ACAT [8]. Over 70% of the newly-synthesized radiosterol is esterified, indicating that the tracer enters the ACAT substrate pool without mixing with the much larger pool of unlabeled C in the plasma membrane. Only a small fraction of the newly synthesized sterol is converted to cholestenone when intact cells are treated with the enzyme cholesterol oxidase [7,8], indicating that most of the sterol tracer resides in intracellular pools that are inaccessible to this enzyme. Even when C esterification is suppressed by an ACAT inhibitor, more than half of the newly synthesized unesterified sterol stays trapped within intracellular compartments. These results suggest that most of the sterol tracer synthesized by growth-arrested, cholesterol-loaded cells is stored within intracellu-

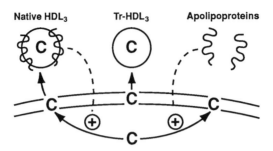

Figure 3. Scheme illustrating how intact HDL$_3$, trypsinized HDL$_3$ (Tr-HDL$_3$) and lipid-depleted apo AI affect cellular cholesterol (C) translocation and efflux.

lar C pools that are in rapid equilibrium with the substrate pool for ACAT.

When quiescent, cholesterol-loaded fibroblasts are pulsed with [3]H-mevalonolactone to selectively radiolabel intracellular pools of sterol and then chased with medium containing unlabeled mevalonolactone to wash out radioactive substrate and prevent further synthesis of radiosterol, the cellular distribution of radiosterol synthesized during the pulse incubation stays relatively unchanged during 4-hour chase incubations in the absence of HDL [7,8]. Most of the sterol tracer remains within intracellular pools that are inaccessible to oxidation by cholesterol oxidase treatment of cells. When HDL$_3$ is added to these cells, however, there is net translocation of radiosterol from intracellular pools to the plasma membrane [7,8,11] (Fig. 3). This movement is mediated by HDL$_3$ apolipoproteins, as evidenced by results showing that trypsin treatment of HDL$_3$ abolishes its stimulatory effects [8] (Fig. 3). Proteolysis of HDL destroys apolipoproteins but does not alter its ability to act as an acceptor of plasma membrane-derived cholesterol [8]. Additional evidence that apolipoproteins mediate the stimulatory effects of HDL$_3$ on sterol translocation was provided by studies showing that lipid-extracted apo AI stimulates this process, even though these lipid-free molecules are poor cholesterol acceptors [11] (Fig. 3). These results suggest that the interaction of HDL apolipoproteins with cells directly stimulates translocation of sterol from intracellular pools to the plasma membrane where it can readily desorb into the medium and be picked up by HDL particles.

If HDL apolipoproteins stimulate C translocation from intracellular pools, this process should deplete intracellular substrate pools for ACAT and thus reduce C esterification. This assumption was borne out by data showing that incubation of cholesterol-loaded cells with either HDL$_3$ or lipid-free apo AI inhibits CE formation, whereas incubation with trypsin-treated HDL$_3$ has no effect [8]. Thus it appears that the stimulatory action of HDL apolipoproteins functions to divert C from intracellular storage sites into an excretory pathway.

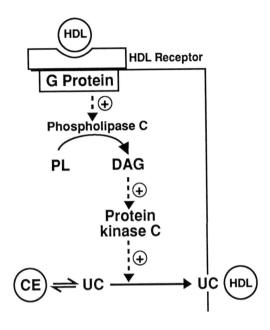

Figure 4. Model for the HDL receptor-mediated signalling pathway.

## STIMULATION OF INTRACELLULAR STEROL TRANSLOCATION BY HDL APOLIPOPROTEINS IS MEDIATED BY A PROTEIN KINASE C SIGNALLING PATHWAY

One possible mechanism for the stimulatory action of HDL on sterol translocation and efflux is that the interaction of apolipoproteins with a plasma membrane receptor activates intracellular signals that modulate sterol trafficking between intracellular compartments and the plasma membrane. Since most receptor-mediated signalling pathways involve activation of one or more of the major classes of protein kinases, we tested the possibility that protein kinase A or C may mediate the stimulatory effects of HDL apolipoproteins. Based on studies using enzyme inhibitors, we concluded that protein kinase A is not involved in this process (Hokland, et al., manuscript submitted). However, several lines of evidence were obtained showing that protein kinase C is the mediator of the stimulatory action of HDL on sterol translocation [11,12]. First, inhibition of protein kinase C by either short-term treatment of cells with sphingosine or chronic treatment with phorbol esters reduces the ability of HDL$_3$ to stimulate translocation and efflux of intracellular sterol. Second, treatment of cells with activators of protein kinase C stimulates sterol translocation, even in the absence of HDL. Third, exposure of cells to HDL$_3$ increases formation of diacylglycerol and activation of protein kinase C.

Based on these results, we propose the model for HDL-mediated sterol translocation and efflux illustrated in Figure 4. This model suggests that HDL apolipoproteins bind to a plasma membrane receptor that activates a signalling pathway, perhaps through the formation of a ligand-receptor complex with a G protein. This complex activates a phospholipase that generates diacylglycerol from hydrolysis of phospholipids. The diacylglycerol activates protein kinase C, which in turn phosphorylates specific proteins involved in modulating C transport between intracellular compartments and plasma membrane domains that allow for rapid desorption of C. Such a pathway would promote continual removal of excess C that enters cells from any source and target this C for removal from the body by the reverse cholesterol transport pathway. Thus this pathway may be the cellular mechanism that underlies some of the antiatherogenic effects of HDL.

## IN SEARCH OF THE PUTATIVE HDL RECEPTOR PROTEIN

The model shown in Figure 4 predicts that HDL-mediated sterol translocation and efflux occurs through a complex pathway involving multiple proteins, including a membrane receptor that transmits signals in response to HDL binding. Using ligand blot analysis, investigators from several laboratories have identified membrane proteins that bind HDL and thus are candidate proteins for an HDL receptor. We have described a 110 kDa HDL binding protein that appears in the membranes of a wide variety of tissues [13]. The expression of this protein increases when cells are either overloaded with cholesterol or growth-arrested [6,13], regulatory properties expected for a receptor that functions to rid cells of excess cholesterol. Using an antibody raised against partially purified 110 kDa HDL binding protein isolated from bovine aortic endothelial cells, we expression-cloned an HDL binding protein (HBP) from a human-dermal fibroblast cDNA library [14]. The deduced amino acid sequence suggests that HBP is synthesized as a 150 kDa protein that contains 14 tandem imperfect repeats of approximately 70 amino acids plus two unique domains at both the N- and C-termini. Each repeat unit comprises two amphipathic stretches, most of which are probably helices, separated by proline-rich $\beta$-turns. The protein does not appear to contain a classic transmembrane spanning domain and thus its structure does not conform to that of known signal-transmitting receptors. Instead, the structure of HBP resembles that of HDL apolipoproteins, and HBP exhibits marginal sequence homology to apo AIV [14].

Transfection of baby hamster kidney (BHK) cells with HBP cDNA led to increased expression of 112 kDa HDL binding protein and an increase in the number of high-affinity HDL binding sites on the cell surface [14]. Ligand blot and immunoblot analyses showed that a major fraction of HBP is associated with the plasma membrane. Cholesterol loading of cells increased HBP mRNA levels and expression of immunoreactive protein. These results suggest that HBP is a novel cell protein that plays a role in modulating cellular cholesterol metabolism, perhaps through its interaction with HDL on the cell surface. However, because of its unusual structure, it can not yet be concluded that this molecule represents the signal-transmitting receptor predicted from the model shown in Figure 4. Work to characterize the function of HBP is in progress in our laboratory.

# CLINICAL IMPLICATIONS OF THE HDL RECEPTOR PATHWAY

The current report summarizes recent data suggesting that HDL apolipoproteins stimulate excretion of intracellular cholesterol from sterol-laden cells by a complex receptor-mediated signalling pathway involving multiple yet unidentified proteins. Mutations in one or more of these proteins could have profound effects on the ability of HDL to clear excess cholesterol from cells of the artery wall. A common indicator of increased risk for coronary artery disease is low levels of circulating HDL cholesterol. It is possible that at least some of these individuals have a genetic defect in the HDL receptor pathway. This pathway also has important implications as a target for drug therapy. A receptor agonist, for example, may enhance the rate of clearance of cholesterol from peripheral cells and reduce deposition of cholesterol in the artery wall, provided that sufficient cholesterol acceptors are present in the extracellular environment to shuttle cholesterol into the reverse cholesterol transport pathway. Thus additional knowledge about the processes involved in the HDL receptor pathway is likely to provide insight into some of the cellular mechanisms that promote atherogenesis and to suggest strategies for therapeutic intervention.

# REFERENCES

1  Brasaemle DL, Attie AD. J Lipid Res 1990;31:103-111.
2  Mahlberg FH, Glick JM, Lund-Katz S, Rothblat GH. J Biol Chem 1991;226:19930-19937.
3  Tabas I, Rosott WJ, Boykow GC. J Biol Chem 1988;263:1266-1272.
4  Rothblat GH, Phillips MC. Curr Opin Lip 1991;2:288-294.
5  Oram JF, Brinton EA, Bierman EL. J Clin Invest 1983;72:1611-1621.
6  Oppenheimer MJ, Oram JF, Bierman EL. J Biol Chem 1988;263:19318-19323.
7  Slotte JP, Oram JF, Bierman EL. Chem 1987;262:12904-12907.
8  Oram JF, Mendez AJ, Slotte JP, et al. Arter and Thromb 1991;11:403-414.
9  Oram JF, Albers JJ, Cheung MC, et al. J Biol Chem 1981;256:8348-8356.
10 Oram JF. Arteriosclerosis 1983;3:420-432.
11 Mendez AJ, Oram JF, Bierman EL. J Biol Chem 1991;266:10104-10111.
12 Mendez AJ, Oram JF, Bierman EL. Arteriosclerosis 1990;10:768a.
13 Graham DL, Oram JF. J Biol Chem 1987;262:7439-7442.
14 McKnight GL, Reasoner J, Gilbert T, et al. J Biol Chem 1992 (In Press).

*High density lipoproteins and atherosclerosis III.*
*N.E. Miller and A.R. Tall, editors.*

Apo A-containing lipoprotein particles : Interactions with HDL binding sites and reverse cholesterol transport

J.-C. Fruchart[a], G. Ailhaud[b] and P. Denèfle[c]

[a] SERLIA & INSERM U.325, Institut Pasteur, 1 rue du Professeur Calmette, 59019 Lille Cédex, France

[b] CNRS, UMR 134, UFR Sciences, Parc Valrose, 06108 Nice Cédex 2, France

[c] Département de Biotechnologie, Rhône-Poulenc Rorer SA, Vitry s/Seine, France

## INTRODUCTION

Apolipoproteins A-I, A-II and A-IV represent 80 to 90% of the total apolipoprotein content of human high density lipoproteins (HDL). In order to evaluate the role of these apolipoproteins in influencing HDL metabolism, particles containing these apolipoproteins were isolated by immunoaffinity chromatography and characterized. Two major subpopulations of HDL particles have been identified in plasma and in interstitial fluid : lipoproteins containing apo A-I and apo A-II (LpA-I:A-II) and lipoproteins containing apo A-I but not apo A-II (LpA-I). These lipoproteins bind specifically and with high affinity the surface of several cell types but differ by their respective ability to promote cholesterol efflux from peripheral cells. Using an "in vitro" approach with complexes containing apo A-I, A-II or A-IV and cultured adipose cells, we have demonstrated the "antagonist" role of apo A-II and the "agonist" role of apo A-I or apo A-IV in cholesterol efflux. The binding of agonists to cell surface binding sites was coupled to a phospholipase mediated hydrolysis of phosphatidylcholine, diacylglycerol production and protein kinase C(s) activation. All three apolipoproteins (A-I, A-II, A-IV) bound to the same recognition sites which are detectable by cross-linking experiments at the cell surface of mouse adipose cells. Both in intact cells and after binding protein purification, 1 mol of apo A-II was bound per 2 mol of apo A-I or A-IV. In order to define how particular structural components of human apo A-I and apo A-IV may be involved in functional biological properties of the entire proteins : (i) we have used monoclonal antibodies selected for their reaction with epitopes spanning most of the apo A-I sequence to inhibit the interaction between apo A-I/POPC complexes and HDL binding sites on HeLa cells and mouse adipose cells ; (ii) we have tested the effect of genetic variants or of variants obtained by site-specific deletion-scanning mutagenesis on adipose cell binding and cholesterol efflux stimulation.

## ISOLATION AND CHARACTERIZATION OF APO A-I CONTAINING LIPOPROTEIN PARTICLES IN HUMAN PLASMA AND INTERSTITIAL FLUID

LpA-I and LpA-I:A-II were isolated from human plasma and interstitial fluid (IF) collected by gentle blister-suction of forearms and analyzed. The concentrations in LpA-I and LpA-I:A-II were significantly lower in IF than in plasma [1] (Table 1).

Table 1
Apolipoprotein and lipid composition of LpA-I and LpA-I:A-II from plasma and interstitial fluid

|  | LpA-I (IF) | LpA-I (P) | LpA-I:A-II (IF) | LpA-I:A-II (P) |
|---|---|---|---|---|
| Apo A-I | 78.34±10.26 | 96.24±1.73 | 69.55±16.12 | 46.35±2.85 |
| Apo A-II | und | und | 29.71±16.29 | 52.56±2.83 |
| Apo A-IV | 16.44±9.39 | 2.25±1.62 | 0.02±0.03 | 0.34±0.31 |
| Apo B | 0.05±0.01 | 0.03±0.03 | 0.02±0.0007 | 0.009±0.009 |
| Apo C-III | 4.56±3.54 | 0.84±0.30 | 0.44±0.26 | 0.35±0.38 |
| Apo E | 0.58±0.44 | 0.59±0.17 | 0.24±0.32 | 0.39±0.27 |
| Cholesterol | 40.05±14.91 | 47.06±10.81 | 48.02±5.25 | 46.94±2.70 |
| Triglycerides | 9.79±2.25 | 6.90±0.53 | 10.39±1.02 | 6.57±0.79 |
| Phospholipids | 50.15±8.88 | 46.02±10.67 | 41.48±3.71 | 46.46±3.50 |
| Concentration (g/L) | 0.08±0.04 | 0.33±0.16 | 0.12±0.04 | 0.54±0.12 |

Three samples of interstitial fluid (IF) (each sample obtained by pooling the interstitial fluid from three patients) were analyzed as well as three samples of plasma (P) obtained from different patients. The results are mean ± range ; they are expressed in mol/100 mol of total apolipoproteins and in mol/100 mol of total lipids. The molecular weights used were : apo A-I : 28391 ; apo A-II : 17412 ; apo A-IV : 46000 ; apo B : 549000 ; apo C-III : 8746 ; apo E : 34145 ; cholesterol : 386 ; triglycerides : 850 and phospholipids : 775.
und : undetectable

Particles differed mainly by their protein composition. LpA-I particles from IF were significantly enriched in apo A-IV as compared to LpA-I from plasma and no apo A-IV is associated to LpA-I:A-II. A preferential association of LCAT activity to LpA-I as compared to LpA-I:A-II was observed (Table 2).

Table 2
LCAT activity in LpA-I and LpA-I:A-II particles from plasma and interstitial fluid

|  | Plasma | Interstitial fluid | IF/P |
|---|---|---|---|
| LpA-I | 8.39±0.01 (80.3) | 0.94±0.03 (79.7) | 0.11 |
| LpA-I:A-II | 2.06±0.32 (19.7) | 0.24±0.12 (20.3) | 0.12 |

Two out of the three samples of interstitial fluid (IF) from Table 1 and two samples of plasma (P) obtained from different patients were used. The results are mean ± range ; they are expressed in % esterified cholesterol/h/mg protein. The percent of LCAT activity determined for each kind of particles is given in parentheses.

A significant enrichment of this activity in plasma particles suggests that cholesterol esterification is a continuous process initiated in IF and becoming more important in plasma, particularly in particles containing apo A-I but not containing apo A-II. Morphographic analysis of IF particle sizes showed a range of diameters reminiscent of that determined in plasma [2] (Figure 1).

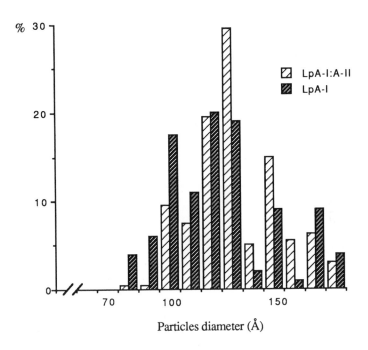

Figure 1. Morphographic analysis of particle diameters.

The observation of a significant proportion (about 10%) of LpA-I of small diameter (70-90 Å) is of interest since, in plasma, a pre-ß-migrating HDL particle of low molecular weight, containing apo A-I, has been proposed as the first cholesterol acceptor of cholesterol-preloaded cells [3].

## BINDING OF APO A-I CONTAINING PARTICLES TO HDL BINDING SITES : ROLE IN CHOLESTEROL EFFLUX

Culture adipose cells have been shown to be a suitable model for the study of reverse cholesterol transport [4]. The ligands which recognize the cell surface HDL binding sites have been identified as apo A-I, apo A-II and apo A-IV [5]. After cholesterol preloading with LDL, the addition of apo A-I or apo A-IV liposomes but not of apo A-II liposomes promoted cholesterol efflux despite the fact that both proteoliposomes were able to bind to the same cell-surface sites of intact cells [5] (Figure 2).

136

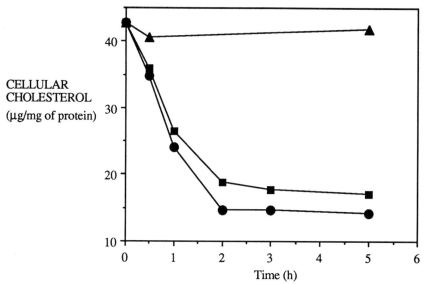

Figure 2. Kinetics of cholesterol efflux from cholesterol preloaded Ob 1771 cells in the presence of various apolipoprotein/DMPC complexes :
Apo A-I DMPC (■) ; Apo A-II DMPC (▲) ; Apo A-IV DMPC (●) complexes.
(J. Steinmetz et al., J. Biol. Chem. 1991, 265/14:7859-7863 - Published by permission)

Exposure to LpA-I or LpA-I:A-II isolated from native plasma and from HDL2 or HDL3 showed that only LpA-I were able to promote cholesterol efflux, despite the fact that both kinds of particles bound to receptor sites within the same range of concentrations (apparent Kd values between 10 and 25 µg/ml) [2] (Figure 3).

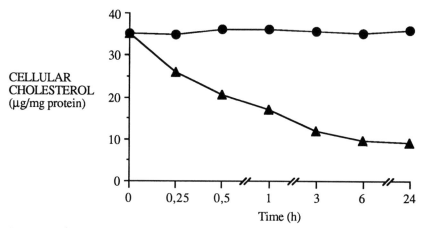

Figure 3. Cholesterol efflux in preloaded Ob 1771 cells exposed to LpA-I (▲) and LpA-I:A-II (●) particles from native plasma depleted of apo E. (A. Barkia et al., Atherosclerosis 1991, 87:135-146 - Published by permission)

The antagonizing and modulating role of apo A-II in preventing LpA-I mediated cholesterol efflux was demonstrated [2]. Slotte et al have suggested that the addition of HDL3 to different cells induces a protein kinase C-dependent translocation of cholesterol from intracellular membranes to the cell surface [6]. We have shown recently that cholesterol efflux from adipose cells is coupled to diacylglycerol production and protein kinase C activation [7]. The fact that the binding of apo A-I liposomes, but not that of apo A-II liposomes, produces diacylglycerol strongly supports the role of apo A-II as an antagonist in the production of cholesterol efflux. Similar results have been obtained by bovine aorta endothelial cells as a model [8] but not with other cells (Table 3).

Table 3
Phosphatidyl-choline breakdown and DAG generation in response to phospholipase C stimulation by proteoliposomes

| | Cellular system | Proteoliposomes containing | |
| | | Apo A-I | Apo A-II |
| --- | --- | --- | --- |
| High efficiency system<br>High phospholipase activity | - Adipocytes<br>- Endothelial cells<br>  from aortic cross | DAG production<br>and efflux<br>+++ | no DAG production<br><br>no efflux |
| Low efficiency system<br>Weak phospholipase activity | - Fibroblasts<br>- Endothelial cells<br>  from the blood<br>  brain barrier | DAG production<br>+ | DAG production<br>+ |

HDL binding sites are detectable by cross-linking experiments at the cell surface of adipose cells [9]. The critical role of these receptor sites in cholesterol efflux was strongly suggested by experiments using cells in which have been induced genetically defined alterations of the growth control mechanism by transferring cloned oncogenes [9]. Culture adipose cells of the Ob17 MT18 clonal line were used for purification of the binding protein [4].

The stoechiometry of binding of the apolipoprotein liposomes during purification of the material was identical for apos A-I and A-IV but only 1 mol of apo A-II was bound per 2 mol of apo A-I or A-IV. The binding activity of apos A-I, A-II and A-IV remained constant during purification, suggesting that a single activity towards these apolipoproteins was present in cell homogenates [4].

138

## STRUCTURAL DOMAIN OF APO A-I AND APO A-IV RECOGNIZED BY HDL BINDING SITES

The characterization of apo A-I epitopes and the matching of their position with the elements of a planar model of apo A-I supersecondary structure has provided evidence for the existence of two structurally distinct regions in apo A-I [10] and major changes in the conformation of apo A-I occurred upon binding to lipids [12]

The knowledge of the exact nature and location of the domain implicated in the interaction of apo A-I containing lipoproteins and the putative HDL receptor is undoubtedly important for understanding the function of apo A-I in cellular cholesterol homeostasis.

To characterize this domain, we have used specific monoclonal antibodies to inhibit the binding of apo A-I/POPC complexes to binding sites of Ob17 mouse adipose cells and HeLa cells [12] (Figure 4).

One antibody (A44) inhibited the binding of apo A-I complexes to HeLa cells by 40% and the cholesterol efflux from Ob17 cells by 30%. The apo A-I epitope recognized by A44 is located in the C-terminal half of the protein and covers sequence 149-186 [12] (Figure 4). By comparison of six different genetic apo A-I variants, it has been found that the apo A-I (Pro 165 → Arg) [13] have a reduction up to 30% of their capacity to promote cholesterol efflux from mouse adipocytes. Further work is needed to confirm that the region 149-186 is responsible for the apo A-I interaction with cells.

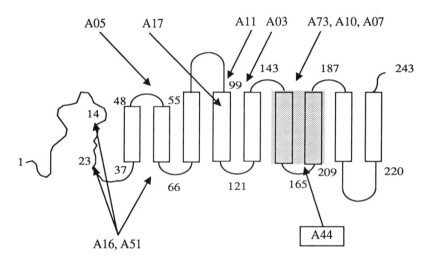

Figure 4. Planar model of apo A-I supersecondary structure in relation to the position of epitopes.

In order to define how particular secondary structural components of human apolipoprotein A-IV (apo A-IV) may be involved in functional biological properties of the entire protein, plasmid constructs have been genetically engineered to yield human apo A-IV derivatives as recombinant proteins in *E.coli*.

Since we started with a partial genomic clone, the strategy we used was to reconstruct a DNA fragment corresponding to the complete coding sequence of mature apo A-IV (isoform 1) preceded by an ATG codon for translation initiation. A useful BamH1 restriction site was also introduced just after the stop codon by site-directed mutagenesis and the sequence was finaly introduced into different constructs under the control of different *E.coli* promoters [14, 15] did not give convincing results in terms of production (not shown), we turned to the T7 system described by Rosenberg et al. [16].

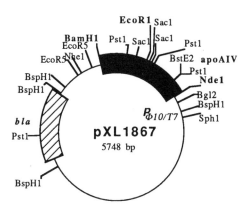

Figure 5. Human apo A-IV expression vector

Even in that case, we observed by pulse-chase experiments that the recombinant apo A-IV could not be stably accumulated within the bacteria. But when we combined the use of a T7 system with that of rifampicin, an antibiotic which inhibits the endogenous RNA-polymerase activity, as early reported by Tabor and Richardson [17], we could this time obtain very stable accumulation of apo A-IV within the bacteria.

Several hundreds mg of the protein could be produced using a 2 1 high-cell density fermentor and the same IPTG-rifampicin system. However, we first observed that the apo A-IV productivity of the bacteria dropped to less than 10% of total proteins instead of a value of about 20-30% in shake-flasks. Secondly, the absorbance of the culture A(610 nm) of the culture also plumetted from 42 to 81 after an incubation of 1 h in the presence of rifampicin. The difference of productivity is probably due to the fermentation conditions that may need some further nutrient optimization. In any case, the expression plasmid was quite stable during all the fermentation process. The dramatic drop in absorbance during the production phase is certainly due to an important lysis of the culture. Whether this bacterial lysis is due to the induction of the prophage DE3 via an SOS response of the bacteria to the apo A-IV expression or to the interaction of apo A-IV with the bacterial membrane remains unanswered. We must stress the point that the lysozyme constitutive expression from pLysS during the whole process appears to be strongly counterselected since less than 0,5% of the clones are still resistant to chloramphenicol at the end of the culture.

Fortunately, recombinant apo A-IV was produced in a soluble form, and an original purification protocol was designed so as to preserve the native conformation of the protein. The low affinity for triglyceride-phospholipids emulsions of apo A-IV did not encourage the design of a lipid extraction of the protein as reported by Protter et al. in the case of apo A-I [18].

To prove that the purified Mr 46.000 polypeptide was indeed recombinant apo A-IV, we determined its amino acid composition, N-terminal sequence, and its reactivity with monoclonal and polyclonal antibodies raised against human apo A-I. We also analysed the mass spectroscopy of the purified material. The aminoacid composition (not shown) correlated rather well with the composition deduced from the DNA sequence [19, 20]. However, an extra Met residue should be expected because of the ATG translation initiation codon which was engineered at the start of the apo A-IV open reading frame. This was both confirmed by amino terminal sequence analysis and mass determination of the protein. This is consistent with the Met-rule predicted by Hirel et al. [21]. All other physico-chemical properties examined so far, PAGE, IEF, or heat stability, showed that human plasma and recombinant apo A-IV have similar behaviour. In addition to this, human plasma and recombinant apo A-IV were indistinguishable either in their respective fluorescence properties or in their reactivity towards four monoclonal antibodies raised against plasma apo A-IV [22].

It was of interest to see if the recombinant apo A-IV would share the same functional properties as the natural apo A-IV isolated from human plasma (A-IV1/A-IV1). Therefore, several functional properties of recombinant apo A-IV were examined and compared to those of this plasma preparation.

Since apo A-IV is known to be active only when it is associated with phospholipids, we could show that reconstituted apo A-IV/PtdCho with several phospholipids were similar with both proteins. As shown by gradient ultracentrifugation analysis, the lipoprotein particles reconstituted either with Myr2GroPCho, L-α-1-palmitoyl-2-oleoylglycero phosphatidylcholine or glycerophosphocholine share exactely the same density when made with natural or recombinant proteins. This suggests identical phospholipid binding properties for both proteins. The results of the lecithin:cholesterol acyltransferase activation assay are totally superimposable when using reconstituted apo A-IV/PtdCho with recombinant or natural proteins. It is interesting to compare the different activation profiles one can obtain when changing the phospholipid component of the reconstituted particle. In fact, the best LCAT activations were always obtained with L-α-1-palmitoyl-2-oleoylglycero phosphatidylcholine as reported before [23].

The results of cellular binding and competition assays with apo A-IV/Myr2GroPCho complexes indicate that natural and recombinant proteins bind with the same affinity to the same site on the surface of mouse adipose cells Ob1771. Moreover, the two types of lipoprotein particles are able to stimulate cholesterol efflux from cholesterol preloaded adipose cells to a comparable extent as isolated human HDL3. It is interesting to note that the amounts of cholesterol, which could be mobilized out of the cells, were quite significant (about 25 μg/mg of cellular protein) and exceeded by far the passive cholesterol transfer which is mediated by Myr2GroPCho alone. The cholesterol efflux experiments were repeated several times and the cellular cholesterol contents were measured either by gas chromatography or by HPLC as recently reported by Araki et al. [24]. The availability of an accurate chromatographic method to perform cholesterol measurements in these concentration ranges should allow us to detect small changes in activity, for instance with apo A-IV variants.

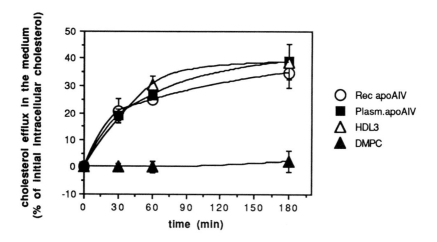

Figure 6. Cholesterol efflux from cholesterol-loaded Ob1771 cells at 37°C.

In conclusion, with the exception of the occurence of an extra methionine at its N-terminus, recombinant apo A-IV and its natural counterpart are quite comparable in their physicochemical properties, in their ability to activate the LCAT enzyme, to bind to murine adipose cells in culture and to stimulate, in a reproductible way, cholesterol efflux from these cells. We therefore provide a powerful tool to further study the role of apo A-IV in reverse cholesterol transport.

The recombinant expression strategy does not only allow to overproduce the protein of interest but also to generate either random or site-directed mutations on the coding sequence so as to study structure-function relationships of the protein.

In the case of human apo A-IV as of many apolipoproteins, there are intriging primary and secondary structural motives which have been conserved through evolution [25]. Our initial strategy was thus to generate deletions of putative secondary structural elements such as helices. Pairs of helices were deleted in order to keep as much as possible the orientation of the remaining helices as predicted on discoidal particles [26]. We also deleted either the 13 first aa or the last 44 aa residues which were not predicted as beeing organized into amphipatic helices. In addition, we introduced a start and a stop codon into the coding sequence at position 183 so as to produce two fragments of the apolipoprotein A-IV which corresponding respectively to the N and C terminal halves of the mature protein.

On the other hand, a fine comparison of the aa sequences of the apo A-IV from human, rat, mouse with those of apo A-I from dog, human and rat allow permitted the identification of some key-residues, which are conserved in all apo A-I or apo A-IV sequences and which seemed important according to predicted local secondary structures. We also started to change these residues. Up to now about twenty mutants of human apo A-IV have been generated successfully. It is remarkable to notice that all the mutants could be produced in *E.coli* with the same efficiency as the original mature sequence.

142

Some of them have already been purified to homogenity and have been assayed for their biological activity [27]. The results so far obtained show that large delections do not affect the biological properties of apo A-IV and suggest that these mutants retain an active conformation.

In conclusion, the deletion scanning approach on apo A-IV (or apo A-I) should allow rapidly to identify its secondary key-components in order to study the structure-function of apo A-IV and related proteins [27].

## REFERENCES

1   Data not published
2   Barkia A, Puchois P, Ghalim N, Torpier G, et al. Atherosclerosis 1991: 87: 135-146.
3   Castro GR, Fielding CJ. Biochemistry 1988: 27: 25-29.
4   Barbaras R, Puchois P, Fruchart JC, Ailhaud G. Biochem Biophys Res Commun 1987: 142: 63-69.
5   Steinmetz A, Barbaras R, Ghalim N, Clavey V, et al. J Biol Chem 1990: 265: 7859-7863.
6   Slotte JP, Oram JF, Bierman EL. J Biol Chem 1987: 262: 12904-12907.
7   Theret N, Delbart C, Aguie G, Fruchart JC, et al. Biochem Biophys Res Commun 1990: 173: 1361-1368.
8   Metelskaya V, Cecchelli R, Bard JM, Fruchart JC. LpA-I but not LpA-II promote cholesterol efflux from bovine endothelial aortic cells. 59th European Atherosclerosis Society Congress, Nice, 17-21 may 1992.
9   Barbaras R, Puchois P, Grimaldi P, Barkia A, et al. Biochem Biophys Res Commun 1987: 149: 545-554.
10  Marcel YL, Provost PR, Koa H, Raffai E, et al. J Biol Chem 1991: 266/6: 3644-3653.
11  Raffai EA, Collet X, Fruchart JC, Marcel YL. J Biol Chem (in press).
12  Castro GR, Luchoomun J, Theret N, Duchateau P, et al. Structural domain of apolipoprotein A-I recognized by high density lipoprotein receptor. 3rd International Symposium on Plasma High Density Lipoproteins and Atherosclerosis, San-Antonio, 4-6 march 1992.
13  Von Eckardstein A, Castro G, Theret N, Duchateau P, et al. J Biol Chem (submitted).
14  Latta M, Philit M, Maury I, Soubrier F, et al. DNA and Cell Biol 1990: 9: 129-137.
15  Denèfle P, Kovarik S, Ciora T, Gosselet N, et al. Gene 1989: 85: 499-510.
16  Rosenberg AH, Lade BN, Chui DS, Lin SW, et al. Gene 1987: 56: 125-135.
17  Tabor S, Richardson CC, Proc Natl Acad Sci USA 1985: 82: 1074-1078.
18  Protter AA, Vigne JL, Mallory JB, Talmage KD, et al. International Patent N°WO 1987: 87/02062.
19  Gordon JI, Bisgaier CI, Sims HF, Sachdev OP, et al. J Biol Chem 1984: 259: 468-474.
20  Yang CY, Gu ZW, Chong I, Xiong W, et al. Biochem Biophys Acta 1989: 1002: 231-237.
21  Hirel PH, Schmitter JM, Dessen P, Fayat G, et al. Proc Natl Acad Sci USA 1989: 86: 8247-8251.
22  Duverger N, Murry-Brelier A, Latta M, Reboul S, et al. Eur J Biochem 1991: 201: 373-383.

23 Steinmetz A, Kaffarnik H, Utermann G. Eur J Biochem 1985: 152: 747-751.
24 Araki N, Horiuchi S, Torab A, Rahim MA, et al. Anal Biochem 1990: 185: 339-345.
25 Elshourbagy NA, Walker DW, Boguski MS, Gordon JI, et al. J Biol Chem 1986: 261: 1998-2002.
26 Vanloo B, Morrison J, Fidge N, Lorent G, et al. J Lipid Res 1991: 32: 1253-1264.
27 Latta M, Duchateau P, Theret N, Murry-Brelier A, et al. Effects of site-specific deletion scanning mutagenesis on adipose cell binding and cholesterol efflux stimulation by recombinant human apolipoprotein A-IV. 59th European Atherosclerosis Society Congress, Nice, 17-21 may 1992.

High density lipoprotein - cell interactions,

C.J. Fielding[ab], P.E. Fielding[ac] and T. Miida[a]

Cardiovascular Research Institute and Departments of Physiology[b] and Medicine[c], University of California, San Francisco, California 94143

## INTRODUCTION

Cholesterol transport between plasma and peripheral cells

It has been difficult to determine unambiguously if the transfer of cholesterol between cell membranes and biological fluids is regulated by physical processes alone, or whether more specific biochemical pathways (for example, cell surface receptors) are also involved. Cholesterol transfers spontaneously through the aqueous phase between lipid surfaces, with kinetics similar to those predicted by Fick's Law for simple diffusion. Predicted diffusion rates depend on experimental values for the diffusion coefficient and true aqueous solubility of free cholesterol; but cholesterol is only slightly soluble (2) and as a result calculated diffusion rates are necessarily approximate. A second approach has been to measure the kinetics of cholesterol transfer under different conditions of donor and acceptor concentration. This can distinguish between diffusion and molecular collision in model systems (1,3). However more complex transfer mechanisms may be consistent with kinetic parameters predicted for diffusion (4).

Diffusion is a physical process depending on the Brownian movement of molecules in solution, and requires only that the solute has a finite solubility in the medium. As a result diffusion must contribute to the total observed transfer of free cholesterol between lipid surfaces. Major characteristics of diffusional net transfer are its lack of specificity, and (for net transfer) dependence on an effective concentration difference between donor and recipient surfaces. Diffusional transfer rates for cholesterol between different surfaces are not necessarily the same, depending on the energy for the desorption of cholesterol from the lipid surface to the aqueous phase, and potentially the presence or absence of a diffusional barrier ("unstirred water layer").

In spite of evidence for diffusional transfer between lipid surfaces in vitro (1-2,4) many laboratories have reported data which suggests that other mechanisms can contribute to overall cholesterol transfer in a more physiological situation when living cells interact with native plasma. This evidence is of several kinds:

a. Specificity. When isotopic cholesterol from cell membranes (5) transfers to plasma, the lipoproteins are not uniformly labeled. At early time points (when intra-lipoprotein transfer does not complicate interpretation; see below) much the greatest part of cell cholesterol is recovered in high density lipoprotein (HDL) (5), even though this makes up only a small part (normally about 25%) of total plasma free cholesterol. In particular, it transfers to a small fraction of HDL, containing only apo A-I and with a prebeta-electrophoretic mobility distinct from that of most other HDL (6.7). The experimental data suggest a difference of up to 30-fold in the ability of different HDL to accept cell-derived cholesterol. Such differences are insufficiently explained on the basis of molecular size or surface curvature.

Consistent with this, when HDL was fractionated by immunoaffinity chromatography instead of electrophoresis, HDL containing only apo-I were the only HDL effective in unloading cholesterol from adipocytes (8). However, not all studies using this technique have found a difference in the cholesterol transport properties of different HDL species (9). Possible reasons for these divergent experimental results are discussed below.

b. Cell specificity. There is now good evidence that many cell types contain HDL binding properties in the plasma membrane, detectable by immunoblotting or by the direct binding of HDL to plasma membrane preparations (10-12). The interaction of HDL with these proteins has many of the properties of a receptor-mediated process. It is saturable and depends on the nature of the HDL protein. The number of binding sites is directly proportional to the cholesterol content of the cell and to the observed rate of efflux. HDL binding is accompanied by the transmission of a protein kinase C-mediate intracellular signal (13). It has not yet proved possible to show that the HDL binding protein, incorporated into a cell membrane (for example following transfection of the corresponding gene) augments cholesterol efflux. As a result it remains possible that the cell signalling data reflects only indirectly the binding of HDL. For example, many HDL preparations are cholesterol-depleted (see below) and could modify the cell plasma membrane by lowering its cholesterol content, possibly stimulating intracellular signalling. Different cell types seem to have different properties in the promotion of cholesterol efflux.

In spite of being very simple in concept, measurements of the mechanism and specificity of the transfer of cholesterol from cells to native plasma or lymph are technically difficult. The following factors contribute to this:

a. Time course. Free cholesterol exchanges very rapidly ($t_{1/2}$ ca 2 min) between HDL subfractions at 37 C (14,15). As a result HDL specificity is observable only over very short incubations. The situation is similar for other lipoproteins, although the rate of exchange is somewhat longer. For example, the exchange of cholesterol from LDL to HDL has a $t_{1/2}$ of about 45 min at 37 C. In spite of this data, in some published studies the incubation period over which efflux was measured was 4-24 h. Under these conditions extensive secondary transfer of cholesterol will occur. Very short incubation times are obviously preferable.

b. Lipoprotein specificity. Centrifugal isolation of HDL removes apo A-I (16) and is associated with the transfer of apo E from native VLDL (17). Free cholesterol is also lost as a result of lecithin:cholesterol acyltransferase (LCAT)activity, with most of the cholesteryl ester generated in vitro retained in the particle unless enzyme action is blocked during the isolation of HDL. HDL purified on immunoaffinity columns have been used in a number of studies. However bound lipoproteins must be dissociated before use from the affinity matrix; the solutions for dissociation (acetic acid, pH 2.5-3 or 3M thiocyanate, pH 7.0) are recognized chaotropic agents sometimes used preparatively to isolate lipid-free apo A-I from HDL (18) and known to inactivate plasma enzymes (19). There may be no currently well-validated technology to isolate native HDL for use in studies of cholesterol efflux. This problem can be circumvented by measuring efflux into native plasma, and only then isolating different HDL, using the precautions described above. Several different techniques are available for HDL separation under mild conditions (5).

c. Disequilibrium of free cholesterol in plasma. LCAT draws part of its substrate cholesterol requirement from cell membranes and part from plasma lipoproteins, particularly LDL. In vivo, newly secreted lipoproteins, some with short circulation times are continually entering the plasma compartment and leaving as triglyceride-depleted remnant lipoproteins. It is unlikely that the free cholesterol in these particles equilibrates fully with that in other lipoproteins and in cell membranes. The equilibrium between cell membranes and lipoproteins is much slower than between different lipoprotein particles (20). The half-time for equilibration at 37 C is usually within the range 6-24 h.

In native plasma LCAT, by sequestering free cholesterol from cell membranes in HDL as its ester, maintains cell-to-plasma cholesterol transport that is in excess of local cholesterogenesis (21). The balance is made up by the uptake of lipoprotein cholesterol (mainly LDL) by receptor-dependent and other pathways. These factors make it likely that plasma and cellular free cholesterol are normally in a complex metastable equilibrium that reflects the continuous entry of nascent lipoproteins of hepatic and intestinal origin, the transfer of free cholesterol from different cell types, and the removal of mature or remnant lipoproteins, mainly by the liver. Because of this, the distribution of free cholesterol between lipoproteins is modified as a function of time as soon as blood plasma is isolated. As a result very short term assays of cholesterol efflux seem to offer the best possibility of measuring the events involved in the interaction of plasma lipoproteins with cell free cholesterol.

EARLY EVENTS IN THE METABOLISM OF CELLULAR CHOLESTEROL IN PLASMA

The following studies were carried out over short periods of incubation (0.5-5 min in different studies), with native plasma from freshly drawn blood, and sometimes with LCAT inhibited before its use in individual experiments. The intention was to retain, as far as possible, the original properties of plasma lipoproteins, particularly labile HDL species involved in the early metabolism of cell-derived cholesterol. Nondenaturing two dimensional electrophoresis was used to separate HDL species (5-8).

Several observations reinforce the concept, discussed above, that the transfer of cell-derived cholesterol to HDL is nonrandom. The esterification of isotopic free cholesterol from labeled cells by LCAT was more efficient than the simultaneous esterification of unlabeled free cholesterol in plasma lipoproteins (6). Also, as described above, there is an early (1 min) accumulation of cell-derived free cholesterol label in a small, prebeta-migrating HDL fraction (prebeta-1 HDL).

<u>Prebeta-1 HDL structure and function.</u> After one dimensional electrophoretic separation, prebeta-HDL appears as a single band, but second-dimensional separation shows that in reality this fraction is made up of several distinct groups of particles, of which three are almost invariably present (prebeta-1, -2 and -3). A even smaller particle is sometimes seen, and may be equivalent to a particle seen in lymph with a molecular weight less than prebeta-1 (22). Two large prebeta-HDL fractions have been detected: a larger lipoprotein (prebeta-2, apparent molecular weight about 300 kDa), with a composition similar to that of a discoidal particle containing 3 apo A-I molecules/disc; and a still larger particle (prebeta-3), apparently a complex of prebeta-2 with LCAT and other proteins (7).

TABLE I. Prebeta HDL - concentration and functions.

| Fraction | % apo A-I | % $^3$H-FC | Ratio |
|---|---|---|---|
| Prebeta-1 HDL | $1.3 \pm 0.8$ | $39 \pm 27$ | $30.3 \pm 5.2$ |
| Prebeta-2 HDL | $2.4 \pm 1.6$ | $14 \pm 16$ | $9.1 \pm 9.3$ |
| Prebeta-3 HDL | $0.5 \pm 0.3$ | $2 \pm 1$ | $1.0 \pm 0.3$ |

Distribution of $^3$H-cholesterol radioactivity among HDL subfractions separated by nondenaturing two-dimensional electrophoresis, after 1 min incubation at 37 C. Data from refs. 6 and 7.

The total apparent molecular weight of prebeta-1 HDL (about 70 kDa) and its lipid and protein composition predict that it contains a single molecule of apo A-I as sole protein, together with phospholipid and a small proportion of free cholesterol. Particles with these properties are not generated by the usual cholate-dialysis techniques used to make synthetic HDL in vitro (23) but an increased concentration of prebeta-1 can be recovered when isolated apo A-I is added to cultured cells in the presence of plasma. Possibly the slow electrophoretic migration rate of prebeta-HDL reflects an unusual apo A-I tertiary structure.

When cultured cell monolayers labeled with $^3$H-cholesterol are incubated (1 min, 37 C) with unlabeled native plasma, about 50% of total label in the plasma is recovered with prebeta-1 HDL, even though this represents on average only about 2% of total HDL (Table I) and contains <0.01% of total plasma free cholesterol. During further incubation some of this free cholesterol label is dissipated by exchange with other HDL fractions as described above, but some is rapidly esterified by LCAT present in the prebeta-HDL fraction, resulting in the approximately 6-fold enrichment of isotopic cholesterol in the cholesteryl ester synthesized by LCAT in native plasma (7).

Comparable results were obtained when isolated apo A-I was incubated with cultured macrophages; except that LCAT was not present, and free cholesterol was retained unesterified in prebeta HDL (24).

Esterification of cell-derived cholesterol. Recent studies are consistent in indicating that much the major part of plasma LCAT is associated with HDL containing apo A-I but not apo A-II. Prebeta-3 HDL contains apo A-I but not apo A-II, and is enriched with labeled cholesterol ester shortly after native plasma is incubated with cells labeled with $^3$H-cholesterol (7). On the other hand when cholesterol label is drawn from LDL, little or no labeled cholesteryl ester was recovered in prebeta-3 HDL (14).

These data indicate that cell-derived cholesterol is compartmentalized within plasma, and that a subfraction of LCAT, identifiable by prebeta electrophoretic mobility, is preferentially active in the esterification of the cell-derived free cholesterol originating in prebeta-1 HDL. Whether prebeta-1 and its free cholesterol is converted by addition of lipids and protein to higher molecular weight prebeta-HDL, or whether the free cholesterol label, perhaps with phospholipid, is transferred from prebeta-1 to prebeta-3 HDL, is not fully understood. What does seem clear is that the prebeta HDL particles act as a shuttle for the preferential transfer and metabolism of cell-derived cholesterol, in contrast to cholesterol derived from plasma lipoproteins (LDL), which is mainly esterified in alpha-HDL.

Transfer of cell-derived cholesterol. It is now clear that a significant, perhaps major, fraction of cholesteryl ester synthesized in plasma by the LCAT reaction from lipoprotein free cholesterol is subsequently transferred to VLDL and LDL. Different studies have estimated rates of cholesteryl ester transfer variously as 0-60% of total LCAT activity (25-27). (Although cholesteryl ester transfer rates increase postprandially, so does LCAT activity and so this proportion probably does not change greatly between the fasting and postadsorptive periods).

When the free cholesterol which is esterified comes from cell membranes, the proportion subsequently transferred to VLDL and LDL is significantly lower (about 10% of total cell cholesterol esterified by LCAT). This finding indicates that relatively little of the cholesterol originating in cell membranes and esterified in HDL as part of the "reverse cholesterol transport" pathway is transferred to VLDL and LDL. A further study showed that this proportion was not dependent upon assay technique (5); the proportion transferred was similarly low when fractionation was by three different techniques.

These results suggest that the metabolism of cell-derived cholesterol is mediated by a specific prebeta-HDL pathway, not shared with plasma lipoprotein cholesterol, and that this compartmentation is maintained by the LCAT reaction, which preferentially esterifies cell-derived free cholesterol. This pathway must be supplemental to that supplied by simple diffusion. The retention in HDL of most of the cholesteryl ester generated from cell-derived cholesterol may indicate that a high HDL cholesterol reflects active and efficient reverse cholesterol transport.

## ACKNOWLEDGEMENTS

The authors' research was supported by the National Institutes of Health through Arteriosclerosis SCOR HL 14237.

## REFERENCES

1  McLean LR, Phillips MC. Biochemistry 1981; 20:2893-2900.
2  Haberland M, Reynolds JA. Proc. Natl. Acad. Sci. (USA) 1973; 70:2313-2316.
3  McLean LR, Phillips MC. Biochemistry 1982; 21:4053-4059.

152

4   Steck TL, Kezdy FJ, Lange Y. J. Biol. Chem. 1988; 263:13023-13031.

5   Francone OL, Fielding CJ, Fielding PE. J. Lipid Res. 1990; 31:2195-2200.

6   Castro GR, Fielding CJ. Biochemistry 1988; 27:25-29.

7   Francone OL, Gurakar A, Fielding CJ. J. Biol. Chem. 1989; 264:7066-7072.

8   Barbaras R, Puchois P, Fruchart J-C, Ailhaud G. Biochem. Biophys. Res. Comm. 1987; 142:63-69.

9   Johnson WJ, Kilsdonk EPC, van Tol A, Phillips MC. Rothblat GH. J. Lipid Res. 1991; 32:1993-2000.

10  Graham DL, Oram JF. J. Biol. Chem. 1987; 262:7439-7442.

11  Tozuka M, Fidge N. Biochem. J. 1989; 261:239-244.

12  Barbbaras R, Puchois P, Fruchart J-C, Pradines-Figueres A, Ailhaud G. Biochem. J/ 1990; 269:367-373.

13  Mendez AJ, Oram JF, Bierman EL. J. Biol. Chem. 1991; 266:10104-10111.

14  Miida T, Fielding CJ, Fielding PE. Biochemistry 1990; 29:10469-10474.

15  Lund-Katz S, Hammerschlag B, Phillips MC. Biochemistry 1982; 21:2964-2969.

16  Kunitake S, Kane JP. J. Lipid Res. 1982; 23:936-940.

17  Castro GR, Fielding CJ. J. Lipid Res. 1984; 25:58-67.

18  Vega GL, Gylling H, Nichols AV, Grundy SM. J. Lipid Res. 1991; 32:867-875.

19  Cheung MC, Wolf AC, Lum KD, Tollefson JH, Albers JJ. J. Lipid Res. 1986; 27:1135-1144.

20  Phillips MC, Johnson WJ, Rothblat GH. Biochim. Biophys. Acta 1987; 906: 223-276.

21  Fielding CJ, Fielding PE. Proc, Natl. Acad. Sci. (USA) 1981; 78:3911-3914.

22  Lefevre M, Sloop CH, Roheim PS. J. Lipid Res. 1988; 29:1139-1148.

23  Nichols AV, Gong EL, Blanche PJ, Forte TM. Biochim. Biophys. Acta 1983; 750:353-359.

24  Hara H, Yokoyama S. J. Biol. Chem. 1991; 266:3080-3086.

25  Castro GR, Fielding CJ. J. Clin. Invest. 1985; 75:874-882.

26  Tall A, Sammett D, Granot E. J. Clin. Invest. 1986; 77:1163-1172.

27  van Tol A, Scheek KLM, Groener JEM. Arterioscl. Thromb. 1991; 11:55-63.

# ANIMAL MODELS OF HDL METABOLISM AND ATHEROSCLEROSIS

# HDL Metabolism: Studies in Transgenic Mice

Jan L. Breslow

Laboratory of Biochemical Genetics and Metabolism, The Rockefeller University, 1230 York Avenue, New York, NY 10021-6399, United States of America

## INTRODUCTION

HDL cholesterol levels are a strong inverse risk factor for coronary heart disease. HDL metabolism is sufficiently complex that a better understanding of the regulation of HDL cholesterol levels and the cholesterol/atherosclerosis susceptibility relationship requires an *in vivo* model. To this end, we have been studying HDL metabolism in transgenic mice expressing various human lipoprotein transport protein genes.

## GENES THAT DETERMINE HDL LEVEL AND PARTICLE SIZE

In our initial experiments, Walsh *et al* introduced the human apo A-I gene with various amounts of flanking sequence into transgenic mice (HuAITg mice) (1). Five lines of animals were established using three different gene constructions. Endogenous mouse apo A-I is expressed equally in liver and intestine, but the transgenic lines expressed human apo A-I only in the liver. These experiments suggested that only 256 bp of 5' flanking sequence was sufficient for liver apo A-I gene expression. However, 5.5 kb of 5' and 3.5 kb of 3' flanking sequence were not sufficient for intestinal expression. In subsequent studies, we have identified the cis-acting region required for intestinal expression of the apo A-I gene. This element resides 3' to the gene in the promoter region of the adjacent but convergently transcribed apo CIII gene (2). From these studies we have concluded that the cis-acting elements determining liver and intestinal apo A-I gene expression are physically distinct.

In several of the HuAITg lines, sufficient apo A-I expression was achieved to affect plasma apo A-I pool sizes. This allowed us to study the effect of human apo A-I gene expression on lipoprotein metabolism (1). The transgenic mice showed an increase in total cholesterol with the vast majority of the increase in the HDL fraction. In different transgenic animals there was a strong correlation of approximately 0.9 between HDL cholesterol and human apo A-I concentrations in plasma. This is roughly the same correlation that we have seen in human clinical studies. The effect on HDL cholesterol levels was quite specific with no significant accompanying change in plasma triglyceride levels. These studies showed for the first time that increasing apo A-I production *in vivo* could actually increase HDL cholesterol levels without major effects on the other lipoprotein fractions.

In further studies we found that the endogenous mouse apo A-I levels in HuAITg mice were reduced by 85% (3). This resulted in over 90% of plasma apo A-I being derived from the human transgene. Thus, in HuAITg animals we had effectively replaced mouse apo A-I with human apo A-I in HDL. Coincidentally, we also detected a change in HDL particle size distribution (3). Mouse HDL is primarily monodisperse with a mean particle diameter of 10.2 nm. Transgenic HDL is polydisperse with populations of mean particle diameters of

11.4, 10.2 and 8.7 nm, corresponding to human $HDL_1$, $HDL_2$ and $HDL_3$, respectively. Thus, the primary sequence of apo A-I appears to determine HDL particle size distribution.

In other studies, we have shown that CETP gene expression *in vivo* can affect HDL cholesterol levels (4). Mouse plasma is normally devoid of CETP activity. In collaboration with Dr. Tall of Columbia, we made a human CETP transgenic mouse. We used a CETP minigene driven by the mouse metallothionein I gene promoter. The specific activity of CETP in the plasma of these animals was comparable to humans. Total CETP activity was also similar to humans with a doubling of activity after adding 10 mM $ZnSO_4$ to the drinking water. HDL cholesterol levels were reduced 20% and 35% and apo A-I levels 2% and 24% before and after Zn stimulation.

## MECHANISMS WHEREBY DIET AND DRUGS INFLUENCE HDL CHOLESTEROL LEVELS

A high fat diet is known to increase HDL cholesterol levels whereas probucol decreases them. In metabolic studies both effects are associated with a change in apo A-I transport rate. Due to the limitations of clinical investigation, further mechanistic studies are precluded. In HuAITg mice we have mimicked both effects and turnover studies indicated that the apo A-I transport rate was involved (5, 6). However, tissue levels of apo A-I mRNA were not altered in either case. Thus far, these studies suggest that high fat diets and probucol affect apo A-I synthesis post mRNA, presumably by altering apo A-I mRNA translation or apo A-I secretion. This is a previously unrecognized level of regulation of apo A-I synthesis and one that is relevant to physiological or therapeutic situations. In addition, a comparison of animals at the extremes of HDL (high fat vs. probucol) showed a 2.5-fold difference in plasma apo A-I levels without a change in the apo A-I fractional catabolic rate. This suggests apo A-I removal is not mediated by a saturable receptor dependent mechanism over the physiological range of apo A-I concentrations.

## PATHWAYS OF HDL CHOLESTEROL ESTER REMOVAL FROM PLASMA

The major tissue site of HDL cholesterol ester removal from plasma is the liver. Physiological studies have indicated three pathways. There is direct uptake of HDL particles, selective removal of HDL cholesterol esters, and CETP-mediated transfer to VLDL with subsequent hepatic removal of IDL and LDL. Through the use of HDL doubly labelled in its protein ($^{125}I$ apo A-I) and cholesterol ester moiety ($^3H$ cholesteryl linoleyl ether), we have studied HDL component clearance in transgenic animals (3). In control mice the $^3H$ cholesteryl linoleyl ether was cleared (fractional catabolic rate) 67% faster than the $^{125}I$ apo A-I, whereas both moieties of HDL had the same clearance in HuAITg mice. These observations suggest that mouse apo A-I containing HDL clear cholesterol ester by particulate and selective uptake mechanisms, whereas human apo A-I containing HDL do so only by particulate uptake. This suggests that the primary structure of apo A-I (in this case mouse versus human) determines selective uptake of HDL cholesterol esters and that this pathway may not be important in humans.

## SUMMARY

The introduction of lipoprotein transport genes into transgenic mice is revealing new information about lipoprotein metabolism. The experiments descrived in this paper with the human apo A-I and CETP genes have provided new insights into the regulation of HDL levels, particle size distribution and metabolism. In the future, we hope to use these animals to better understand the role of HDL in cholesterol metabolism and atherosclerosis susceptibility.

## REFERENCES

1. Walsh A, Ito Y, Breslow JL. J Biol Chem 1989; 264:6488-6494.
2. O'Connell A, Walsh AM, Azrolan N, Breslow JL. Circulation 1990; 82:1717.
3. Chajek-Shaul T, Hayek T, Walsh A, Breslow JL. Proc Natl Acad Sci USA 1991; 88:6731-6735.
4. Agellon LB, Walsh A, Hayek T, Moulin P, Ziang XC, Shelanski S, Breslow JL, Tall AR. J Biol Chem 1991; 266:10796-10801.
5. Ito Y, Hayek T, Verdery RB, Azrolan N, Chajek-Shaul T, Walsh A, Breslow JL. J Clin Invest 1992; Submitted.
6. Hayek T, Chajek-Shaul T, Walsh A, Azrolan N, Breslow JL. Arteriosclerosis and Thrombosis 1991; 11:1295-1302.

# High Density Lipoprotein Subpopulation Distribution

S. Eisenberg

Department of Medicine, Hadassah University Hospital, POB 12000
i191120 Jerusalem, Israel

## I. HDL POPULATIONS

High density lipoprotein (HDL) exists in plasma in multiple forms. Populations of HDL that differ in density, composition, electrophoretic mobility and apolipoprotein profile have been identified when different techniques have been applied to the study of HDL. HDL populations differ not only in chemical and physical properties, but perhaps also in function. Various metabolic activites were assigned to specific HDL particle populations, including cholesterol esterification by the LCAT enzyme; neutral lipid transfers by the cholesterol ester transfer protein (CETP); reverse cholesterol transport; protection against atherosclerotic diseases; delivery of cholesterol to the liver and many others. Yet, virtually nothing is known about pathways that regulate the levels, distribution, origin and catabolism of the different HDL populations.

Studies in our laboratory during the last decade focused on one form of HDL heterogeneity – density populations – with an attempt to elucidate pathways that determine the levels and distribution of these HDL particles. Classification of HDL to density population – $HDL_2$ and $HDL_3$ – was the first identified heterogeneity of this lipoprotein, described already in the earliest papers by Gofman, Lindgren and Nichols (1). These investigators also found an association between HDL levels, in particular $HDL_2$, and ischemic diseases (2), a forgotten observation that was rediscovered in the 1970s.

$HDL_2$ and $HDL_3$ can be separated by a variety of ultracentrifugation methods. In our laboratory we use predominantly the rate zonal ultracentrifugation method described by Patsch et al(3). With this method, it is clear that HDL comprised of a discontinued spectrum of particles and that $HDL_2$ and $HDL_3$ are almost totally separated from each other, with a "dip" of mass between the two. We speculated that this macro-heterogeneity of the HDL system represents a "quantum jump" between two stable states ($HDL_3$ and $HDL_2$) possibly reflecting the difference of one apo A-I molecule between the two (4). Micro-heterogeneity also exists within each population and perhaps accounts for the ability to further separate $HDL_2$ and $HDL_3$ into subpopulations, e.g. $HDL_2a$ and $HDL_2b$ or $HDL_3a$ and $HDL_3b$. Comparing $HDL_2$ to $HDL_3$, a major difference between the two can be found: $HDL_2$ carries about 2-3 more cholesterol per one apo A-I than $HDL_3$, 20-30 molecules and 8-12 molecules respectively. This observation alone suggests that $HDL_2$ levels in plasma will predominate in conditions where relatively more cholesterol is carried in HDL.

Plasma levels of $HDL_2$ and $HDL_3$ are related to total plasma HDL in a distinctly different fashion. While $HDL_3$ levels are constant over a large range of plasma HDL (except levels below 30 mg cholesterol/dl), $HDL_2$ is almost not detected when plasma HDL cholesterol is below 40 mg/dl but accounts for virtually all the additional HDL mass in subjects with higher HDL levels. This phenomenon, known for many years, was most elegantly demonstrated by Andersen et al., in a large group of male and female subjects and was especially pronounced for the lighter $HDL_2$ fraction, $HDL_2b$ (5). This observation again supports the concept that $HDL_2$, with its higher capacity to transport cholesterol, accumulates in plasma when HDL cholesterol levels are high.

The observational data described above strongly indicate that the $HDL_2$ and $HDL_3$ are metabolically related to each other and are possibly in a metabolic equilibrium that reflects processes that regulate cholesterol transport in the HDL system. This consideration prompted us to initiate a series of in vitro studies on possible conversion ($HDL_3 \rightarrow HDL_2$) and reverse-conversion ($HDL_2 \rightarrow HDL_3$) processes in human plasma (6,7). Indeed, both processes could be demonstrated in the test tube. Conversion of small size and dense HDL populations (e.g. $HDL_3$) to large size and less dense HDL was shown under situations where redundant phospholipids, cholesterol and apoproteins from the surface of lipolyzed triglyceride-rich lipoproteins are transferred to $HDL_3$. These light, $HDL_2$-like particles are unstable, but we hypothesized that when cholesteryl esters are formed by the LCAT reaction and are displaced to the lipid core of the particle, true $HDL_2$ is formed. Reverse-conversion of large size and high HDL populations (e.g. $HDL_2$) to small size and dense HDL was also demonstrated in our in vitro studies. The reverse-conversion process, in our model, also occurs in two steps. First, a hetero-exchange of HDL-cholesteryl esters for VLDL or chylomicrons-triglycerides takes place in the presence of the cholesterol ester transfer protein (CETP). This reaction produces replacement of the core-cholesteryl esters in the $HDL_2$ by triglycerides but does not modify the size or density of the particles. When acted upon by lipases however, the transferred triglycerides are hydrolized and small size and dense HDL that resembles $HDL_3$ is formed. The two processes combined can therefore modulate $HDL_2$ and $HDL_3$ particle distribution and account for their relative levels in the plasma. Indeed, this hypothesis agrees extremely well with observations in human subjects with dyslipidemia and in experimental animals. A few examples are the predominance of small size and dense HDL in patients with low lipoprotein lipase activity and especially high plasma triglyceride levels (8). The two conditions are associated with lower transfer of "surface remnants" from the triglyceride-rich lipoproteins to HDL and accelerated hetero-exchange of the HDL cholesteryl esters for triglycerides combined with normal or even high hepatic lipase activity. Predominance of $HDL_2$ is observed in human subjects that lack CETP activity (9) or with abetalipoproteinemia (10) when triglyceride-rich lipoproteins are absent from the plasma. It is also observed in animal species that lack CETP, e.g. rats (11). Thus, it is reasonable to assume that the pathways shown to affect the HDL size and density in vitro also regulate HDL subpopulation distribution in vivo.

## II. ORIGIN OF HDL POPULATIONS

The data and hypotheses presented above do not provide a clue to the origin of $HDL_2$ and $HDL_3$. Unlike the triglyceride-rich lipoproteins and their metabolic products - VLDL, IDL and LDL - HDL is not secreted into the plasma as a spherical lipoprotein but rather as a discoidal precursor that matures in the plasma to form the circulating HDLs. Graphic representation of three possible routes to explain the origin of HDL is shown in Figure 1.

# Origin Of HDL Population

HDL-2          HDL-3

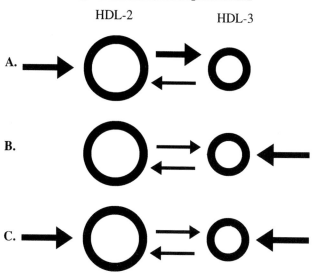

Figure 1. Possible routes of the origin of HDL populations

A. HDL$_2$ is formed initially from the precursor particles and through the reverse-conversion process is converted to HDL$_3$. B. HDL$_3$ is the primary plasma HDL particle but some, or much of the HDL$_3$ is converted to HDL$_2$. C. HDL$_2$ and HDL$_3$ are formed simultaneously at an arbitrary concentration and are quickly remodelled in plasma by the metabolic pathways that are responsible for the conversions and reverse-conversion processes.

Investigations on the origin of HDL populations in plasma are scarce. This perhaps reflects methodological difficulties inherent in such studies. Since all HDL consituents rapidly distribute and equilibrate between particles, it is almost impossible to label a lipid or apoprotein constituent and through this technique to follow the metabolic fate of the particle. In humans, for example, if HDL$_2$ is labeled in any constituent and is re-injected, it is impossible to determine whether labels appearing in HDL$_3$ reflect exchange processes or a true reverse conversion of the particle. This consideration prompted us to investigate plasma HDL particles metabolism in vivo in an experimental animal, the rat. Because rats lack cholesterol ester transfer activity we reasoned that by using HDL populations labeled in their cholesteryl ester moiety it would be possible to follow the fate of particles rather than lipid or apoprotein constituents (12). As in humans, rat plasma contains two HDL populations: apo A-I rich HDL$_2$ and apo E-rich HDL$_1$. When the rats were injected with labeled HDL$_1$, radioactivity did not appear in HDL$_2$. Thus, in the absence of CETP activity, reverse-conversion did not take place. When the rats were injected with HDL$_2$ however, considerable amount of radioactivity was gradually built up in HDL$_1$ and by 24 hours after the injection the amount of radioactive cholesteryl esters in HDL$_1$ was greater than in HDL$_2$. Thus, conversion of HDL$_2$ - the smaller and denser HDL population in rats - to

HDL₁ did take place. In a subsequent study, rats were injected with human HDL₃ labeled with [³H]cholesteryl esters (13). Within 60 min of the injection all the HDL₃ was converted to HDL₂ and thereafter conversion of some, but not all the HDL₂ to HDL₁ was found. Since these conversions could not be reproduced during in vitro incubations, we concluded that in vivo a true conversion cascade along the HDL spectrum - HDL₃ -> HDL₂ -> HDL₁ - is a physiological phenomenon. Of interest, injection of the rats with human CETP had no effect on the rapid conversion of HDL₃ to HDL₂ but caused a significant decrease of the amount of [³H]cholesteryl esters that followed the HDL₂ -> HDL₁ conversion.

Can these observations be extrapolated to humans? We do not know. They indicate, however, that pathway B in Figure 1 exists in vivo and strongly support the assumption that HDL may initially be formed as a small size and dense spherical particle that enters a conversion process, presumably by accumulating cholesteryl ester, addition of one apo A-I molecule and re-arrangement of the surface domain. Data that this route actually occurs in humans, however, is unavailable. Of interest, the effects of two drugs that increase HDL cholesterol levels - nicotinic acid and fibrates - on HDL₂ and HDL₃ distribution is very different. Nicotinic acid specifically increases HDL₂ (14) while fibrates, HDL₃ (8). The mechanism(s) responsible for the divergent effects of the two drugs on HDL populations is unknown. Nicotinic acid decreases fatty acid transport and VLDL formation, while fibrates increase lipoprotein lipase activity. Neither drug appears to affect CETP activity. Thus, additional, as yet unidentified metabolic processes may have important effects on HDL population origin and plasma distribution.

## III. CATABOLISM OF HDL POPULATIONS

The site of catabolism of HDL particles and the mechanisms responsible for uptake and degradation of HDL by cells are unclear. Even less is known about processes involved specifically with the removal from plasma of defined HDL populations. Several investigators have shown that some, or much of the HDL is not removed from the plasma as spherical particles but rather individual lipid and protein constituents are independently taken up by tissue cells. For example, in rats, HDL cholesteryl esters are preferentially removed from the particles in tissues such as liver and adrenal while lipid-poor apo A-I molecules may be filtered in the kidneys (15). Other HDL particles, however, appear to be catabolized as particles.

One mechanism by which HDL may be removed from the plasma is after interactions of apo E-containing HDL particles with the LDL-receptor or apo E-receptors. That indeed appears to be the major catabolic route for apo E-HDL from cholesterol-fed animals (16). Whether this mechanism accounts for catabolism of significant amounts of HDL in humans or experimental animals on normal diet is, however, doubtful. Although apo E-rich human HDL interacts with high affinity with the LDL-receptor (e.g. apo E-rich HDL from patients with abetalipoproteinemia (17)), HDL levels are not high in patients with homozygous familial hypercholesterolemia who lack the LDL-receptor. HDL levels in such patients are usually low. Direct evidence that apo E-rich HDL is not catabolized at an accelerated rate in vivo was obtained in studies in rats (12). In the study, the turnover of rat plasma lipoproteins labeled by biological procedures with [³H]cholesteryl esters was determined. The decay from plasma of apo E-rich $HDL_1$ was the slowest. When compared to LDL, the circulating lifetime of $HDL_1$ was 50-100% longer. In a further study we indeed found that the uptake and degradation of the apo E-rich $HDL_1$ by cultured fibroblasts is considerably less than that of LDL (unpublished). Clearly, interaction of apo E-containing HDL with cellular receptors appears to be insufficient to account for catabolism of significant amounts of HDL.

Regardless of the mechanisms responsible for catabolism of HDL particles in general, at least three potential routes for catabolism of HDL populations can theoretically be suggested. The three routes are shown schematically in figure 2: A. as $HDL_3$, B. as $HDL_2$ and C. both. There is no

## Catabolism Of HDL Population

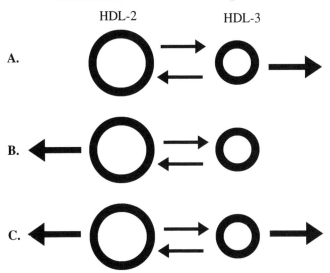

Figure 2. Possible routes of the catabolism of HDL populations

direct evidence to support any of the three routes as a major pathway for the tissue clearance of HDL. In principal, arguments can be put forward in favor of each of the three routes. For example, it can be argued that when HDL accumulates excess cholesterol and becomes $HDL_2$ or even $HDL_1$, the particle is removed from the plasma (route B). Conversely, it can be argued that when HDL becomes smaller and denser the particles are destabilized and degraded (route A). It is of course possible that HDL is cleared from plasma indiscriminatively as either large or small particles (route C). This question, as discussed in detail by Dr. Brinton in another chapter of the book, has received a partial answer in recent studies carried out at the Rockefeller University (18,19). It appears that in humans, HDL and apo A-I levels are determined predominantly by the fractional catabolic rate (FCR) of apo A-I. Apo A-I FCR in turn is determined largely by the size and density of HDL, estimated by the ratio of HDL-cholesterol to the sum of the mass of apo A-I and apo A-II. Thus, it must be assumed that apo A-I catabolism occurs predominantly from the density range of $HDL_3$. While

164

these observations still do not fully answer the question whether apo A-I is catabolized in a lipid-poor form or is a signal for whole particle catabolism, they indirectly support route A. Evidently, new approaches and techniques should be developed in order to further elucidate the mechanisms and routes of HDL catabolism.

**IV. HDL POPULATION METABOLISM**

The data and considerations presented above lead us to suggest a general scheme of HDL population metabolism (figure 3). According to the hypothesis presented in the figure, $HDL_3$ plays a central role in the processes involved with HDL population metabolism. It is suggested that nascent HDL are either small spherical particles that belong to the $HDL_3$ density range or, when spherical particles are formed from the discoidal HDL precursors

## Metabolism Of HDL Population

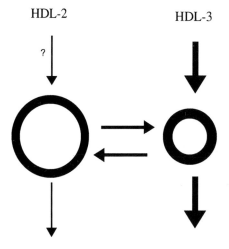

Figure 3. An hypothetical scheme of HDL population metabolism

the initial product is a small and dense $HDL_3$. These small spherical $HDL_3$ particles contain apo A-I regardless of their origin, primary secretory products of cells or particles formed from discoidal structures. Whether $HDL_2$ can also be formed, is not known. $HDL_3$ may follow one of two routes: conversion to $HDL_2$ or catabolism. We suggest that the catabolism of HDL occurs also predominantly, but not exclusively, from the density of $HDL_3$. We however also suggest that there is also catabolism of HDL particles from the $HDL_2$ density range. In the absence of detailed information on the pathways responsible for the catabolism of HDL in general, we suggest that all HDL particles are taken up by cells by the same mechanism, regardless of density. In essence, there is no evidence to indicate that $HDL_2$ and

HDL$_3$ are catabolized by different routes. However, the "sensitivity" and/ or affinity of the catabolic site towards different HDL populations, is low for HDL$_2$ but high for HDL$_3$. When conditions in plasma favor high HDL cholesterol levels, more HDL$_3$ is converted to HDL$_2$ and the reverse-conversion of HDL$_2$ to HDL$_3$ is slow. Under these conditions, HDL$_2$ accumulates, may become the predominant HDL population and the overall catabolic rate of HDL apoproteins A-I and A-II (and presumably of whole HDL particles) is low. The opposite situation is found in subjects in whom transport of cholesterol in HDL is low and total HDL cholesterol levels are also low.

The scheme shown in figure 3 is obviously speculative but appears to be compatible with most, if not all observations on the HDL system in humans and experimental animals. It explains not only the observations on the distribution of the populations in plasma but also the results of the metabolic studies. Yet, it is a purely hypothetical scheme that must await testing and verification.

## REFERENCES

1. Lindgren FT, Elliot HA, Gofman JW. J Phys Colloid Chem 1951; 55: 80-93.
2. Gofman JW, de Lalla O, Glazier F, Freeman NK, Lindgren FT. Plasma 1954; 2: 413-484.
3. Patsch JR, Sailer S, Kostner G, Sandhofer F, Holasek A, Braunsteiner H. J Lipid Res 1974; 15: 356-366.
4. Eisenberg S. J Lipid Res 1984; 25: 1017-1058.
5. Anderson DW, Nichols AV, Pan SS, Lindgren FT. Atherosclerosis 1987; 29: 161-179.
6. Patsch JR, Gotto AM, Olivecrona T, Eisenberg S. Proc Natl Acad Sci USA 1978; 75: 4519-4523.
7. Deckelbaum RJ, Eisenberg S, Oschry Y, Granot E, Sharon I, Bengtsson-Olivecrona G. J Biol Chem 1986; 261: 5201-5208.
8. Eisenberg S, Gavish D, Oschry Y, Fainaru M, Deckelbaum RJ. J Clin Invest 1984; 74: 470-482.
9. Brown ML, Inazu A, Hester CB, Agellon LB, et al. Nature 1989; 342: 448-451.
10. Deckelbaum RJ, Eisenberg S, Oschry Y, Cooper M, Blum C. J Lipid Res 1982; 23: 1274-1282.
11. Oschry Y, Eisenberg S. J Lipid Res 1982; 23: 1099-1106.
12. Eisenberg S, Oschry Y, Zimmerman J. J Lipid Res 1984; 25:121-128.
13. Gavish D, Oschry Y, Eisenberg S. J Lipid Res 1987; 28: 257-267.
14. Olsson AG, Walldiens G, Wohlberg G. In: Shepherd J, Packard CJ, eds. Pharmacological Control of Hyperlipidaemia. Barcelona: JR Prous Science Publishers, 1987; 217-230
15. Glass CK, Pittmam RC, Keller GA, Steinberg D. J Biol Chem 1983; 258: 7161-7170.
16. Pitas RE, Innerarity TL, Arnold KS, Mahely RW. Proc Natl Acad Sci USA 1979; 76: 2311-2315.
17. Blum CB, Deckelbaum RJ, Witte LD, Tall AR, Cornicelli J. J Clin Invest 1982; 70: 1157-1169.
18. Brinton EA, Eisenberg S, Breslow JL. J Clin Invest 1989; 84: 262-269.
19. Brinton EA, Eisenberg S, Breslow JL. J Clin Invest 1991; 87: 536-544.

Lipoproteins and Atherosclerosis in Transgenic Mice Expressing HDL Associated Apolipoproteins

Edward Rubin, M.D., Ph.D.

Cell and Molecular Biology, Lawrence Berkeley Laboratory, University of California, Berkeley, California 94720

Apolipoprotein AI (apoAI), the primary protein component of high density lipoproteins (HDL), is suspected of having a major effect on the levels of HDL in plasma, the structure of the HDL particle, and on the susceptibility of an individual to develop atherosclerosis. In this study, we examined the in vivo effect of over expression of apoAI by introducing the human apoAI gene into the atherosclerosis susceptible inbred mouse strain C57BL/6. The human apoAI DNA fragment (a kind gift of S. Karathanasis) introduced into the mice is diagrammed in Figure 1. This particular construct is expressed primarily in the livers of transgenic animals, slightly in gonadal tissues, and not at all in the intestine.

## ApoAI

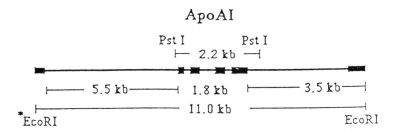

**Figure 1.**
*Human apoAI genomic sequence used in creating the apoAI transgenic mice.*

In two independent human apoAI transgenic lines, plasma levels of total apoAI and HDL were increased to twice that of non-transgenic litter mates (Table 1). Surprisingly the level of endogenous mouse apoAI in plasma from the transgenic animals is markedly reduced, up to 10 fold, and contributes only 4% to the total plasma apoAI mass. To investigate a possible mechanism for this decrease RNA was isolated from various tissues of transgenic and control animals and murine apoAI levels were quantitated (Table 1). Murine apoAI message was detected exclusively in the liver and the intestine of both groups of animals. Approximately equal amounts of mouse apoAI mRNA was detected in the expressing tissues of the transgenic and control animals, indicating that the marked decrease in murine apoAI in the plasma of the human apoAI transgenic mice is occurring at a post transcriptional step. This decrease of murine apoAI has recently been confirmed by Chajek-Shaul et. al. (2) using a different human apoAI construct in a different strain of mice, suggesting that this is a general effect of high level expression of human apoAI in transgenic mice.

TABLE 1
Apoliprotein in Transgenic and Control Mice

|  | Human AI Copy # | Mouse AI* Liver | Mouse AI* Intestine | Mouse AI° mg/dl | Human AI° mg/dl |
|---|---|---|---|---|---|
| C57BL/6 Control | 0 | 1. | 1. | 112.1 ± 10 | 0 |
| ApoAI Transgenic A2 | 25 | 0.84 | 0.89 | 6.5 ± 2.2 | 245 ± 9.6 |
| ApoAI Transgenic A16 | 5 | 0.88 | 0.92 | 17.3 ± 8 | 156 ± 4.0 |

*Relative mouse apoAI mRNA levels. This was derived utilizing the C57BL/6 control mouse apoAI/cytochromoxidase ratio as an internal reference.
°Plasma protein levels

Our current model to explain the 10 fold decrease in murine AI plasma levels is one that proposes that a hybrid HDL particle containing both human and mouse apoAI is unstable. This model which we have named a hybrid suicide model, is illustrated in cartoon form in Figure 2. Murine apoAI (denoted by *AI*) is synthesized in the liver and intestine of the control animals, and the transgenics while human apoAI (denoted by *aI*) is synthesized exclusively in the livers of the transgenic mice at extremely high levels. We postulate that in the transgenics, due to the relative abundance of human apoAI, HDL composed exclusively of human apoAI is the primary stable HDL species, while HDL composed entirely of mouse apoAI is a minor coponent. According to this model the majority of mouse apoAI is rapidly catabolized due to its aborted interaction with human apoAI. Our failure to detect hybrid HDL particles containing both human and murine apoAI is consistant with this model.

## Hybrid Suicide

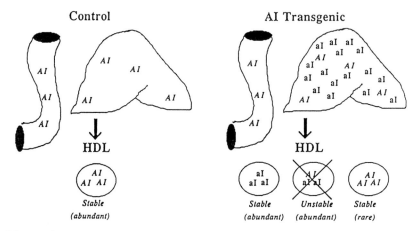

Figure 2.

169

Although the sequence of mouse apoAI has not been published, rat apoAI differs by more than 60% from that of the human protein (3). Since HDL sizes differ significantly between mice and humans, the human apoAI transgenic animals serve as a unique substrate in which to investigate the role of apoAI sequence in determining HDL size. The transgenic mice exhibit two distinct HDL populations, identical in size to the human size subclasses HDL2b and HDL3a, instead of the distinct single-sized HDL population present in control mice (Figure 3). This HDL size distribution is indistinguishable from the size distribution HDL isolated from the plasma of humans which contains only apoAI. These results suggest a dominant role for the human apoAI primary amino acid sequence in determining the size of HDL regardless of whether the lipoprotein particles are formed in the plasma of humans or mice (1). (Again these results have recently been confirmed by Chajek-Shaul et. al. (2) using a different human apoAI construct in a different strain of mice.)

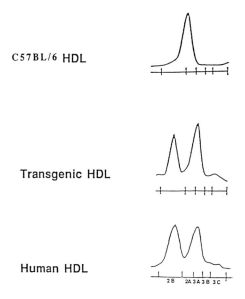

C57BL/6 HDL

Transgenic HDL

Human HDL

**Figure 3.**
*Densitometric scans of isolated HDL separated on 4 - 30 % non-denaturing gradient gels (4). The lower panal is apoAI without apoAII HDL isolated by immunoaffinity chromatography from human plasma.*

In parallel with these in vivo studies (in collaboration with Alex Nichols and Elaine Gong), we have assembled model apolipoprotein/lipid complexes in vitro using human or murine apoAI. Under the exact same in vitro conditions we observed that the size distribution of complexes formed using human apoAI differed markedly from those formed using murine apoAI. The size distribution of the model complexes formed with human or mouse apoAI somewhat mimicked that seen in plasma. Although apoAI comprises significantly less than half of total HDL mass, both in vivo and in vitro studies suggest the importance of apoAI primary amino acid sequence in determining the size of this macromolecule.

We next examined the effect that the changes in apoAI and HDL in the transgenic mice had on their susceptibility to diet induced atherosclerosis. In mice atherosclerosis susceptibility is a polygenic trait (5). Presently three murine atherosclerosis susceptibility genes, *ath1* (6), *ath2* (7), and *ath3* (8), have been identified none of which map to the murine apoAI gene. The C57BL/6 mice used for these studies are homozygous for atherosclerosis susceptibility alleles at all three of these loci, and thus are exquisitely sensitive to diet induced atherosclerosis. The lipoprotein profile of the C57BL/6 strain differs from that of strains resistant to diet induced atherosclerosis by its lower HDL concentrations when fed a high fat diet. The C57BL/6 transgenic mice expressing the human apoA1 transgene differed from control animals in their HDL response to the high fat diet (Table 2). The VLDL and LDL of transgenic and control animal did not differ significantly. Analysis of the atherogenic response to the high fat diet is shown in Table 2. Clearly the transgenic animals are significantly protected from the development of diet induced atherosclerosis when compared to their non-transgenic C57BL/6 litter mates (9).

TABLE 2
*A quantitative assessment of lipoproteins and atherogenesis in transgenic and control mice fed a high fat (15%) and high cholesterol (1.0 %) diet for 18 weeks (9). The lipoprotiens and area of lipid staining material per section per animal was assessed for over 14 animals in each group.*

| Animals | Cholesterol | | Mean Atherosclerotic lesion area |
| | HDL | LDL + VLDL | (μm per section per animal) |
| --- | --- | --- | --- |
| C57BL/6 ApoAI | $34 \pm 4$ | $86 \pm 5$ | $1607 \pm 195$ |
| Transgenics | $86 \pm 6$ | $72 \pm 15$ | 0 |

All studies were conducted on 7 or more animals after an 18 week exposure to 15% fat (primary source is dairy butter), 1% cholesterol, 5% Sodium Cholate, and 20% Casein (9).

These results in mice transgenic for human apoA1 indicate: 1) the existence of a post transcriptional mechanism that alters the plasma level of endogenous mouse apoAI, 2) the importance of apoAI in determining the level and particle size of HDL, and 3) that high plasma concentrations of human apoAI protects C57BL/6 mice from developing atherosclerosis. This last finding addresses a yet unresolved issue concerning whether the association in humans of high apoAI and HDL levels and protection from atherosclerosis is a direct effect or an indirect association. The present study demonstrates that high human apoAI and HDL concentrations in mice directly inhibits a polygenic form of atherosclerosis in this organism. These results support the hypothesis that apoAI and HDL have direct anti-atherogenic effects and that therapeutic interventions which raise their plasma levels may decrease the risk of atherosclerosis.

In conjunction with these studies we have recently characterized the effect of high level expression of the other major HDL associated apolipoprotein,

apolipoprotein AII (apoAII), in several human apoAII transgenic lines of mice. Unlike what we observed in the human apoAI transgenic mice, increases up to 4 fold in plasma apoAII had little effect on the endogenous murine apoAI or apoAII levels or on the plasma HDL concentrations of these mice (10). The apoAII transgenic mice contain the major sized HDL population present in control C57BL/6 mice but in addition have a population of smaller human apoAII only HDL particles. Transgenic mice expressing high levels of both human apoAI and human apoAII had HDL concentrations similar to those of mice expressing high levels of human apoAI further supporting a primary role for apoAI in determining HDL concentration. The HDL size profile of transgenic mice expressing both human apoAI and human apoAII bore little resemblance to either the apoAI or apoAII transgenic mice alone, but rather displayed a complex pattern of discrete sized HDL particles. These results suggest that human apoAII in the plasma of mice has little effect on HDL levels but does participate in determining HDL size, especially when interacting with human apoAI. Presently the atherosclerosis susceptibility of apoAI transgenic and apoAI + apoAII transgenic mice with similar HDL levels but differing HDL size profiles is being examined to investigate the anti-atherogenic properties of various HDL subclasses.

## ACKNOWLEDGEMENTS

This work was supported by the National Dairy Research and Promotion Board, and was conducted at the Lawrence Berkeley Laboratory (Department of Energy Contract DE-AC03-76SF00098 to the University of California).

## REFERENCES

1  Rubin, E, Ishida, BY, Clift, SM, Krauss, RM.  Proc. Natl. Acad. Sci., U.S.A. (1991); 88: 434-438.
2  Chajek-Shaul, T, Hayek, T, Walsh, A, Breslow, J.  Proc. Natl. Acad. Sci., U.S.A. (1991); 88: 6731-6735.
3  Haddad, IA, Ordovas, JM, Fitzpatrick, T, Karathanasis, SK.  J. Biol. Chem. (1986); 261: 13268-13277.
4  Nichols, AV,.Krauss, RM, Musliner, TA.  Methods Enzymol. (1986); 128: 417-431.
5  Ishida, B, Paigen, B.  In: Genetic Factors and Atherosclerosis: Approaches and Model Systems  (eds Lusis, A. and Sparks) 198-222 (Karger, Basel 1989).
6  Paigen, B, Mitchell, D, Reue, K, Morrow, A, LeBoeuf, R.  Proc. Natl. Acad. Sci., U.S.A. (1987); 84: 3763-3767.
7  Paigen, B, Nesbitt, MN, Mitchell, D, Albee, D, LeBoeuf, R.  Genetics (1989); 122: 163 168.
8  Stewart-Philip, J, Lough, J, Skomene, E.  Clin. Invest. Med. (1989); 12; 121-126.
9  Rubin, E, Krauss, R, Spangler, E, Verstuyft, J, Clift, S.  Nature. (1991); 353: 265-267.
10  Schultz, J, Clift, S, Rubin, E.  Circulation 1585A (1992).

# REVERSE CHOLESTEROL TRANSPORT AND PHYSIOLOGY

# Apolipoprotein E: Structure-function correlations

K. H. Weisgraber[a], S. Lund-Katz[b], and M. C. Phillips[b]

[a]Gladstone Institute of Cardiovascular Disease, Cardiovascular Research Institute, Department of Pathology, University of California, San Francisco, P.O. Box 419100, San Francisco, California, U.S.A. 94141-9100

[b]Department of Physiology and Biochemistry, Medical College of Pennsylvania, Philadelphia, Pennsylvania, U.S.A. 19129

## INTRODUCTION

Apolipoprotein (apo-) E is one of the best-characterized human plasma apolipoproteins with respect to structure-function relationships. It is associated with several classes of plasma lipoproteins, and because of its interaction with the low density lipoprotein (LDL) receptor, apo-E plays an important role in cholesterol and triglyceride metabolism (for review, see Ref. 1). In addition, apo-E binds to the LDL receptor-related protein (LRP) [2], which has been identified as the $\alpha_2$-macroglobulin receptor [3] and which appears to play a role in chylomicron remnant clearance [2, 4]. The high density lipoprotein (HDL) subclass enriched in apo-E (HDL-with apo-E) has been suggested to play a role in the reverse cholesterol transport process [5], particularly in species with low cholesteryl ester transfer activity, such as dogs, rats, and pigs [6].

Apolipoprotein E (299 amino acids, $M_r$=34,200) contains two independently folded domains that are approximated by two thrombolytic fragments (residues 1-191 and 216-299) [7, 8] and are involved in different functions of the protein. The receptor binding function of the protein resides in the amino-terminal, 22-kDa fragment [9]. Although the amino-terminal fragment associates with phospholipid vesicles, forming discoidal complexes [9], the carboxy-terminal, 12-kDa fragment represents the major lipid-binding region of the protein [10, 11]. The region of the 22-kDa fragment that interacts with the LDL receptor has been localized to the vicinity of residues 134 to 150 (for review, see Ref. 1). It has been postulated that the basic residues contained in this region interact with the clusters of acidic residues that are present in the ligand-binding domain of the LDL receptor [12].

Another important characteristic of the amino-terminal fragment of apo-E is its relatively high free energy of stabilization compared with other apolipoproteins and the carboxy-terminal fragment of apo-E [7]. With respect to receptor binding activity, it is interesting to note that phospholipid association is required for apo-E to bind to the LDL receptor with high affinity [13]. These results suggest that apo-E undergoes a conformational change when associated with lipid such that it can interact effectively with the LDL receptor.

Recently, the three-dimensional structure of the lipid-free apo-E 22-kDa receptor-binding fragment has been determined to 2.5-Å resolution by X-ray crystallography [14]. The fragment contains a four-helix bundle in which the helices are arranged in an antiparallel manner. The helices are unusually elongated compared with other proteins with this folding motif. The helices are amphipathic and are arranged such that the hydrophobic faces are directed toward the interior of the bundle. It has been postulated that in apolipoproteins, amphipathic helices are the structures that mediate their interaction with lipids [15, 16].

Determination of the three-dimensional structure of the lipid-free form of the 22-kDa fragment of apo-E represents a major advance in understanding apolipoprotein structure. However, because lipid association is required for high-affinity binding of this fragment to the LDL receptor, a complete understanding of the structure of apo-E will require determining the relationship of the lipid-free and the lipid-associated structures, as well as the effect that lipid association has on the conformation of the protein. Toward this first goal, we examined the surface properties of the 22-kDa fragment of apo-E at an air/water interface. This approach has been used extensively to model the interaction of apolipoproteins with lipid [17-20].

## RESULTS

As shown in Figure 1, the four-helix bundle of the 22-kDa fragment of apo-E can be viewed as a roughly rectangular box in which each helix corresponds to a long edge. As calculated from the crystal structure, the dimensions of the box are approximately $65 \times 20 \times 20$ Å. To determine the organization of the four-helix bundle at an air/water interface, the 22-kDa fragment was spread as a monomolecular film in a Langmuir trough and the surface pressure-molecular area isotherm determined as previously described [20, 21]. The isotherm for apo-A-I was measured for comparison. The molecular areas at the collapse pressures were determined to be ~16 Å$^2$/residue for both the 22-kDa fragment and apo-A-I. The value for apo-A-I is in agreement with that obtained previously by other investigators [17, 18, 22, 23] and is in the range reported for α-helical homopolypeptides (13-19 Å$^2$/residue) [24].

The surface-active behavior of the 22-kDa fragment was examined by measuring the kinetics of its adsorption to the air/water interface. Serum albumin and apo-A-I were included for comparison as examples of a highly water-soluble globular protein and a surface-active apolipoprotein, respectively. As shown in Figure 2, the 22-kDa fragment caused a rapid increase in surface pressure that reached a plateau at approximately 21 dynes/cm within 30 to 40 min. The surface-active apo-A-I also resulted in an increase in surface pressure, with a plateau at approximately the same pressure as the 22-kDa fragment (~21 dynes/cm); however, apo-A-I was slightly slower in exerting its maximal surface pressure than the 22-kDa fragment. In marked contrast, the globular albumin molecule adsorbed relatively slowly and had a 4-fold smaller effect on surface pressure than either the 22-kDa fragment or apo-A-I. These results indicate that the 22-kDa fragment is highly surface-active and that its surface-active properties are comparable to those of apo-A-I.

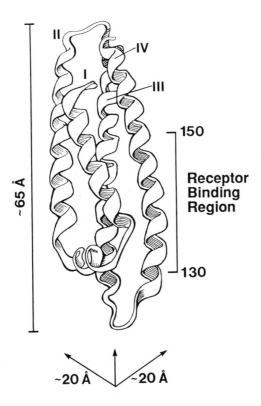

Figure 1. Ribbon model of the 22-kDa fragment of apo-E as determined by X-ray crystallography [14]. The approximate dimensions of the four-helix bundle were determined from the crystal structure.

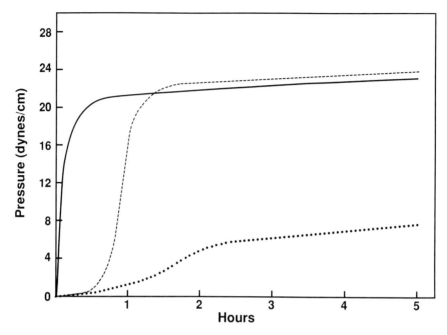

Figure 2. Comparison of the kinetics of adsorption of the 22-kDa fragment of apo-E, apo-A-I, and serum albumin at the air/water interface. Protein was injected into the subphase, and the increases in surface pressure with time were monitored. The time courses are representative of at least two experiments that did not differ significantly. (——), the 22-kDa fragment of apo-E; (- - -), apo-A-I; (· · ·), bovine serum albumin.

## DISCUSSION

The agreement of the limiting molecular areas of apo-A-I and the 22-kDa fragment (approximately $16\text{Å}^2$/residue) indicates that these proteins adopt a similar conformation at an air/water interface. These values are in basic agreement with those for model peptides whose helices lie co-planar with the interface [24]. In previous studies using the air/water interface as a model system for lipid interaction, it has been postulated that the amphipathic helices of apo-A-I and other apolipoproteins lie co-planar with the surface such that the hydrophobic face is directed toward the air and the hydrophilic face is toward the water [23].

A molecular area of $16\text{ Å}^2$/residue implies that one molecule of the 22-kDa fragment (191 residues) occupies an area of approximately $3000\text{ Å}^2$ at the interface surface. This value is consistent with the four-helix bundle undergoing a major rearrangement in structure as it associated with the interface. For example, if the bundle associated with the interface only along a major face without rearrangement, it would occupy only a molecular area of ~1300 Å$^2$ (20 × 65 Å). But if the structure of the bundle underwent a conformational change in interacting with the interface such that the bundle "opened up" or unfolded, it would be predicted to occupy ~2600 Å$^2$ (20 × 130 Å), in closer agreement with what was observed experimentally. Thus, we conclude that the four-helix bundle undergoes a structural reorganization at the interface surface. In this reorganization, the hydrophobic faces of the four helices, which are shielded from the aqueous environment by being sequestered in the interior of the bundle, would be predicted to be oriented toward the air in order to remain in a hydrophobic environment.

Extrapolating these results to a lipid surface, we suggest that the 22-kDa fragment undergoes a similar rearrangement in associating with a phospholipid vesicle to form a discoidal complex. The unfolding of the 22-kDa fragment when binding to phospholipid to form a discoidal complex would be consistent with two known physical measurements of the lipid-free fragment relative to the phospholipid-complexed fragment. First, there is no significant change in the helical content of the 22-kDa fragment when it is complexed to phospholipid [8]. In the case of all other apolipoproteins that have been examined, there is always a significant increase in helical content upon lipid association [16]. Second, there is no shift in the wavelength of tryptophan fluorescence when the fragment associates with lipid [8], indicating that the four trytophan residues (residues 20, 26, 34, and 39), three of which are contained in helix I, are maintained in a hydrophobic environment in both states. If the four-helix bundle simply unfolds at the interface without disruption of the α-helices, the α-helical content of the fragment would remain unchanged. Also, the hydrophobic environment of the tryptophan residues would be maintained in both states, *i.e.*, in the interior of the bundle in the lipid-free state or in proximity to the fatty acyl side chains of the phospholipid in a discoidal complex.

In summary, our determination of the surface properties of the 22-kDa fragment of apo-E indicates that the fragment is highly surface-active and that the four-helix bundle undergoes a major conformational change at an air/water interface. In this structural change, we propose that the bundle unfolds such that the four helices are co-planar with the surface. It is likely that the fragment undergoes a similar change in conformation when the fragment combines with lipid to form a discoidal complex. The results from the present study support the hypothesis that a major change in conformation of the 22-kDa fragment of apo-E occurs at an interface and that this change is likely to contribute to the increase in receptor binding activity that occurs with lipid association.

## ACKNOWLEDGMENTS

The authors wish to thank Sheila Benowitz, Yvonne Newhouse, and Lynne Shinto for excellent technical assistance; Kerry Humphrey for manuscript typing; Tom Rolain and Charles Benedict for graphic arts; and Al Averbach for editorial assistance.

This work was supported in part by National Institutes of Health Grants HL41633 and HL22633.

## REFERENCES

1  Mahley RW. Science 1988; 240: 622-630.
2  Kowal RC, Herz J, Weisgraber KH, Mahley RW, Brown MS, Goldstein JL. J Biol Chem 1990; 265: 10771-10779.
3  Strickland DK, Ashcom JD, Williams S, Burgess WH, Migliorini M, Argraves WS. J Biol Chem 1990; 265: 17401-17404.
4  Hussain MM, Maxfield FR, Más-Oliva J, Tabas I, Ji ZS, Innerarity TL, Mahley RW. J Biol Chem 1991; 266: 13936-13940
5  Mahley RW, Weisgraber KH, Bersot TP, Innerarity TI. In: Gotto Jr AM, Miller NE, Oliver MF, eds. High Density Lipoproteins and Atherosclerosis. Amsterdam: Elsevier/North-Holland Biomedical Press, 1978; 149-176.
6  Tall AR. J Lipid Res 1986; 27: 361-367.
7  Wetterau JR, Aggerbeck LP, Rall Jr SC, Weisgraber KH. J Biol Chem 1988; 263: 6240-6248.
8  Aggerbeck LP, Wetterau JR, Weisgraber KH, Wu CSC, Lindgren FT. J Biol Chem 1988; 263: 6249-6258.
9  Innerarity TL, Friedlander EJ, Rall Jr SC, Weisgraber KH, Mahley RW. J Biol Chem 1983; 258: 12341-12347.
10  Rall Jr SC, Weisgraber KH, Mahley RW. J Biol Chem 1982; 257: 4171-4178.
11  Weisgraber KH. J Lipid Res 1990; 31: 1503-1511.
12  Mahley RW, Innerarity TL, Hui DY, Rall Jr SC, Weisgraber KH. In: Fidge NH, Nestel JP, eds. Atherosclerosis VII. Amsterdam: Elsevier Science Publishers, 1986; 119-123.
13  Innerarity TL, Pitas RE, Mahley RW. J Biol Chem 1979; 254: 4186-4190.
14  Wilson C, Wardell MR, Weisgraber KH, Mahley RW, Agard DA. Science 1991; 252: 1817-1822.
15  Segrest JP, Jackson RL, Morrisett JD, Gotto Jr AM. FEBS Lett 1974; 38: 247-253.
16  Sparrow JT, Gotto Jr AM. CRC Crit Rev Biochem 1982; 13: 87-107.
17  Phillips MC, Sparks CE. Ann NY Acad Sci 1980; 348: 122-137.

18  Shen BW, Scanu AM. Biochemistry 1980; 19: 3643-3650.

19  Camejo G, Muñoz V. In: Day CE, ed. High-Density Lipoproteins. New York: Marcel Dekker Inc, 1981; 131-147.

20  Phillips MC, Krebs KE. Methods Enzymol 1986; 128: 387-403.

21  Phillips MC, Chapman D. Biochim Biophys Acta 1968; 163: 301-313.

22  Yokoyama S, Kawai Y, Tajima S, Yamamoto A. J Biol Chem 1985; 260: 16375-16382.

23  Krebs KE, Ibdah JA, Phillips MC. Biochim Biophys Acta 1988; 959: 229-237.

24  Malcolm BR. Progress in Surface and Membrane Science, Vol. 7. New York: Academic Press, 1973; 183-229.

# Mice lacking apolipoprotein A-I and apolipoprotein E made by gene targeting

## Nobuyo Maeda

Department of Pathology and Curriculum in Genetics,

University of North Carolina at Chapel Hill, Chapel Hill, NC 27599-7525

## Targeted modification of genes in mouse embryonic stem cells

With the use of gene targeting methods, alterations can now be introduced into specific genes in the genome of mice to allow studies of the consequence of the alterations in whole animals.

Homologous recombination between a native target chromosomal gene and exogenous DNA to modify the target locus in a preplanned fashion in cultured mammalian cells was first demonstrated by Smithies et al (1985)[1]. The incoming DNA was designed to contain a region of sequence identity to the target gene to facilitate homologous recombination within the region. The exogenous DNA introduced into the cells was integrated in the target locus.

The other essential element in this gene targeting technology for altering genes in animals was the establishment of mouse embryonic stem cells (ES cells) by Evans and Kaufman (1981)[2]. ES cells are derived from the inner cell mass of mouse blastocysts and can be maintained in culture without differentiation and without losing their pluripotentiality. They can colonize both somatic and germ-cell lineages of chimeric mice following their reintroduction into host blastocysts (Bradley et al., 1984[3]).

The capability of replacing a normal gene with a specifically engineered mutant version by the use of homologous recombination in cultured ES cells able to re-enter the germline has opened a new way to investigate the in vivo function of many interesting genes. This technique is especially valuable when the phenotype to be investigated is so complex that it can only be realized in the whole animal. Making transgenic animals by the use of ES cells having specific pre-determined genotypes has two main advantages over conventional pronuclei injection. First, the genes modified by homologous recombination are present in their own natural chromosomal context, so that any resulting phenotypes are due only to the specific mutation introduced and not to a variable chromosomal location. Second, modification of the gene by homologous recombination can replace the normal gene so that the effects of mutant genes expected to behave in a recessive fashion can be studied.

The gene targeting technique has been applied to various gene systems. It has, for example, assisted in gaining an understandings of the developmental roles played by genes such as oncogenes and homeobox genes

(McMahon and Bradley, 1990[4]; Mucenski et al., 1991[5]; Schwarzberg et al., 1991[6]; Soriano et al., 1991[7]; Chisaka and Capecchi, 1991[8]). It has also increased our knowledge of the immunological importance of molecules such as ß$_2$ microglobulin (Koller et al., 1990[9]; Zijlstra et al., 1990[10]) and interleukin-4 (Kuhn et al., 1991[11]).

## Gene targeting as a means of identifying disease-causing mutations

Current effects in human genome analysis using positional cloning techniques show great promise for allowing scientists to map and identify new genes, or specific mutations in known genes that are involved in human genetic disorders. For some disorders the connection between mutation and phenotype can be obvious, but in many cases the causative nature of a specific mutation may require proof. Gene targeting provides the means to differentiate whether a given mutation is truly causative of the disease condition, or is merely an accidental companion that is linked to the disease-causing gene.

When the disease under study is caused by a single gene defect, elucidation of the genotype/phenotype relationships can be straightforward. However, if the disease is caused by multiple genetic factors, and particularly when it is also strongly influenced by environmental factors, the genotype/phenotype relationships can be very complex. Gene targeting experiments can, nonetheless, still provide an approach to unravelling the complex etiology of the multifactorial disease. Individual candidate genes can be modified, and their isolated effects in the living animal can be determined in controlled environments. Even more powerfully, single gene modifications can be combined by breeding so that eventually the genetics of the multifactorial disease can be deciphered.

## Gene targeting and atherogenesis

In order to obtain a better understanding of the relationships between atherogenesis and genetically controlled molecular variability, my laboratory has been working towards making mice carrying mutations in various lipid metabolism-related genes. We have produced mice lacking apolipoprotein E (Piedrahita et al, 1992[12]), and others lacking apolipoprotein A-I (R. Williamson, D. Lee, J. Hagaman, and N. Maeda; submitted).

## Mice lacking apolipoprotein E

Apolipoprotein E (apoE) is a constituent of very low density lipoprotein (VLDL) and of a subclass of high density lipoproteins (HDL). ApoE mediates high affinity binding of apoE-containing lipoprotein particles to the low density lipoprotein (LDL) receptor and is thus responsible for the cellular uptake of these particles. ApoE is also a major protein constituent of chylomicron remnants. Following transport of dietary cholesterol and triglycerides by chylomicrons, the chylomicron remnants are taken up by the liver by an apoE dependent receptor mediated mechanism (Mahley, 1986[13]). In humans a variant form of apoE that is defective in binding to the LDL receptor is associated with type III hyperlipoproteinemia, characterized by increased plasma triglyceride and cholesterol levels, xanthomas and atherosclerosis. ApoE deficiencies in humans are reported to cause a rare form of type III hyperlipoproteinemia (Ghiselli et al, 1981[14]). Mice lacking apo-E are, therefore, expected to show the similar phenotypes.

## Targeting strategy and gene targeting of the apoE gene

Figure 1 illustrates two targeting plasmids, pJPB69 (b) and pNMC109 (e), used for our experiments. Both plasmids were constructed so that parts of the coding sequences were deleted and replaced with the neomycin phosphotransferase (neo) gene driven by a thymidine kinase promoter and a mutated polyoma enhancer (pMCneopolA, Thomas and Capecchi, 1987[15]). The neo gene confers G418 resistance on cells that have incorporated the targeting plasmids into their genomes.

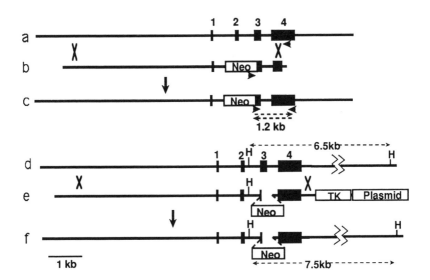

Figure 1. Strategy for targeting the mouse apoE gene. a,d; endogenous mouse apoE locus, b; targeting fragment of pJPB69, e; linealized targeting plasmid pNMC109, c,f; The apoE locus after homologous recombination. Arrow heads indicate the locations of PCR primers. H, HindIII site.

The pJPB69 (Figure 1b) contained 4.9 kb of uninterrupted sequence in the 5' region, and 700bp in the 3' region to facilitate the homologous recombination. Two primers (one specific to the neo gene in the targeting DNA, and the other specific to genomic sequences 3' to the apoE gene that are not included in the targeting DNA) were designed for use with the polymerase chain reaction (PCR) in screening for cells in which homologous recombination has occurred at the apo-E locus (Kim and Smithies, 1988[16]).

The second plasmid, pNMC109 (Fig. 1e), was designed so as to be able to use positive-negative selection (Mansour et al., 1988[17]). For this purpose, a copy of the herpes simplex virus thymidine kinase (TK) gene was placed at the 3' end of the construct. This allows enrichment of the targeted cells by ganciclovir selection, which kills cells expressing the TK gene. Because homologous recombination eliminates nonhomologous sequences (including the TK gene) that are outside of the region of homology, cells correctly targeted will not be killed by the ganciclovir. The plasmid contained 6.4 kb and 1.2 kb of uninterrupted sequences in the 5' and 3' regions.

Mouse ES cells (E14T2a, Hooper et al., 1987[18]) were electroporated with linearized DNA, and selected with G418 only, or with G418 and ganciclovir, for approximately 12 days. PCR analysis of G418-resistant cells obtained after treatment with pJPB69 was carried out in pools containing 4 or 6 colonies. Six of 128 pools analyzed gave a positive PCR signal as judged by amplification of the 1.2 kb fragment diagnostic of the targeted locus (Fig. 1c). From these six pools, four individuals clones were isolated, and the occurrence of the targeted disruption of the apoE gene was confirmed by Southern blot analysis. The overall frequency of finding the targeted cells in G418 resistant cells from in these four experiments was 0.07% (5/648).

In the experiments using pNMC109, the occurrence of targeting was investigated directly by Southern blot analysis of HindIII digests of DNA isolated from colonies doubly resistant to G418 and ganciclovir. An unmodified apoE locus will yield a 6.5kb HindIII fragment after hybridization to an apoE probe. If homologous recombination takes place between the endogenous apoE locus and the plasmid pNMC109, the size of the HindIII fragment hybridizing to the apoE probe will be increases by 1.0 kb (see Fig. 1f). Thus the presence of a 7.5 kb band in the Southern blot analysis can be used to diagnose homologous recombination. In this way, we identified 39 targeted colonies, at a combined frequency of targeting of 22% of the doubly resistant colonies (39/177 analyzed). The overall targeting frequencies at the mouse apoE locus using pJPB69 and pNMC109 are respectively 2.6 and 10 in $10^7$ treated cells.

## Production of chimeras and germline transmission of the modified apoE gene

Six different ES cell lines targeted at the apoE locus were tested for the production of chimeras after injection into C57BL/6J blastocysts. Average 50 embryos were used to test each line, and all six generated chimeras. The degree of chimerism, as determined by coat color, ranged from very weak (less than 10% of the coat corresponding to the ES cells) to very strong (greater than 80 %). One male chimera transmitted the ES cell genome to 100 % of his offspring. Southern blots of tail DNA from his pups revealed that 14 of 30 pups had inherited the disrupted copy of the apoE gene.

## Mice homozygous for the disrupted apoE gene

By mating animals heterozygous for the disrupted apoE gene, we have obtained animals homozygous for the modified apoE locus, as identified by Southern blot of their tail DNAs. Ouchterlony double immunodiffusion using a rabbit anti-rat apoE antiserum showed that plasma samples from animals that are homozygous for the modified apoE gene gave no detectable immunoprecipitate with anti-apoE antibody, although precipitation is clearly visible with plasma from animals heterozygous or homozygous for the normal gene. This establishes at the protein level that we have succeeded in generating mice that lack apoE protein. Preliminary analysis of the plasma lipoproteins shows (S. Zhang, J. Piedrahita and N. Maeda, unpublished data) a marked increase of total plasma cholesterol levels in the homozygous animals; the levels are approximately 4 to 5 fold normal. In contrast to human type III hyperlipoproteinemia, however, triglycerides were not significantly increased in plasma of homozygous mutants fasted overnight. The lipoprotein levels in plasma of animals heterozygous for the disrupted gene were similar to normal. Heterozygous and homozygous mutants appear healthy at age 6 and 4 months, respectively.

## Mice lacking apolipoprotein A-I

Apolipoprotein A-I (apoA-I) is the major protein component of HDL particles, elevated levels of which are inversely correlated with the risk of coronary atherosclerosis in humans (Gordon & Rifkind, 1989[19]). Several cases of mutations in the apoA-I gene in humans have been characterized, and individuals deficient in apoA-I appear to show premature coronary heart diseases (reviewed by Breslow, 1989[20]). The importance of apoA-I in atherogenesis has also been demonstrated by the protective effects against high dietary lipids afforded by apoA-I overexpression in transgenic mice (Rubin et al, 1991[20]), which leads to as much as three fold higher levels of total and HDL cholesterol (Rubin et al, 1991[21]; Walsh et al, 1989[22]). Mice having their apoA-I gene inactivated by gene targeting are, therefore expected to have reduced levels of HDL cholesterol, and may have an increased susceptibility to atherosclerosis.

188

## Targeted disruption of the mouse apoA-I gene

A positive/negative selection strategy was used in the experiments with the apoA-I gene as illustrated in Figure 2. The targeting DNA contains a neo gene, which replaces exon 2 of the apoA-I gene, together with 3 kb and 5.5 kb of uninterrupted mouse genomic sequences in the 5' and 3' regions. The TK gene was placed either at the 5' or 3' end of the construct.

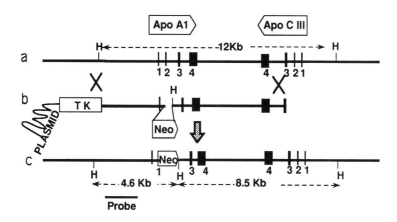

Figure 2. Strategy for targeting the mouse apoA-I gene. a; endogeous apoA-I and apoC-III loci, b; targeting construct, c: a correctly targeted locus. H; HindIII sites.

DNA was linearized and introduced into ES cells by electroporation. DNA samples from ES cell colonies resistant to G418 and ganciclovir were assayed for targeting by Southern blotting. The presence of the 4.6 kb HindIII band in the target locus compared to 12kb of the endogenous apoA-I locus was used for initial diagnosis (Figure 2). The frequency of targeting the mouse apoA-I locus was very high, ranging from 46% to 82% of the colonies that survived double selection. The overall frequency of targeting the apoA-I gene in mouse ES cells was 1 in $10^5$ of the treated cells, about ten times the best seen with the apoE gene.

## Generation of mice homozygous for the mutated apoA-I gene

When injected into blastocysts, the targeted cell lines varied in the extent of chimerism that they produced in the resulting offspring, as was the case in the apoE modified cells described above. Two of nine lines injected have produced four germline- competent chimeras that transmit the inactivated apoA-I gene to their offspring.

Animals homozygous for the modified apoA-I gene were generated from matings of heterozygotes. The homozygotes lack apoA-I protein in their plasma, as judged by Ouchterlony double immunodiffusion tests against rabbit anti-mouse apoA-I antiserum. At the lipid level, we find that the total cholesterol in the plasma from homozygous mutants at 8 weeks of age is approximately one third that of normal animals. HDL cholesterol is reduced to an even greater extent, to 17% of normal. Total cholesterol and HDL cholesterol levels are also reduced to 54% and 40% respectively of the levels in normal animals. Both the heterozygous and homozygous mutants appear healthy at 5 and 3 months respectively.

## Conclusions

We have used gene targeting to produce mice lacking apoE and apoA-I. The fact that the homozygous animals have been born at the expected frequency, and that they appear healthy is important. It demonstrates that lack of these proteins is compatible with normal development, and the survival of the animals provides new tools for studying the roles of these proteins in lipid metabolism and in atherogenesis. As described above, mice homozygous for the inactivated apoE gene have four to five fold elevated plasma cholesterol levels, while those homozygous for the inactivated apoA-I gene have HDL cholesterol levels reduced to one fifth of normal. Considering the importance of these proteins, as suggested by the phenotypes of the rare cases of human individuals deficient in them, it will be of great interest to determine whether the mouse mutants will develop atherosclerosis spontaneously as they age. Their response to atherogenic diets will be equally interesting.

We anticipate that both the inactivated apoA-I gene and the inactivated apoE gene will have different effects in different genetic backgrounds. Currently we are backcrossing the mutant animals to normal C57BL/6J animals so that we can study the effects of the mutations in the C57BL/6J background, which itself is associated with some susceptibility to dietary-induced atherosclerosis (Paigen et al., 1985[23]). We have also commenced breeding the animals carrying the null apoA-I allele to mice carrying the null apoE allele. Combination of these two defects should greatly increase the likelihood that animals will be obtained that develop atherosclerosis spontaneously, even when fed a normal diet.

Three other sets of experiments aimed at generating mice carrying an inactivated hepatic lipase gene, an inactivated apolipoprotein CIII gene, and a modified apolipoprotein B gene are also in progress in my laboratory (G. Homanics, T. Smith and N. Maeda, unpublished work). Studies of the effects of combining five different mutations each with some atherogenic potential will therefore be possible in the near future. We hope, in this way, to be able to decipher the complex multifactorial genetics that determine individual risks of developing atherosclerosis.

190

## Acknowledgements

The author thanks to Dr. Jorge Piedrahita, Dr. Roger Williamson, and Ms. Sunny Zhang for their hard work in carrying out the gene targeting experiments, Ms. Denise Lee for assistance in tissue culture, Mr. John Hagaman and Ms. Paula Oliver for embryo manipulations, and Dr. Oliver Smithies for continuous encouragement. This work was supported by an NIH grant, HL42630.

## References

1. Smithies O, Gregg RG, Boggs SS, Koralewski MA, Kucherlapati RS. Nature 1985;317:230-234.
2. Evans MJ, Kaufman MH. Nature 1981;292:154-156.
3. Bradley AK, Evans M, Kaufman MH, Robertson E. Nature 1984;309:255-256.
4. McMahon AP, Bradley A. Cell 1990;62:1073-1085.
5. Mucenski ML, McLain K, Kier AB, Swerdlow SH, Schreiner CM, Miller TA, Pietryga DW, Scott WJ Jr, Potter SS. Cell 1991;65:677-689.
6. Schwarzberg PL, Stall AM, Hardin JD, Bowdish KS, Humaran T, Boast S, Harbison ML, Robertson EJ, Goff SP. Cell 1991;65:1165-1175.
7. Soriano P, Montgomery C, Geske R, Bradley A. Cell 1991;64:693-702.
8. Chisaka O, Capecchi MR. Nature 1991;350:473-479.
9. Koller BH, Marrack P, Kappler JW, Smithies O. Science 1990;248:1227-1230.
10. Zijlstra M, Bix M, Simister NE, Loring JM, Raulet DH, Jaenish R. Nature 1990;344:709-711.
11. Kühn R, Rajewsky WP, Müller W. Science 1991;254:707-710.
12. Piedrahita J, Zhang SH, Hagaman JR, Oliver P, Maeda N. Proc Natl Acad Sci USA (in press).
13. Mahley RW. Clin Inves Med 1986;9:304-308.
14. Ghiselli GE, Schaefer EJ, Gascon P, Brewer HB. Science 1981;214:1239-1241.
15. Thomas KR, Capecchi MR. Cell 1987;51:503-512.
16. Kim H-S, Smithies O. Nucl Acids Res 1988;16:8887-8903.
17. Mansour SL, Thomas KR, Capecchi MR. Nature 1988;336:348-352.
18. Hooper M, Hardy K, Handyside A, Hunter S, Monk M. Nature 1987;326:292-295.
19. Gordon DJ, Rifkind BM. N Eng J Med 1989;321:1311-1316.
20. Breslow JL. In: Scriver CR, Beaudet AL, Sly WS, Valle D, eds. The metabolic basis of inherited diseases. New York:McGraw-Hill, 1989;1251-1266.
21. Rubin EM, Krauss RM, Spangler EA, Verstuyft JG, Clift SM. Nature 1991;353:256-267.
22. Walsh A, Ito Y, Breslow JL. J Biol Chem 246;1989:6488-6494.
23. Paigen B, Morrow A, Brandon C, Michell C, Homes P. Atherosclerosis 1985;57:65-73.

High density lipoproteins and atherosclerosis III.
N.E. Miller and A.R. Tall, editors.

# IS CHOLESTEROL EFFLUX FROM TISSUES REGULATED BY LIPOLYSIS OF TRIGLYCERIDE-RICH LIPOPROTEINS?

NORMAN E. MILLER

Department of Internal Medicine, Bowman Gray School of Medicine, Winston-Salem, North Carolina, U.S.A.

## INTRODUCTION

Fractionation of plasma high density lipoproteins (HDL) by immunochemical procedures has revealed that there are two major apolipoprotein AI-containing subclasses: one which also contains apo AII (LpAI w AII) and another which does not contain apo AII (LpAI w/o AII) [1,2]. The latter fraction is of particular interest, as a reduction in its concentration appears to underly the low plasma total apo AI concentration present in many coronary heart disease victims [3].

The LpAI w/o AII fraction also contains the primary acceptors of cell membrane cholesterol when cultured fibroblasts or adipocytes are exposed to plasma lipoproteins [4,5]. These particles are members of a quantitatively minor subclass, which differs from the majority of LpAI w/o AII in having pre-ß mobility on electrophoresis, and they have been termed preß₁LpAI [5]. They contain only one molecule of apo AI, are rich in phospholipid, and contain little or no core lipid (i.e., cholesteryl ester, CE, or triglyceride, TG [5-7]). In most humans the total preßLpAI class accounts for 1-10% of plasma apo AI [5-9], while the preß₁ subclass comprises on average about 2% [5]. Total preßLpAI concentration is negatively correlated with plasma lecithin: cholesterol acyltransferase (LCAT) activity [9], and is increased in various forms of hyperlipidemia [7-9], in familial LCAT deficiency [7], and (in mice and dogs) by a diet rich in saturated fat and cholesterol [10,11]. They are present in human tissue fluids, including those of the artery wall [10,12-14].

As the preß₁LpAI are the smallest apo AI-containing particles [5,10,12], it is likely that they cross vascular endothelia more readily, and have a larger volume of distribution in the extracellular matrix, than do other HDL. These properties, combined with their avidity for cell membrane cholesterol, make it likely that the preß₁LpAI function as the principal acceptors of cell-derived cholesterol in tissue fluids. Accordingly, there is the possibility that the rate of their delivery to peripheral cells may significantly influence the efficiency of reverse cholesterol transport.

## ORIGINS OF PRE-BETA₁ LpAI PARTICLES

Current evidence suggests that these particles may be produced by two types of process: synthesis in hepatocytes, and remodeling of other HDL in plasma and/or tissue fluids.

Table 1
PUTATIVE MECHANISMS OF PRE-BETA$_1$ LpAI PRODUCTION

---

A. Synthesis in hepatocytes
B. Remodeling of HDL:
    (i)     Hydrolysis of HDL-PL in tissue fluids
    (ii)    Transfer of PL from cells to HDL in tissue fluids
    (iii)   Fusion of HDL particles in presence of LCAT
    (iv)   Hydrolysis of HDL-TG by HL
    (v)    Transfer of PL from TG-rich lipoproteins to HDL during lipolysis

---

PL, phospholipid: HL, hepatic endothelial lipase. See text for details and references.

Evidence for production by hepatocytes has been provided by studies of cultured human Hep G2 hepatoma cells [15] and cultured monkey hepatocytes [16], although the possibility that they are produced by interaction of other HDL with HL and/or LCAT in the culture medium has not been excluded. Proposed mechanisms of HDL remodeling to release small apo AI-phospholipid particles include hydrolysis of HDL phospholipid in tissue fluids [13,17]; fusion of HDL particles under the influence of LCAT [18]; and the creation of a surplus of surface phospholipid on HDL, as a consequence either of the hydrolysis of HDL triglyceride by HL [19-21] or of the transfer of phospholipid to HDL from cells or triglyceride-rich lipoproteins (TGRLs) [22-26].

## HEPARIN-RELEASABLE LIPASES AND PRE-BETA$_1$ LpAI

The possibility that one or both of the two heparin-releasable endothelial-bound lipases, lipoprotein lipase (LPL) and HL, play important roles in preß$_1$LpAI production from larger HDL in humans is suggested by the increases in the concentration of preß-migrating apo AI [8,9], and in the number of small spherical lipoprotein particles [22], that have been seen in plasma collected after induction of intravascular lipolysis by i.v. heparin. A similar increase in preßLpAI concentration occurred during incubation of human post-heparin plasma *in vitro* [9]. On the basis of their studies with purified HL *in vitro*, Barter and co-workers [19-21] suggested that hydrolysis of HDL core triglyceride (transferred to HDL from TGRLs in exchange for CE) by HL leads to a reduction in particle size and consequent dissociation of redundant surface phospholipid in combination with apo AI. Neary et al [9] found that triglyceride lipase from Pseudomonas also increased the preßLpAI concentration when added to HDL *in vitro*. Both groups felt that hydrolysis of HDL phospholipid by HL is unlikely to play a role, as incubation of HDL with other phospholipases (A$_2$ or C) *in vitro* appeared not to have a similar effect [9,27,28]. These results do not necessarily conflict with those of Gebhardt et al [13,17], as the substrate HDL for phospholipases in tissue fluids may differ from those in plasma.

The interpretation of the foregoing results from *in vitro* experiments is complicated by possible effects of product accumulation (e.g., fatty acids, lysolecithin), decreases in substrate concentrations, and absence of the normal synthesis and catabolism of lipoproteins and their components that occur *in vitro*.

## LIPOPROTEIN LIPASE AND PERIPHERAL PRE-BETA$_1$ LpAI PRODUCTION

Clearly a mechanism of preß$_1$LpAI production that requires both CE/TG transfer protein activity and HL cannot operate efficiently in species that are deficient in one or the other (e.g., rats, rabbits). Presumably, therefore, alternative mechanisms are possible. Studies by Lefevre et al [29] have shown that the concentration of preßLpAI in canine peripheral lymph normally exceeds that in plasma, indicating that a peripheral mechanism must exist in dogs, either in tissue fluids or at the blood-endothelium interface. Nichols et al [18] proposed that fusion of HDL particles, under the influence of LCAT, may be important. Other studies [23,24] have documented the dissociation from bovine and human HDL of small particles, composed of one molecule of apo AI in association with phospholipid, during incubation of HDL with dimyristoylphosphatidylcholine. At the same time large square-packing HDL were also formed (24). As square-packing HDL are present in human lymphedema fluid, it was suggested that a similar process occurs in tissue fluids, as a result of the transfer of phospholipid from cells to filtered plasma HDL.

Substantial amounts of phospholipid are transferred to HDL during lipolysis of TGRLs [30,31]. Tall and Small [25] discussed the physical chemistry of this process, and pointed out that one consequence might be dissociation of apo AI from the HDL surface. If this does indeed occur, it might provide a mechanism whereby reverse cholesterol transport is driven by the catabolism of TGRLs, the principal source of cholesterol-rich particles destined for receptor-mediated uptake by cells (Figure 1). Such a mechanism has theoretical appeal, as it would presumably generate cholesterol-acceptor particles where and when they are most needed: on site in those peripheral tissues with high LPL activity.

Several lines of evidence accord with this concept. First, phase diagram analysis of the lipid compositions of the cores and surface monolayers of TGRLs by Miller and Small [32] suggested that lipolysis is accompanied by an influx of unesterified cholesterol (UC), which is ultimately recovered in HDL. Second, if apo AI is normally catabolized principally as a component or HDL-with apo E [33], it offers an explanation for the associations of apo AI fractional catabolic rate (FCR) with VLDL apoB FCR and LPL activity [34-36]. Third, diets rich in fat raised plasma preßLpAI concentration in dogs [29] and mice [11]. Fourth, Neary et al [9] found that the increase in preßLpAI after intravenous heparin was augmented postprandially and in endogenous hypertriglyceridemia. It is also noteworthy that Castro and Fielding [37] found that the net rate of transport of cholesterol from cultured fibroblasts was greater when the cells were exposed to postprandial, rather than to fasting, plasma, though the mechanism favored by the authors was a decrease in the UC/phospholipid ratio of non-HDL lipoproteins.

194

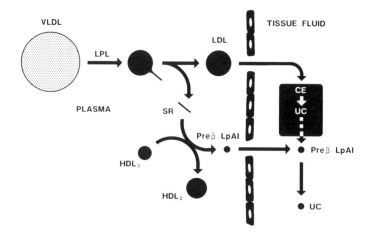

Figure 1.

Putative mechanism by which lipolysis of triglyceride-rich lipoproteins may generate preßLpAI particles, and thereby facilitate reverse cholesterol transport. LPL, lipoprotein lipase; UC, unesterified cholesterol; CE, cholesteryl ester; SR, surface remnants.

## LIPOPROTEIN LIPASE AND HDL CHOLESTEROL PRODUCTION IN MUSCLE

Support for the concept was also provided by the results of a recent study by Kiens and Lithell [38], who measured arterio-venous differences in plasma lipoprotein lipid concentrations across the knee extensor muscles in humans. At rest trained muscles hydrolyzed 15% of VLDL-TG in a single pass. In the same subjects arterial VLDL-cholesterol averaged 186 $\mu$mol/l, of which about 30% (56 $\mu$mol/l) would have been UC [39]. As Chajek and Eisenberg [31] have shown that 15% hydrolysis of VLDL-TG by LPL in the perfused rat heart leads to the transfer of about 8% of VLDL-UC to HDL, lipolysis would have increased HDL cholesterol on average by about 5 $\mu$mol/l in the subjects studied by Kiens and Lithell. However, the actual increase which occurred was 55 $\mu$mol/l, the residual 50 $\mu$mol/l presumably reflecting cholesterol transport from muscle and other cells.

The same study showed that the rate of HDL cholesterol production in exercising muscle was linearly related to the rate of VLDL-TG degradation. However, the slope of the regression line relating the two variables was about 0.9, when on the basis of the foregoing considerations a slope of only 0.1 would be expected if lipolysis were the only contributing factor. It appears, therefore, that the contribution of tissue cholesterol to the arterio-venous increment in HDL cholesterol across the muscles increased with increasing LPL activity. As no arterio-venous difference in LDL cholesterol was detected, this presumably was not a passive consequence of increased cholesterol influx into muscle tissue, but of increased efficiency of reverse cholesterol transport.

In recent studies we have tested the lipolysis-preßLpAI-cholesterol efflux hypothesis in two experimental systems. In rabbits, a species which under normal dietary conditions is deficient in HL [40], the effect on the transfer of cholesterol from peripheral cells to plasma of acutely stimulating lipolysis with intravenous heparin was studied [41]. In humans with low HDL cholesterol levels, the long-term effects of treatment with gemfibrozil, a drug known to raise LPL activity [42,43], on apo AI and cholesterol concentrations in peripheral lymph were investigated [44].

## EFFECT OF HEPARIN-INDUCED LIPOLYSIS OF TRIGLYCERIDE-RICH LIPOPROTEINS ON TISSUE CHOLESTEROL EFFLUX IN RABBITS

Non-fasted New Zealand White rabbits (n=28), maintained on laboratory chow, were infused intravenously with 0.5-1.0 mCi of [³H]cholesterol to label tissue cholesterol pools. Several weeks later (mean, 69 d) each was given 1000 units of bovine lung heparin intravenously. Blood samples were collected at timed intervals from an ear vein, and HDL cholesterol mass and radioactivity were quantified after chemical precipitation of apoB-containing lipoproteins. Induction of lipolysis of TGRLs was evidenced by rapid decreases in plasma triglycerides. Plasma HDL cholesterol concentration increased, reaching a peak value of 120-160% of baseline after 12-24 h. This was associated with increases in the specific radioactivities of HDL cholesterol, and to a lesser extent, of plasma total cholesterol.

## EFFECTS OF GEMFIBROZIL ON CONCENTRATIONS OF APO AI AND CHOLESTEROL IN HUMAN PERIPHERAL LYMPH

If lipolysis of TGRLs leads indirectly to dissociation of apo AI from plasma HDL at the blood-endothelium interface, and in consequence to increased transfer of apo AI from plasma to tissue fluids, apo AI concentration in peripheral lymph would be expected to be increased by a drug that raises LPL activity. This was tested in men with hyperlipidemia and HDL cholesterol levels below 35 mg/dl. Lymph was collected for 3-5 h by cannulation of a lymph trunk in the dorsum of the foot. Apo AI was measured by immunoelectrophoresis against a polyclonal antiserum. Two cannulations were performed, off and on gemfibrozil treatment, separated by an interval of six or more weeks. In preliminary unpublished data from three men, gemfibrozil increased both plasma and lymph apo AI concentrations. In each subject the increase in lymph apo AI was proportionately much greater than that in plasma apo AI, producing a rise in the lymph/plasma ratio. These changes were associated with a rise in lymph cholesterol, in spite of a decrease in plasma cholesterol concentration.

DISCUSSION

The results of our two studies strengthen the hypothesis that the catabolism of TGRLs increases apo AI dissociation from HDL, and in consequence cholesterol efflux from peripheral cells.

As apo AI is not synthesized in human peripheral cells, the increase in lymph/plasma apo AI ratio observed during gemfibrozil must have reflected an increase in the rate of net transfer of apo AI from plasma to tissue fluids, a reduced rate of movement in the opposite direction, or a decrease in the volume of distribution of apo AI in tissue fluids. The rise in lymph cholesterol concentration in the presence of a reduction of plasma cholesterol is noteworthy, as plasma and lymph cholesterol are normally positively correlated, and is consistent with an increase in the rate of cholesterol efflux from tissues. However, it could also have reflected an increased rate of transfer of cholesterol-rich lipoproteins from plasma to tissue fluids or a decrease in the distribution volume of lipoproteins in the extracellular matrix. Pending studies of the effects of gemfibrozil on apo AI and cholesterol kinetics in human plasma and peripheral lymph, it is not yet possible to distinguish between these possibilities.

In the rabbit experiments the early part of the rise in HDL cholesterol concentration can be attributed to the well documented [30,31] transfer of surface material from lipolyzed TGRLs to HDL. However, the continued slower rise for a further 10-20 h cannot readily be explained on this basis. The accompanying increase in cholesterol specific radioactivity was compatible with augmented mobilization of cholesterol of high specific radioactivity from peripheral tissues into HDL. Theoretically, this effect on specific radioactivity could also have reflected an increased rate of bi-directional exchange of UC between HDL and the plasma membranes of cells, without net transfer of cholesterol mass. However, an increase in cholesterol mobilization is considered to be the more likely, as kinetic studies have indicated that the UC in plasma membranes belongs largely to the same pool as that in plasma [26].

REFERENCES

1.  Koren E, Puchois P, Alaupovic P, et al. Clin Chem 1987;33:38-43.
2.  Cheung MC, Albers JJ. J Biol Chem 1984;259:12201-12209.
3.  Puchois P, Kandoussi A, Fievet P, et al. Atherosclerosis 1987;68:35-40.
4.  Barbaras R, Puchois P, Fruchart J-C, Ailhaud G. Biochem Biophys Res Commun 1987;142:63-69.
5.  Castro GR, Fielding CJ. Biochemistry 1988;27:25-29.
6.  Kunitake ST, La Sala KJ, Kane JP. J Lipid Res 1985;26:549-555.
7.  Ishida BY, Frolich J, Fielding CJ. J Lipid Res 1987;28:778-786.
8.  Daerr WH, Minzlaff U, Greten H. Biochim Biophys Acta 1986;879:134-139.
9.  Neary R, Bhatnagar D, Durrington P, et al. Atherosclerosis 1991;89:35-48.
10. LeFevre M, Sloop CH, Roheim PS. J Lipid Res 1988;29:1139-1148.
11. Ishida BY, Albee D, Paigen B. J lipid Res 1990;31:227-236.

12. Reichl D, Sterchi JM, Miller, NE. Eur J Clin Invest. (In Press)
13. Gebhardt DOE, Beintema A, Reman FC, Van Gent CM. Clin Chim Acta 1979;94:93-100.
14. Smith EB, Ashall C, Walker JE. Biochem Soc Trans 1984;12:843-844.
15. McCall MR, Forte TM, Shiere VG. J Lipid Res 1988;29:1127-1137.
16. Castle CK, Pape ME, Marotti KR, Melchior GW. J Lipid Res 1991;32:439-447.
17. Gebhardt DOE, Hogeweg M, Post M. Exp Eye Res 1983;36:381-388.
18. Nichols AV, Gong EL, Blanche PJ, et al. J Lipid Res 1987;28:719-732.
19. Hopkins GJ, Chang LBF, Barter PJ. J Lipid Res 1985; 26:218-229.
20. Hopkins GJ, Barter PJ. J Lipid Res 1986;27:1265-1277.
21. Clay MA, Newnham HH, Barter PJ. Arteriosclerosis 1991;11:415-422.
22. Forte TM, Krauss RM, Lindgren FT, et al. Proc Natl Acad Sci U.S.A. 1979;76:5934-5938.
23. Nichols AV, Gong EL, Forte TM, et al. Lipids 1978;13:943-950.
24. Forte TM, Ren CL, Nordhausen RW, et al. Biochim Biophys Acta 1985;834:386-395.
25. Tall AR, Small DS. N Engl J Med 1978;299:1232-1236.
26. Reichl D, Miller NE. Arteriosclerosis 1989;9:785-797.
27. Newnham HH, Hopkins GJ, Devlin S, et al. Atherosclerosis 1990;82:167-176.
28. Perret BP, Chollet F, Durand S, et al. Eur J Biochem 1987;62:279-286.
29. Le Fevre M, Sloop CH, Roheim PS. J Lipid Res 1988;29:1139-1148.
30. Redgrave TG, Small DM. J Clin Invest 1979;64:162-171.
31. Chajek T, Eisenberg S. J Clin Invest 1978;61:1654-1665.
32. Miller KW, Small DM. J Clin Invest 1983;258:13772-13784.
33. Sherill BC, Innerarity TL, Mahley RW. J Biol Chem 1982;255:11442-11447.
34. Magill P, Rao SN, Miller NE, et al. Eur J Clin Invest 1982;12:113-120.
35. Brinton EA, Eisenberg S, Breslow JL. J Clin Invest 1989;84:262-269.
36. Goldberg IJ, Blaner WS, Vanni TM, et al. J Clin Invest 1990;86:463-473.
37. Castro GR, Fielding CJ. J Clin Invest 1985;75:874-882.
38. Kiens B, Lithell H. J Clin Invest 1989;83:558-564.
39. Sata T, Havel RJ, Jones AL. J Clin Invest 1972;13:757-768.
40. Clay MA, Hopkins GJ, Ehnholm CP, et al. Biochim Biophys Acta 1989;1002:173-181.
41. Miller NE, Nanjee MN. FEBS Lett 1991;285:132-134.
42. Nikkila EA, Ylikahri R, Huttunen JK. Proc R Soc Med 1976;69(Suppl 2):58-63.
43. Saker K, Gartside PS, Hynd BA, et al. J Clin Invest 1985;75:1702-1712.
44. Reichl D, Sterchi JM, Miller NE. In preparation.

Interstitial Fluid Lipoprotein Metabolism

P.S. Roheim, B.F. Asztalos, M. Lefevre, C.H. Sloop and L. Wong


Division of Lipoprotein Metabolism and Pathophysiology, Department of Physiology, Louisiana State University Medical Center, 1542 Tulane Avenue, New Orleans, LA 70112 USA

ABSTRACT
We have studied interstitial fluid lipoprotein composition and metabolism using dog prenodal peripheral lymph, an acceptable model of interstitial fluid. We have observed changes in lipid and apolipoprotein composition, as well as biological characteristics of interstitial fluid. Changes of chemical composition are responsible for functional differences between plasma and interstitial fluid high density lipoproteins (HDL). In agreement with the literature, plasma HDL produced free cholesterol efflux from cells in contrast to interstitial fluid HDL which donated free cholesterol to cells in tissue culture. Two-dimensional electrophoresis studies of apoA-I-containing HDL subpopulations in plasma and interstitial fluid have revealed lipoproteins with faster electrophoretic mobilities than albumin (preα).
These preα particles have not been recognized previously. In the interstitial fluid, a major change of HDL subpopulations takes place. The predominant particles in interstitial fluid have preα and preβ mobilities, while the majority of plasma HDL have α mobility. It is postulated that as a result of these changes in subpopulations of interstitial fluid, the filtered plasma HDL will be converted from cholesterol acceptor to cholesterol donor.

INTRODUCTION
We have to consider the anatomical compartmentalization of lipoprotein metabolism. In the first compartment are the organs where synthesis and secretion, as well as uptake and catabolism of lipoproteins take place, i.e. liver and intestine. The second compartment represents the intravascular space, where remodeling of lipoproteins occurs. The third compartment is the interstitial space where lipoproteins interact with peripheral cells initiating reverse cholesterol transport.

It is necessary to recognize that interstitial fluid, and not plasma, is the media which is in direct contact with the peripheral cells. In order to understand the early events in reverse cholesterol transport, information on the composition and biological characteristics of interstitial fluid is necessary.

When we compare the composition of interstitial fluid with plasma, we must consider the different factors which influence interstitial fluid composition.

Interstitial fluid lipoprotein composition is influenced by:

• The composition of plasma lipoproteins

• Efficiency of lipoprotein transport (filtration and diffusion) across the capillary

• Interaction of filtered lipoproteins with -

  a) the capillary wall

  b) interstitial space matrix

  c) peripheral cells

All of these factors establish the final composition and metabolic behavior of interstitial fluid lipoproteins.

### RESULTS AND DISCUSSION
One can only obtain interstitial fluid by micropuncture, which does not provide enough material for chemical analysis and/or metabolic studies. Therefore, we use another method to obtain interstitial fluid - dog prenodal peripheral lymph [1]. Lipoproteins in the peripheral lymph are the end products of the interaction of plasma lipoproteins with peripheral cells just before reentry into the general circulation.

Since high density lipoproteins (HDL) are the key lipoproteins in reverse cholesterol transport, we concentrated our studies on the characteristics of these lipoproteins in the interstitial fluid.

Table I summarizes the major findings of our previous studies [1]:

TABLE I
Summary of Previous Studies

| |
|---|
| • Interstitial fluid HDL is enriched in free cholesterol |
| • Interstitial fluid contains nascent lipoproteins rich in apoE and apoA-IV |
| • Interstitial fluid is enriched in lipid poor (preβ) apoA-I |
| • Interstitial fluid HDL is structurally modified |
| • Interstitial fluid HDL is a poor substrate for LCAT |

Based on changes in chemical composition of interstitial fluid, we postulated that the functional characteristics of interstitial fluid HDL would be different from plasma HDL. To test this hypothesis, we measured the ability of interstitial fluid and plasma HDL to influence the flux of cholesterol from peripheral cells.

We first used the bidirectional flux measurement of radiolabeled cholesterol as described by Johnson *et al*. [2], to compare *in vitro* cholesterol flux between the cells and the media. In this system, one simultaneously measures the rate constant for the movement of radiolabeled HDL cholesterol to cells, i.e., cholesterol influx, and the movement of cellular cholesterol to HDL, i.e., cholesterol efflux. We observed that incubation of normal fibroblasts or macrophages with plasma HDL results in a net efflux of cholesterol from peripheral cells to media. In contrast, incubation of interstitial fluid HDL causes a net movement of cholesterol from the media to the cells.

We also measured the change in free cholesterol mass in the media during incubation of fibroblasts with plasma or interstitial fluid HDL. The findings from these studies were consistent with the kinetic data. We found a decrease in media free cholesterol content in incubation with interstitial fluid HDL, while there was an increase of free cholesterol concentration in incubation with plasma HDL.

In an effort to understand those factors responsible for determining the direction of net cholesterol flux between cells and HDL, we plotted net cholesterol flux for each pair of plasma and peripheral lymph samples versus either the free cholesterol/apoA-I ratio (FC/AI) or the free cholesterol/phospholipid ratio (FC/PL).

Our data showed that the change in the FC/PL ratio of the lipoprotein particle is an important determinant for the direction of net cholesterol flux and is consistent with the data in the literature [3]. In contrast, the FC/AI ratio did not influence cholesterol flux.

Our results demonstrate that a remodeling of plasma HDL takes place during the passage through the capillary wall and through interaction with the peripheral cells and interstitial space matrix. This remodeling is responsible for the differences in chemical composition and physiological characteristics between interstitial fluid and plasma lipoproteins. Interstitial fluid HDL becomes a cholesterol donor to cells as opposed to plasma HDL, which is a cholesterol acceptor. We also confirmed that the FC/PL ratio is an important parameter influencing the direction of cholesterol flux.

We also analyzed how these compositional and functional differences between plasma and interstitial fluid HDL are related to structural changes. Previously, Fielding, *et al. [4]*, showed that specific HDL subpopulations have different physiological functions. We used a modified technique of two-dimensional electrophoresis to examine differences in HDL subpopulations in detail.

Agarose electrophoresis is run in the first dimension, followed by nondenaturing electrophoresis on a 2 to 35% polyacrylamide gradient gel. After completion of electrophoresis, proteins are transferred to nitrocellulose and probed with antiapoA-I antibody. We characterized our samples according to their mobility relative to albumin and according to the size based on internal standards run simultaneously with the sample. In plasma, most of the apoA-I was found in particles with α-mobility. In contrast, interstitial fluid showed a shift to particles with preα-mobility, i.e., particles having mobilities faster than albumin. We also observed an increase in interstitial fluid of particles with preβ-mobilities.

We also quantitated apoA-I distribution and used the PhosphorImager (Molecular Dynamics, Sunnyvale, CA) which directly determines the amount of radioactivity present in different areas. Utilizing this instrument, several lipoprotein subpopulations containing apoA-I were identified. An accurate definition of these particles is necessary to compare plasma and interstitial fluid lipoproteins. We describe these subpopulations using a coordinate system. In the agarose dimension, we defined mobilities relative to albumin ($R_f$ = 1.0). The second dimension is described according to the size of the particle. Using this system in dog plasma and interstitial fluid, we recognized the following major apoA-I-containing subpopulations:

preβ$_1$ particles ($R_f$ ~ 0.4 and modal diameter ~ 5 nm)

α$_1$ particles ($R_f$ ~ 0.9 and modal diameter ~ 12 nm)

α$_2$ particles ($R_f$ ~ 0.9 and modal diameter ~ 10 nm)

preα$_1$ particles ($R_f$ ~ 1.2 and modal diameter ~ 12 nm)

preα$_2$ particles ($R_f$ ~ 1.2 and modal diameter ~ 10 nm)

Although plasma and interstitial fluid have similar apoA-I-containing particles, the distribution between the plasma and interstitial fluid subpopulations was very different. A major shift of apoA-I from α-migrating particles occurs toward preα and preβ particles, consequently α-migrating particles decrease substantially in the interstitial fluid.

From these data, we can conclude that a major change of HDL subpopulations occurs in the interstitial fluid. Using the two-dimensional electrophoresis method, we have shown that the majority of interstitial fluid HDL migrates with preα-mobility, while the majority of plasma HDL migrates with α-mobility. In contrast to plasma, a significant portion of interstitial fluid HDL migrates with preβ-mobility. We postulate that the structural characteristics of interstitial fluid HDL may explain the functional differences between these particles and those of plasma.

We believe it will be important to study the mechanisms responsible for these changes in apoA-I subpopulations in interstitial fluid. To understand these processes, we need to isolate sufficient quantities of different subpopulations for determining the chemical basis responsible for their modifications.  We also would like to learn how these structural changes in interstitial fluid lipoproteins reflect physiological function and subsequent metabolism of these particles.

Using the above described two-dimensional method, we can identify and quantitate subpopulations of apoA-I, preβ, α and preα mobilities in human plasma.

The existence of a preα HDL subpopulation has not been described previously. It will be important to extend the studies of HDL subpopulations using the two-dimensional electrophoresis system to include pathological conditions. Application of this methodology may help our understanding of the mechanisms of disorders of lipoprotein metabolism.

REFERENCES

1. Sloop C, Dory L, Roheim P.  J Lipid Res 1987; 28:225-237

2. Johnson W, Bamberger M, Latta R, Rapp P, et al.  J Biol Chem 1986; 281:5766-5776.

3. Johnson W, Mahlberg F, Rothblat G, Phillips M. 1991; Biochim Biophys Acta 1085:273-298.

4. Castro G, Fielding C.  Biochemistry 1988; 27:2

ACKNOWLEDGMENTS

This study was supported by NIH Grant No. HL25596.

# HUMAN HDL METABOLISM AND GENETICS

# DETERMINANTS OF HDL METABOLISM IN SUBJECTS WITH LOW HDL-C LEVELS

Eliot A. Brinton[a,b], Shlomo Eisenberg[c], and Jan L. Breslow[a]

[a]The Rockefeller University, New York, New York 10021

[b]Current address: Bowman Gray School of Medicine, Medical Center Boulevard, Winston-Salem, NC 27157-1047

[c]Hadassah University Hospital, Jersalem, Israel

## INTRODUCTION

Considerable epidemiologic evidence suggests that low plasma levels of high-density lipoprotein cholesterol (HDL-C) are linked to elevated risk of atherosclerosis [1]; however, the metabolic mechanisms underlying a low HDL-C are somewhat unclear. HDL turnover studies of subjects with normal HDL levels have found that apo A-I FCR correlates inversely with HDL-C [2]. Studies from this laboratory have confirmed this finding both on high fat and low fat intake [3] and in women with high HDL-C [4]. Studies of patients with low HDL-C levels and hypertriglyceridemia (HTG) have shown an elevated fractional catabolic rate (FCR) of the major HDL apolipoproteins apo A-I [5] and apo A-II [5,6]. It was concluded that HTG itself was the cause of the low HDL-C level and the increase in HDL apolipoprotein FCR, yet these studies lacked the crucial comparison group of patients with low HDL-C and normal TG levels. Only one HDL turnover study has directly compared low HDL-C patients with normal or high TG [7]. In that study, the low-HDL-C, normal TG subjects had normal apo A-I FCR but low TR, whereas the low-HDL-C, HTG subjects had elevated apo A-I FCR and TR. This implied a striking contrast in the metabolism of apo A-I between low HDL-C patients with or without HTG. Because the comparison groups were small, however, and there was incomplete control over the subjects' diets, we have chosen to reexamine this important issue.

We have studied the turnover of apo A-I and apo A-II on a standard 42% fat diet under metabolic ward conditions in subjects with low-HDL-C and normal or high-plasma TG compared to control subjects with normal HDL-C and TG levels. We find that elevated HDL apolipoprotein FCR is the major metabolic mechanism of low HDL-C levels in both normal-TG and HTG subjects, suggesting that HTG is not a unique cause of the elevated FCR. Rather, we find that HTG is one of several factors that combine, possibly in an additive manner, to account for the increased FCR in patients with low HDL-C levels. Results of these studies are summarized here and have been published in full detail elsewhere [8].

METHODS

Twelve male and 16 female subjects were recruited for HDL metabolic studies from three sources: (a) clinic patients; (b) healthy, adult volunteers from the community; (c) undergraduate students. The subjects were classified into three groups by age and sex-corrected percentiles of fasting HDL-C and TG levels from values obtained on the study diet. Group 1 had HDL-C below the 20th percentile and TG below the 90th percentile. Group 2 had HDL-C below the 20th percentile and TG at or above the 90th percentile. Group 3, the normal control group, had an HDL-C level from the 20th to the 79th percentile and a TG level below the 90th percentile. All subjects were free from hepatic, renal, thyroid, and immunologic disorders by history and laboratory screening. One subject had been taking an oral hypoglycemic, glyburide, 5 mg daily for a few years at the time of the study. None of the other subjects were taking medications known to alter glucose or lipid levels. The studies were approved by the Institutional Review Board of the Rockefeller University, and informed consent was obtained from the subjects. The subjects were admitted to the Rockefeller University Hospital for 4 wk in the inpatient ward and kept on a natural food metabolic diet of 42% fat, 43% carbohydrate, and 15% protein, a polyunsaturated-to-saturated fat (P/S) ratio of 0.1 and with 215 mg cholesterol per 1,000 calories. No alcohol intake was allowed and subjects were instructed to maintain their usual level of physical activity.

After 2 wk on the metabolic diet, the subjects received radioiodinated apo A-I and apo A-II (10-25 $\mu$Ci of $^{125}$I and $^{131}$I), by intravenous bolus. Apolipoproteins A-I and A-II were purified from healthy donor plasma and radioiodinated by the iodine monochloride method as previously outlined [4]. To allow for thorough mixing of the tracers with HDL in the plasma compartment, the first blood sample was taken after 10 min. Blood was then taken at 4, 12, 14, and 36 h and then daily until 14 d. Each sample was handled and counted as outlined previously [4]. The radioactive decay curve was plotted directly from the die-away of plasma counts, and the FCR was calculated from this curve as previously [4]. Absolute transport (production or synthetic) rate (TR) was calculated by multiplying the FCR by the plasma pool (apolipoprotein level times plasma volume) and dividing by the body weight. Plasma volume was determined by isotope dilution. To show that the iodinated apo A-I and apo A-II associated with HDL, in each study extra aliquots of plasma were taken 10 min and 7 and 14 d after injection. Three fractions were prepared by ultracentrifugation, $d < 1.063$, $1.063 < d < 1.21$, and $d > 1.21$. The density distribution of radiolabel was calculated as a percentage of total counts, and the results for the 10-min 7- and 14-d samples were averaged. On days 1, 3, 7, 10, and 14 of the turnover period, lipid, lipoprotein, and apolipoprotein levels were measured after an overnight fast. Lipids and lipoproteins were measured by enzymatic methods as previously described [4], while Apo A-I levels were measured by ELISA and apo A-II levels by radioimmunoassay [8]. Three d before isotope injection, a postheparin lipase test was performed. Blood was drawn 15 min after an intravenous bolus dose of heparin, 60 U/kg body weight, and the plasma activities of lipoprotein lipase (LPL) and hepatic lipase (HL) were measured as described previously [8]. Linear regression analysis was performed by the least squares method and group differences were evaluated by Neumann-Keuls, both at a $P$ value $< 0.05$. Calculations were performed on The Rockefeller University Hospital CLINFO system.

RESULTS

The sex, age, body mass index, and lipoprotein profiles were determined for each subject. The mean and standard deviation of these variables were calculated for low-HDL-C subjects with normal TG (group 1) and HTG (group 2), and were compared by ANOVA to that of a group of subjects with normal HDL-C and TG levels (group 3) who were studied under identical conditions. Mean age did not differ among the groups. Variation among groups in body mass index was confined to two obese subjects. Total cholesterol and LDL-C did not differ among the groups. As expected, VLDL-C was higher in the HTG subjects of group 2 than in the normal-TG subjects of groups 1 and 3. By selection, the mean HDL-C levels were lower in groups 1 and 2 compared with group 3. Also by selection, the mean TG level of group 2 was much higher than values of groups 1 and 3., which did not differ significantly from each other.

Apo A-I levels of groups 1 and 2 were both significantly lower than group 3 and they did not differ significantly from each other. The FCR of apo A-I was equally elevated in groups 1 and 2 compared to group 3. The apo A-I TR did not differ significantly among the groups. The apo A-II parameters were in partial contrast to those of apo A-I. Apo A-II levels did not differ significantly among the three groups. The mean apo A-II FCR did not differ significantly between groups 1 and 2; however, compared to group 3, group 2 was significantly higher whereas group 1 was not significantly so. The TR of apo A-II varied in that it was 37% higher in group 2 than in group 3, whereas group 1 did not differ significantly from either group 2 or 3.

Mean LPL activity in group 2 was 29% lower than group 3, but group 1 did not differ significantly from either group 2 or 3. In contrast, there was no significant difference in HL among the groups. Because LPL and HL are reported to have opposing effects on HDL-C levels, we calculated the LPL/HL ratio. An identical 50% lowering of LPL/HL was seen in both groups 1 and 2 compared to group 3. An index of HDL composition was obtained by calculating the HDL-C/apo A-I + apo A-II molar ratio from plasma levels. All three groups differed significantly from each other, with group 1 being 18% lower and group 2 being 32% lower than group 3. The percent of each tracer found in the $d < 1.063$, $1.063 < d < 1.21$ (HDL), and $d > 1.21$ g/ml fractions of plasma was determined. The percent of tracer in the $d < 1.063$ fraction was very small ($< 2\%$) and varied little. The percent of the tracer in the $d > 1.21$ fraction is an indicator of the amount of lipid-poor HDL (VHDL), relative to more lipid-rich HDL fractions $HDL_2$ and $HDL_3$ . The percent of apo A-I tracer in the $d > 1.21$ fraction was elevated in groups 1 and 2 compared to group 3. The percent of apo A-II tracer in $d > 1.21$ fraction was less in every subject than for the apo A-I tracer; however, it was also elevated in groups 1 and 2.

To further explore the mechanisms of low HDL-C levels across the range of TG levels studied, we evaluated interrelationships among HDL-C levels, its metabolic parameters, and TG levels by linear regression analysis. HDL-C had a strong inverse correlation with the FCR of apo A-I and apo A-II, but HDL-C did not correlate with apo A-I TR. Although HDL-C did correlate with apo A-II TR, this correlation explains little more than half as much of the variance in HDL-C as does the correlation with either FCR. As expected,

HDL-C correlated inversely with TG in single linear regression; however, in stepwise multivariate linear regression TG did not add significantly to the prediction of HDL-C variability by the FCR of apo A-I or of apo A-II. We next tested for the reported relationship between FCR and TG. Univariate linear regression analysis revealed a positive correlation between apo A-I FCR and plasma TG; however, the significance of this relationship depended upon inclusion of the normal subjects. Apo A-II FCR also correlated significantly with TG levels, and this relationship was independent of the normal subject group. Given the significant differences among the three subject groups in lipase activity, the HDL/apo A-I + apo A-II ratio and density distribution of tracer, we tested for possible relationships of FCR and TR of apo A-I and apo A-II with these factors. The FCRs of apo A-I and apo A-II had inverse relationships of borderline and moderate significance, respectively, with LPL activity. The TRs of apo A-I and apo A-II also had inverse correlations of borderline and high significance, respectively, with LPL activity. In contrast, the FCRs of both apo A-I and apo A-II correlated positively with HL activity but neither the TR of apo A-I nor of apo A-II correlated with HL activity. The FCRs of apo A-I and apo A-II correlated well with the LPL/HL ratio, perhaps more strongly than with HL. The TRs of apo A-I and apo A-II had an absent or borderline correlation, respectively, with LPL/HL. The FCRs of apo A-I and apo A-II correlated strongly and inversely with the HDL-C/apo A-I + apo A-II ratio. The TRs of apo A-I and apo A-II also had borderline and strong inverse correlations, respectively, with the HDL-C/apo A-I + apo A-II ratio. The FCR, but not the TR, of apo A-I correlated with the percent of apo A-I tracer found in the $d > 1.21$ fraction.

Due to the importance of the FCR in predicting HDL-C, we explored the interrelationships of FCR with other study parameters by stepwise multivariate linear regression analysis. The HDL-C/apo A-I + apo A-II ratio was the strongest univariate predictor of apo A-I FCR, and the LPL/HL ratio made the largest addition to this correlation. TG levels, as a third parameter, did not add significantly to this prediction of apo A-I FCR by HDL-C/apo A-I + apo A-II and LPL/HL. LPL/HL was a strong univariate predictor of apo A-I FCR, and plasma TG did contribute significantly to this prediction. The percent of apo A-I tracer in the $d > 1.21$ fraction was also a univariate predictor of apo A-I FCR and added significantly to the prediction of apo A-I FCR by plasma TG. Tracer distribution did not, however, add to the prediction of apo A-I FCR by LPL/HL or HDL/apo A-I + apo A-II, separately or together. Given the importance of the HDL-C/apo A-I + apo A-II ratio as a single and multivariate predictor of apo A-I FCR, we tested for correlations of this ratio with factors expected to influence HDL composition. TG was the strongest univariate predictor of HDL-C/apo A-I + apo A-II. The LPL/HL ratio also was a strong univariate predictor of HDL-C/apo A-I + apo A-II and LPL/HL added strikingly to the prediction of that ratio by TG. The percent apo A-I tracer in $d > 1.21$ also correlated with the HDL-C/apo A-I +apo A-II ratio but it did not add significantly to the prediction of this ratio by TG or LPL/HL separately or together in multivariate analysis. Finally, we compared the female and male subjects from the low HDL-C groups. Age, BMI, and the lipid and lipoprotein values did not differ. The women had higher HDL-C levels, as expected. Also, the women had higher levels of apo A-I and apo A-II. Interestingly, despite these differences in the HDL-C, apo A-I, and apo A-II levels there were no significant differences in any of the metabolic parameters nor in any of the other measured parameters.

## DISCUSSION

The major goal of this study was to elucidate the metabolic mechanisms of low HDL-C levels. In particular we wished to explore the role of HTG, with which low HDL-C is often, but not always, associated. Only one previously published study has directly addressed the question of the interaction between low HDL-C and HTG in HDL metabolism [7]. Apo A-I turnover was performed in patients with low HDL-C and normal TG, patients with low HDL-C and elevated TG, and subjects with normal HDL-C and normal TG. In that study, by ANOVA the low HDL-C, normal TG group was found to have a low TR and a normal FCR compared to controls, whereas the HTG group was found to have high TR and FCR. Although the low TR and the lack of elevated FCR in the low-HDL-C normal TG group contrast with the current paper, when we performed linear regression analysis of the data in that report, we found at least three important parallels with our own results. Those data revealed a strong inverse correlation between HDL-C and apo A-I FCR, a strong direct correlation between TG and apo A-I FCR, and the lack of a correlation between HDL-C levels and apo A-I TR. By this analysis, those data support our conclusion that FCR is more important than TR in determining HDL-C levels.

Previously, men and women with normal HDL-C levels have been found to differ both in FCR and TR of HDL apolipoproteins [2]. In our study, among control subjects the women had a lower FCR of apo A-I and apo A-II than the men. In contrast, among our low-HDL-C subjects we found no differences in HDL metabolism between the men and women. Despite having the expected higher levels of HDL-C, apo A-I, and apo A-II, these women had values indistinguishable from their male counterparts both for the metabolic parameters (FCR and TR) and for the other measured factors. The apparent paradox of unequal plasma levels but comparable metabolism is explained by the finding of lower plasma volume as a percent of body weight in the women. That is, production of the same amount of HDL apolipoprotein per kilogram body weight into a smaller plasma volume resulted in higher plasma levels in the women.

We evaluated the relationship of HDL-C to parameters of HDL apolipoprotein metabolism and related factors in subjects with low HDL-C with or without HTG. We found hypercatabolism of apo A-I to a comparable degree in both low HDL-C groups; thus, elevated FCR of the principal HDL apolipoprotein appears to be characteristic of low HDL-C, regardless of TG levels. We found a strong positive relationship between FCR and TG by univariate linear regression analysis; however, the correlation between apo A-I FCR and TG depended upon the inclusion of the normal subjects. That is, looking solely with the low-HDL-C group, TG levels did not correlate with apo A-I FCR.

Given the apparent importance of the FCR of apo A-I and apo A-II in determining HDL-C levels, we carefully explored potential determinants of FCR in addition to plasma TG levels. Two indices of HDL size, density or composition, the HDL-C/apo A-I + apo A-II ratio, and the percent of apo A-I tracer in the $d > 1.21$ fraction, both correlated strongly with the apo A-I FCR, inversely and directly, respectively. We previously found an inverse correlation between FCR and the HDL-C/apo A-I + apo A-II ratio in women with high

HDL-C levels [4], similar to the correlation in this report. That study and this one together strongly suggest that HDL composition is an important determinant of FCR across the usual range of HDL-C levels. The single best predictor of apo A-I FCR was the HDL-C/apo A-I + apo A-II ratio. This ratio, in turn was best predicted (over 70% of the variability in multiple linear regression) by TG and LPL/HL. The LPL/HL ratio highlights reciprocal changes in LPL and HL activity. A coordinate role of elevated TG levels may be the promotion of removal of poorly catabolized cholesteryl ester in exchange for TG in the HDL core. This TG is readily hydrolyzed by HL, causing depletion of HDL core lipid. Thus, we hypothesize that TG levels and the LPL/HL ratio are important determinants of HDL size and composition, which appear to be major determinants of apo A-I and apo A-II FCR, which, in turn, may determine HDL-C levels (see Fig. 1, source: Reference #8).

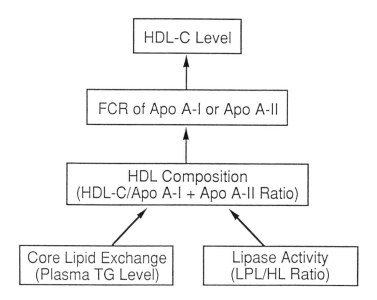

Figure 1. Hypothetical schema of the factors influencing the metabolism and levels of HDL. Determinants of HDL composition, its effect on the FCR of apo A-I and apo A-II, and the effect of FCR on HDL-C level are illustrated (from reference #8, used with permission).

In summary, we have demonstrated that high apo A-I and apo A-II FCR is the major metabolic mechanism of low HDL-C, regardless of the presence or absence of HTG. Nevertheless, HTG can contribute to lowering of HDL-C levels, and this may occur via an effect of TG levels on FCR. The promotion of FCR by HTG may be additive to the effect of a low LPL/HL ratio, and both of these factors appear to be mediated through lipid depletion of HDL. Given the importance of low HDL-C levels as predictors of atherosclerosis risk, we suggest that elevated FCR of apo A-I and apo A-II may constitute an important metabolic mechanism underlying such a susceptibility. Furthermore, as potential determinants of FCR, TG levels, postheparin lipase activity, and HDL composition may also play important mechanistic roles in atherogenesis.

## REFERENCES

1.  Miller GJ, and Miller NE, 1975. Lancet. i:16-19.

2.  Shaefer EJ, Zech, LA, Jenkins LL, Bronzert TJ, Rubalcaba EA, Lindgren FT, Aamodt RL, and Brewer HB, Jr. 1982. J Lipid Res. 23:850-862.

3.  Brinton EA, Eisenberg S, and Breslow JL. 1990. J Clin Invest. 85:144-151.

4.  Brinton EA, Eisenberg S, and Breslow JL. 1989. J Clin Invest. 84:262-269.

5.  Saku K, Gartside PS, Hynd BA, Mendoza SG, and Kashyap ML. 1985. Metab Clin Exp. 34:754-764.

6.  Rao SN, Magill PJ, Miller NE, and Lewis B. 1980. Clin Sci (Long.). 59:359-367.

7.  Le N-A, and Ginsberg HN. 1988. Metab Clin Exp. 37:614-617.

8.  Brinton EA, Eisenberg S, and Breslow JL. 1991. J Clin Invest. 87:536-544.

© 1992 Elsevier Science Publishers B.V. All rights reserved.
High density lipoproteins and atherosclerosis III.
N.E. Miller and A.R. Tall, editors.

Role of the Kidney in Increased Clearance of Apolipoprotein A-I in Subjects with Reduced High Density Lipoprotein Cholesterol Concentrations.

Barry S. Horowitz[1], Ira J. Goldberg[1], Jacques Merab[1], Theresa Vanni[1], Rajasekhar Ramakrishnan[2], Henry N. Ginsberg[1].

Departments of Medicine[1] and Pediatrics[2], Columbia University College of Physicians and Surgeons and the Columbia Presbyterian Medical Center, New York, N.Y. 10032.

## INTRODUCTION

Individuals with low plasma levels of HDL cholesterol also have reduced concentrations of apolipoprotein (apo) A-I. Reduced plasma levels of apoA-I could result from decreased secretion into plasma or increased removal from plasma of this apolipoprotein. Most studies utilizing radiolabeled HDL tracers have demonstrated that accelerated HDL apoA-I fractional catabolic rates (FCRs), and not reduced rates of apoA-I secretion into plasma, are associated with low apoA-I concentrations. Recent studies indicate that high apoA-I FCRs are associated with low HDL levels independent of plasma triglyceride concentrations.

The mechanisms underlying accelerated fractional catabolism, including the sites of increased removal of apoA-I from plasma, have not been clearly delineated. ApoA-I can exchange among lipoprotein particles in vivo, indicating that it has the ability to associate with and dissociate from HDL (as well as other lipoproteins). Indeed, "free" apoA-I has been identified in plasma by several investigators (1-4). Glass et al. (5), demonstrated that the kidney can accumulate apoA-I without core lipid components and apoA-I has also been measured in urine from nephrotic patients (6,7). Furthermore, increased "free" apoA-I is present in plasma of patients with renal failure (8). The recent studies of Goldberg et al. (9), which demonstrated that increased apoA-I FCRs in hypertriglyceridemic monkeys were associated with increased renal catabolism of apoA-I, suggest the quantitative importance of the kidney in apoA-I catabolism.

These data raise the possibility that increased fractional catabolism of apoA-I in subjects with low plasma HDL cholesterol levels results from increased dissociation of apoA-I from HDL particles and subsequent increased clearance of "free" apoA-I by the kidney. We have carried out studies to identify and characterize the metabolism of more readily dissociable apoA-I. HDL was either directly radiolabeled with 125-I (whole-labeled) or exchange-labeled with pure 131-I-apoA-I and these tracers were used to determine apoA-I FCR in individuals with high and low HDL cholesterol. Renal uptake of HDL isolated from subjects with low and high HDL cholesterol concentrations was compared in isolated perfused rabbit kidneys. HDL that was modified by triglyceride-enrichment, followed by exposure to lipoprotein lipase (LPL) and hepatic triglyceride lipase (HTGL), was also used to study renal metabolism of apoA-I. Our results suggest that subjects with low HDL cholesterol have increased apoA-I FCRs because they have more loosely bound, easily exchanged apoA-I that is more rapidly cleared by the kidney.

## METHODS

Subjects: Men with either low or high plasma HDL cholesterol concentrations prior to any dietary intervention were studied. Subjects with low HDL cholesterol had been eating an American Heart Association (AHA) Step 1 diet for at least several months. None were receiving any lipid-lowering agents at the time of the study. Some of these men had previously been treated with lipid-altering agents, which stopped at least six weeks prior to study. Subjects with high plasma HDL cholesterol levels were instructed in the AHA diet by one of our research dieticians 2-3 weeks prior to study. None of these men had ever received a lipid-altering drug. None of the study subjects in either group had any other disease, nor were they taking any other medication known to affect lipid metabolism.

<u>Turnover Protocol:</u> Plasma was isolated after a 12-14 hour fast and HDL (d:1.063-1.210) was isolated by sequential ultracentrifugation using sterile techniques (10). HDL was *whole-radiolabeled* with 125-I (11). Homologous apoA-I was radiolabeled with 131-I and *exchange-radiolabeled HDL* was prepared by incubating the 131-I-apoAI with a separate aliquot of the subject's HDL at 37°C for thirty minutes, followed by reisolation of the HDL by ultracentrifugation. The incubation was carried out so that there was no excess of apoA-I particles (12). The two radiolabeled HDL tracers were injected within 24 hrs of preparation.

One day prior to injection with the radiolabeled lipoproteins, subjects were admitted to the General Clinical Research Center (GCRC) . A sample of blood was obtained after an overnight fast, and 25 $\mu$Ci of 131-I-apoA-I-HDL and 75 $\mu$Ci of 125-I-HDL were injected intravenously. Samples were then obtained at 0.5, 1, 2, 6, 12, 24 and 36 hours, followed by daily blood samples during the next two weeks. Subjects consumed the AHA Step 1 diet during the entire study. All subjects received a saturated solution of potassium iodide, twice daily, starting the day prior to tracer injections, and continuing throughout the study period.

Plasma obtained from each blood sample and HDL was isolated by sequential ultracentrifugation in a 50.3 Ti rotor (10). VLDL, IDL and LDL were removed together by ultracentrifugation at 39,000 rpm for 24 hrs at d:1.063. This was followed by a second centrifugation at the same density. HDL (d:1.063-1.210) was isolated by ultracentrifugation at 39,000 rpm for 48 hrs at d:1.210. The isolated HDL was recentrifuged at the same density for 24 hrs. The exchange-labeled specific radioactivity of HDL apoA-I in each sample was calculated from the 131-I-apoA-I-HDL radioactivity in each sample and the protein concentration as assayed by the method of Lowry et al. 125-I-AI (whole-labeled) specific radioactivity was calculated as follows: An aliquot of each HDL sample was delipidated, redissolved in 6M urea, and apoA-I isolated from other apolipoproteins by FPLC (13). The pooled fractions of pure apoA-I were then counted and protein concentration determined. FPLC purification of apoA-I was necessary for whole-labeled specific radioactivity determinations because several apolipoproteins are labeled by the ICl method. The specific radioactivity data were then used to estimate the fractional catabolic rates of exchange- and whole-labeled HDL apoA-I, using a two-pool model (10). Radioactivity in the density greater than 1.210 fraction as a percent of total plasma radioactivity was also determined. ApoA-I mass in the density greater than 1.210 fraction was also measured.

<u>In vitro studies:</u> To determine if 125-I and 131-I had different effects on the integrity of the tracers used in the *in vivo* studies, a longterm *in vitro* incubation protocol was carried out. HDL was both whole- and exchange-labeled with both 125-I and 131-I, thus creating four separate tracers. Two separate incubations were performed with plasma, using 131-I whole-labeled tracer and 125-I exchange-labeled tracer in one incubation, and 125-I whole-labeled tracer and 131-I exchange-labeled tracer in the other. Each incubation was performed at 37°C for two weeks, with an aliquot taken every two days for ultracentrifugation at d.1.210 for 24 hours. Radioactivity in the d<1.210 and d>1.210 fractions was examined to assess any radiation damage to particles that might have occurred over the two-week period.

<u>Kidney perfusion studies:</u> Kidneys were isolated from New Zealand white rabbits and perfused according to the method of Maack (14). Whole-labeled 125-I-HDL (density

1.063-1.210) from subjects with either low or high HDL cholesterol levels was first incubated with excess VLDL for 24 hrs at 37°C to allow labeled HDL apoCs and apoE to exchange with unlabeled apolipoproteins in VLDL. The reisolated 125-I-HDL was enriched in radiolabeled apoA-I (>80% of the radioactivity as determined by SDS PAGE). It was injected into the perfusate and, after thirty minutes, the kidney was washed with five volumes of fresh perfusate to rinse out unincorporated label. Aliquots of venous effluent were collected at five and thirty minutes, as well as after the wash-out period. The kidney was weighed at the end of the experiment, and sections of renal cortex, papilla and perinephric fat cut out for gamma counting. Uptake of apoA-I by the kidney was quantified by determining the activity in the cortex, expressed per gram tissue, as a percent of radioactivity in the perfusate after five minutes of perfusion.

Modification of HDL: Radiolabeled HDL (d:1.063-1.210) obtained from subjects with high HDL cholesterol levels were incubated with VLDL for 24 hours at 37°C to diminish apoC and E labeling. The resiolated HDL were incubated a second time for 24 hours at 37°C with VLDL and d>1.210 fraction (as a source of cholesteryl ester transfer protein (CETP)). The reisolated triglyceride-enriched HDL were incubated a third time for 24 hours at 37°C in the presence or absence of purified LPL and HTGL. After one final reisolation by ultracentrifugation, the modified HDL were injected into the isolated kidney as described above.

Assays: Plasma and lipoprotein triglyceride and cholesterol levels were determined using enzymatic methods on an ABA-100 automated spectrophotometer (Abbott, Chicago IL). Our laboratory is standardized by the Centers for Disease Control and we participate in their ongoing quality control program. Apolipoprotein A-I was measured by radioimmunoassay (15) in plasma, HDL and d>1.210 fractions.

Statistics: Comparisons between whole- and exchange-labeled tracers were done using paired t-tests. Comparisons between groups with low and high HDL cholesterol levels were done using unpaired t-tests.

**RESULTS**

Subjects: The clinical characteristics of the study patients are depicted in Table 1. Plasma lipids at the time of referral to our clinic, or at the time of recruitment for the study, are also presented in this table. By design, all of the subjects in the low HDL cholesterol group had values below the 25th percentile for their age, whereas subjects in the high HDL cholesterol group had values above the 90th percentile for their age. Mean HDL cholesterol concentrations were $31\pm4$ mg/dl and $72\pm5$ mg/dl in the two groups. While total and low density lipoprotein cholesterol values were similar in each group, triglyceride measurements were higher in the group with low HDL cholesterol ($372\pm275$ mg/dl vs $92\pm24$ mg/dl).

HDL turnover studies: In every subject, whether in the low or high HDL cholesterol group, the exchange-labeled FCR (pools/d) was greater than the whole-labeled FCR. The mean ($\pm$SD) exchange-labeled FCR ($0.306\pm0.088$) was significant greater than the mean whole-labeled FCR ($0.213\pm0.054$) $p<0.0004$.

In every patient, whether from the low or high HDL cholesterol group, there was more radioactivity in the d>1.210 fraction derived from the exchange-labeled than from the whole-labeled tracer ($12.55\pm4.95\%$ vs $1.02\pm0.38\%$; $p<0.003$). In addition, there was significantly more exchange-labeled d>1.210 radioactivity in the low HDL cholesterol (16.5%) than in the high HDL cholesterol group (8.6%; $p<0.02$). There was also more than a two-fold greater proportion of apoA-I measured by radioimmunoassay in

218

*Table 1. Clinical characteristics of study patients.*

| Subject # | Age* | %IBW** | TC*** | TG | HDLC | LDLC |
|---|---|---|---|---|---|---|
| Low HDLC | | | | | | |
| 1 | 26 | 95.5 | 194 | 241 | 33 | 113 |
| 2 | 42 | 133.2 | 355 | 269 | 30 | 271 |
| 3 | 41 | 90.4 | 171 | 101 | 35 | 116 |
| 4 | 57 | 118.0 | 215 | 353 | 31 | 109 |
| 5 | 62 | 109.0 | 176 | 174 | 34 | 107 |
| 6 | 28 | 112.3 | 238 | 897 | 22 | 58 |
| 7 | 40 | 131.2 | 194 | 569 | 31 | 49 |
| x | 42 | 112.8 | 220 | 372[+] | 31[++] | 118 |
| ±sd | 13 | 16.3 | 64 | 275 | 4.3 | 73 |
| High HDLC | | | | | | |
| 8 | 45 | 108.5 | 217 | 115 | 72 | 122 |
| 9 | 25 | 89.3 | 145 | 67 | 68 | 64 |
| 10 | 35 | 84.5 | 192 | 95 | 77 | 96 |
| x | 35 | 94.1 | 185 | 92 | 72 | 94 |
| ±sd | 10 | 12.7 | 37 | 24 | 4.5 | 29 |

* Age in years

** Percent Ideal Body Weight

*** All lipids in mg/dl: TC=total cholesterol; TG=total triglycerides; HDLC=high density lipoprotein cholesterol; LDLC=low density lipoprotein cholesterol.

[+] P<0.03, low vs high HDLC. [++] P<0.0001, low vs high HDLC.

d>1.210 fraction, as a percent of HDL apoA-I concentration, in the low versus the high HDL cholesterol groups. These data suggest that exchange-labeled apoA-I traces a more easily dissociated pool of apoA-I and that this pool makes up a greater proportion of total apoA-I in subjects with low HDL cholesterol than in subjects with high HDL cholesterol.

We conducted two turnover studies (subjects 2 and 5) with the tracers reversed. The FCRs of these two low HDL cholesterol subjects fell well within the range of the rest of the group. In each case, the exchange-labeled tracer was removed more rapidly than the whole-labeled tracer, and the difference in the FCRs for the exchange- and whole-labeled tracers in subjects 2 ($\Delta$=0.068) and 5 ($\Delta$=0.161) were comparable to the mean for the group with low HDL cholesterol levels described above. In one kinetic study in which we injected both homologous and autologous exchange-labeled tracers into a low HDL individual, the FCRs of the two exchange-labeled tracers were virtually identical; the autologous and homologous HDL apoA-I FCRs were both 0.31 pools/day.

In vitro studies: The two-week incubation study comparing exchange- and whole-labeled HDL tracers with either isotope revealed no significant differences in the amount of radioactivity in the different fractions over the two-week period. In addition, there were no significant differences between tracers. These results indicate that the in vivo observations did not result from methodologic artifacts related to labeling techniques or "isotope effects".

Kidney perfusion studies: When kidneys were injected with HDL from low HDL cholesterol subjects, twice as much apoA-I radioactivity accumulated in the rabbit kidney cortex during the perfusion compared to that accumulated during perfusion of HDL from high HDL cholesterol subjects. In two sets of kidneys, a ten-fold greater amount of tracer was added to the perfusion and the percent of renal cortical uptake was similar to that using less tracer. Therefore, at the amounts of tracer used, renal uptake was not saturated. These studies indicate that apoA-I associated with low HDL cholesterol particles is taken up by the kidney to a greater extent than apoA-I associated with high HDL cholesterol particles.

Modification of HDL: When the triglyceride-enriched HDL, which had been exposed to both lipases, was added to the kidney perfusate, three-fold more apoA-I was accumulated in the cortex compared to the unmodified preparation. Triglyceride-enrichment of HDL alone did not significantly affect uptake. These results paralleled those obtained when we perfused HDL from low and high HDL cholesterol subjects, and suggest that triglyceride-enrichment of HDL followed by lipolysis could be important factors *in vivo*.

Modified and unmodified HDL were also subjected to ultracentrifugation at d:1.210 to determine whether the degree of dissociation of apoA-I was affected by triglyceride-enrichment and lipolysis. Exposing unmodified HDL from high HDL cholesterol subjects to lipases did not alter the amount of radioactivity found in the d < 1.210 and d > 1.210 fractions. Similarly, triglyceride-enrichment alone did not affect the distribution of radioactivity. However, when triglyceride-enriched HDL was exposed to LPL, significantly more radioactivity was found in the d > 1.210 fraction. This effect was increased by using a combination of LPL and HTGL. Therefore, triglyceride-enrichment of HDL and the addition of lipase resulted in the greatest dissociation of apoA-I in the ultracentrifuge.

## DISCUSSION

Although the majority of individuals with low levels of HDL cholesterol and apoA-I have increased fractional clearance of apoA-I from plasma (10,16,17), the exact mechanisms underlying accelerated HDL apoA-I catabolism have not been delineated. Because apoA-I can exchange between lipoproteins (18), and can exist "free" in plasma (1-4), we proposed that (a) apoA-I can bind to HDL with a spectrum of affinities, and (b) that individuals with low plasma HDL cholesterol levels have a greater proportion of their apoA-I in an easily dissociable pool. We tested this hypothesis in subjects with low and high levels of plasma HDL cholesterol utilizing a dual-tracer approach. Whole-labeling of HDL was used to trace the kinetics of metabolism of all of the apoA-I molecules on each HDL particle; exchange-labeling of HDL was used in an attempt to preferentially trace the kinetics of the least tightly bound, most easily dissociable apoA-I molecules.

Exchange-labeled HDL had a higher FCR than whole-labeled HDL in every subject studied, whether they had high or low HDL cholesterol. Ultracentrifugation was associated with greater dissociation of exchange-labeled apoA-I from HDL particles than of whole-labeled apo A-I as well. These results supported the view that we could distinguish between pools of apoA-I with different biologic and physical characteristics.

The exchange-labeled apoA-I FCR was greater in the low HDL cholesterol group than in the high HDL cholesterol group. Similarly, the proportion of apoA-I dissociating from HDL during ultracentrifugation of exchange-labeled tracer was much greater than that of whole-labeled tracer in the low versus the high HDL cholesterol group. These results were compatible with the hypothesis that individuals with low levels of HDL cholesterol have a greater proportion of their apoA-I in an easily dissociable form. The finding that a greater proportion of HDL apoA-I, measured by radioimmunoassay, was in the d > 1.210 fraction in the low HDL cholesterol group supported further our hypothesis.

Several groups of investigators have studied the catabolism of whole- and exchange-labeled HDL, and published results are conflicting (12,18,19). Each of the previous studies was done with different methods, and we are unable, therefore, to explain results that conflict with ours. We believe, however, that neither radiation damage, nor the use of homologous apoA-I (as opposed to autologous apolipoprotein) played roles in the differences we observed in apoA-I FCRs with whole- and exchange-labeled tracers.

We carried out a series of studies using an isolated kidney perfusion system to address questions relevant to both the mechanisms underlying the presence of a rapidly cleared pool of "free" apoA-I in HDL from subjects with low HDL cholesterol levels, and to the site of catabolism of this apoA-I. The results of the kidney perfusion studies with HDL from low and high HDL cholesterol subjects, and with modified HDL suggest that individuals with small, relatively triglyceride-enriched HDL particles have more "free" apoA-I available to be cleared by the kidney. The incubation studies suggest that increased renal clearance of apoA-I occurs when HDL that is cholesterol depleted and relatively enriched in triglycerides interacts with plasma LPL and/or HTGL. We believe that the reduction in HDL size resulting from such interactions leads to increased apoA-I dissociation from HDL. This conclusion is consistant with our observation that more radioactivity was found in the d > 1.210 fraction when triglyceride-enriched, hydrolyzed HDL (originally isolated from subjects with high HDL cholesterol levels) was subjected to ultracentrifugation.

The role of the kidney in apoA-I metabolism was first noted by Glass et al. (5) who reported that the rat kidney could accumulate apoA-I without necessarily taking up the entire HDL particle. Studies by Kashyap and colleagues (6) demonstrated that isolated kidneys could filter and reabsorb apoA-I. More recently, we demonstrated that monkeys made acutely hypertriglyceridemic by inhibition of lipoprotein lipase developed marked reductions in HDL cholesterol and apoA-I levels, and that increased apoA-I radioactivity was accumulated in the kidneys of those animals (9). Neary and Gowland reported increased plasma "free" apoA-I in individuals with either renal disease (8) or hypertriglyceridemia (1).

The present studies demonstrate that individuals with low plasma levels of HDL cholesterol have increased apoA-I FCRs because thay have an increased proportion of their HDL apoA-I in a more easily dissociable pool that can be more rapidly cleared by the kidney. The predisposition to dissociate results, in turn, from the hydrolysis of a triglyceride-enriched HDL core by HTGL (20) and/or LPL. Finally, triglyceride-enriched HDL is generated by the action of cholesteryl ester transfer protein in the presence of increased VLDL triglyceride. This scheme links abnormalities of triglyceride or apoprotein-containing lipoproteins to reduced levels of HDL cholesterol and, therefore, to increased risk for coronary heart disease (21-23).

REFERENCES

1. Neary, R.H. and Gowland, E. Clin. Chem. 1987; 33:1163-1169.

2. Schonfeld, Z., Bailey, A., Steelman, R. Lipids 1978; 13:951-959.

3. Gebhardt, D.E, Schicht, I.M., Paul, L.C. Ann. Clin. Biochem 1984; 21:301-305.

4. Daerr, W.H., Minzlaff, U. Greten, H. Biochem. Biophys. Acta 1986; 879:134-139.

5. Glass, C., Pittman, R.C., Civen, M. and Steinberg, D. J. Biol. Chem 1985; 261:744-

6. Mendoza, S.G., Kashyap, M.L., Chen, C.Y. et al. Metabolism 1976; 25: 1143-1149.

7. Shore, V.G., Forte, T., Licht, H., et al. Metabolism 1982; 31: 258-268.

8. Neary, R.H. and Gowland, E. . Clinica Chimica Acta 1988; 171: 239-246.

9. Goldberg, I.J., Blaner, W.S., Vanni, T.M., Moukides,M., and Ramakrishnan, R. J.Clin. Invest 1990; 86:463-473.

10. Le, N.A. and Ginsberg, H.N. Metabolism 1988; 37:614-616.

11. McFarlane, A.A. Nature 1958; 182:183.

12. Shepherd, J., Gotton, A.M., Jr., Taunton, O.D., Caslake, M.J., and Farish, E. Biochim. Biophys. Acta 1977; 489:486-501.

13. Polecek, D., Edelstein, C. Scanu, A.M. Lipids 1981; 16:927-929.

14. Maack, T. Am. J. Physiol. 1980; 238:F71-F78.

15 Smith, S.J., Cooper, G.R., Henderson, L.O., et al. Clin. Chem. 1988; 33:2240-9.

16. Nicoll A, Miller NE, Lewis B. High density lipoprotein metabolism Adv in Lipid Res. Vol 17. Academic Press, Inc. 1980;54-106.

17. Brinton, E.A., Eisenberg, S., and Breslow, J.L. J. Clin. Invest. 1991; 87:536-544.

18. Schaefer, E.J., Foster, D.M., Jenkins, L.L., Lindgren, F.T., Berman, M., Levy, R.I. and Brewer, H.B., Jr. Lipids 1979; 14:511-522.

19. Vega, G.L., Gylling, H., Nichols, A.V., Grundy, S.M. J. Lipid Res. 1991; 32:867-875.

20. Clay, M.A., Newnham, H.H., and Barter, P.J. Arteriosclerosis and

Thrombosis 1991; 11:415-422.

21. Miller, N.E., Thelle, D.S., Forde, O.H., Mjos, O.D. Lancet 1977; I:965-968.

22. Castelli, W.P., Garrison, R. J., Wilson, P.W. et al. J. Am. Med. Assoc 1986; 256:2835-2838.

23. Gordon, K.J., Knoke, J., Probstfield, J.L. et al. Circulation 1986; 74:1217-1225.

# DRUGS, HORMONES AND EPIDEMIOLOGY

# Interrelated Changes of HDL and LDL Subclasses Induced by Variation in Dietary Fat Intake

Ronald M. Krauss, M.D. and Darlene M. Dreon, Dr.P.H.

Lawrence Berkeley Laboratory, University of California, Berkeley, California 94720

## INTRODUCTION

The absence of significant correlations between HDL- and LDL-cholesterol (HDL-C and LDL-C) has led to the conclusion that these lipoproteins contribute independently to coronary disease risk (1). However, measurements of HDL and LDL subclasses in our laboratory have established that levels of $HDL_2$ are positively correlated with levels of larger, more buoyant LDL particles (LDL-I), and negatively correlated with levels of smaller, denser LDL (primarily LDL-III) as well as with levels of triglyceride-rich lipoproteins (2, 3). While variations in plasma levels of HDL-C are associated with changes in $HDL_2$, levels of LDL-C are poorly correlated with levels of individual LDL subclasses. Therefore, potentially important relationships of LDL and HDL components are obscured by simple measurements of LDL- and HDL-C.

Recently, studies employing non-denaturing gradient gel electrophoresis of HDL subclasses have extended these observations by demonstrating that a component within $HDL_3$, designated $HDL_{3b}$, is inversely correlated with levels of $HDL_2$ (4). Thus, levels of $HDL_{3b}$ are positively associated with levels of small, dense LDL as well as with levels of triglyceride-rich lipoproteins (4).

The metabolic factors responsible for these interrelationships are poorly understood. Evidence has been presented elsewhere that factors affecting the metabolism of triglyceride-rich lipoproteins may be in part responsible for reciprocal variations of $HDL_2$ and smaller, denser LDL (5-9). However, both cross-sectional and longitudinal studies in healthy subjects (2, 3) have indicated that concordant changes in levels of $HDL_2$ and LDL-I are independent of changes in plasma triglyceride concentrations, suggesting that other metabolic factors may contribute to this relationship.

Changes in content of dietary fat and cholesterol have been shown to result in parallel reductions in LDL- and HDL-C, although generally the degree of reduction in LDL exceeds that of HDL (10-12). The aim of the present study was to determine whether levels of specific LDL and HDL subclasses are influenced by variation in amount of dietary fat intake, and whether these changes reflect interrelationships among these subclasses that have been described previously.

## METHODS

Subjects consisted of 105 healthy men who were randomly assigned to outpatient treatment with diets containing high (46%) and low (24%) fat content for six weeks each in a double cross-over design. Dietary fat content was changed by substitution of carbohydrate without significant change in other major dietary variables, including total energy, cholesterol (150 mg/1000 kCal), dietary fiber (4-5 g/1000 kCal), total protein (15% energy), and ratio of polyunsaturated to saturated fat (0.7). An equal ratio of simple and complex carbohydrates was chosen to minimize possible divergent effects of these two nutrients on plasma lipoprotein profiles (13, 14). Participants were instructed on the experimental diets by registered dietitians and given menus demonstrating number and size of servings. The subjects were non-smokers and abstained from alcohol throughout the study.

Dietary assessment was obtained from 4-day food records (Thursday to Sunday) of measured and weighed food intake (15). Nutrient calculation was performed using Minnesota Nutrition Data System software (16). The Food Database and Nutrient Database Versions 2.1 were employed (17, 18). As described elsewhere (Dreon, D., Miller B., Krauss R., unpublished), the averages for intake of all dietary components as assessed by these measures were extremely similar to the prescribed intake of these nutrients.

Laboratory measurements were obtained at the end of each six week dietary period. Blood samples were collected in chilled tubes containing $Na_2EDTA$, 1.4 mg/ml following a 12-16 hour overnight fast. Plasma was separated by low speed centrifugation within two hours and stored for no more than 5 days before laboratory analyses were carried out. Plasma total cholesterol and triglycerides were determined by enzymatic procedures on a Gilford Impact 400E analyzer. These measurements were consistently in control as monitored by the NHLBI-CDC standardization program. HDL-C was measured after heparin sulfate and magnesium chloride precipitation of plasma (19) and LDL-C was calculated from the formula of Friedewald et al. (20). ApoA-I and apoB concentrations in plasma were determined by maximal radial immunodiffusion (21, 22).

Analytical ultracentrifugation of the d<1.063 g/ml and d<1.21 g/ml ultracentrifugal fractions of plasma was used to determine concentrations of lipoprotein total mass as a function of Svedberg flotation rate (23). Very low density lipoproteins (VLDL) were measured as the sum of 11 intervals from flotation rate ($S_f$) 20-400, and intermediate density lipoproteins as the sum of 4 intervals from $S_f$ 12-20. For LDL ($S_f$ 0-12), mass was measured in intervals from $S_f$ 7-12 (LDL-I), $S_f$ 5-7 (LDL-II), $S_f$ 3-5 (LDL-III), and $S_f$ 0-3 (LDL-IV). HDL mass was measured as the sum of 15 intervals from flotation rate ($F_{1.2}$) 0-9, and divided into intervals which have been shown to be most closely related to $HDL_{2b}$ ($F_{1.2}$ 3.5-9), $HDL_{2a}$ ($F_{1.2}$ 2.5-3.5), $HDL_{3a}$ ($F_{1.2}$ 1.5-2.5), and $HDL_{3b+c}$ ($F_{1.2}$ 0-1.5) as assessed by non-denaturing gradient gel electrophoresis (4).

Statistical procedures (t-tests, Spearman correlations, regression analyses) were carried out using the Statview II Software package. Due to the number of correlation analyses performed, only correlation coefficients significant at p<0.01 or less are presented.

## RESULTS

Table I shows mean levels of plasma lipids, lipoprotein cholesterol, and apoproteins for both both the high- and low-fat diets and for the difference (low-fat minus high-fat). Overall, the change between the high- and low-fat diets resulted in significant increases in triglycerides (average 40%) and reductions in total cholesterol, LDL-C, HDL-C, and apoprotein (apo)B and A-I (average 12%, 14%, 10%, and 9%, respectively).

**Table 1**

Lipid, lipoprotein cholesterol and apoprotein concentrations in 105 men on high- and low- fat diets.

|  | HIGH-FAT | LOW-FAT | DIFFERENCE Low-fat minus high-fat |
|---|---|---|---|
|  | | mg/dl ± S.D. | |
| Triglyceride | 100±48.8 | 140±77.7 | 40.3±59.2* |
| Cholesterol | 212±38.0 | 196±34.9 | -15.4±21.0* |
| LDL-Cholesterol | 143±33.8 | 126±32.0 | -16.6±19.6* |
| HDL-Cholesterol | 49±10.0 | 42±8.5 | -7.0±06.5* |
| ApoB | 110±25.7 | 109±24.6 | -1.08±13.7 |
| ApoA-I | 126±17.2 | 115±15.1 | -11.1±13.1* |

* Difference significant, P<0.0001

Measurements of lipoproteins by analytic ultracentrifugation (Table 2) reveal diet-induced changes in total VLDL, LDL, and HDL mass that parallel those observed for plasma triglyceride, LDL-C, and HDL-C, respectively. Among the four major LDL subclasses, significant reductions on the low-fat diet were observed for LDL-I and LDL-II, and significant increases in mass of LDL-III and LDL-IV. Within the HDL particle spectrum, the major significant reduction was seen in $HDL_{2b}$, with smaller reductions in particles of progressively higher density.

**Table 2**

Lipoprotein Mass Concentration in 105 men on high-fat and low-fat diets

|  |  | HIGH-FAT | LOW-FAT | DIFFERENCE Low-fat minus high-fat |
|---|---|---|---|---|
|  |  |  | mg/dl ± S.D. |  |
| VLDL | ($S_f$ 20-400) | 91.8±78.2 | 175±88.7 | 83.3±77.8* |
| IDL | ($S_f$ 12-20) | 32.9±16.5 | 33.3±16.8 | 0.37±13.7 |
| LDL-Total | ($S_f$ 0-12) | 325±80.1 | 299±76.7 | -26.5±40.5* |
| LDL-I | ($S_f$ 7-12) | 196±61.3 | 93.0±39.6 | -103±48.2* |
| LDL-II | ($S_f$ 5-7) | 123±38.4 | 107±35.3 | -15.7±32.3* |
| LDL-III | ($S_f$ 3-5) | 60.0±37.9 | 80.8±40.2 | 20.8±33.0* |
| LDL-IV | ($S_f$ 0-3) | 11.0±10.3 | 17.9±15.3 | 6.88±12.1* |
|  |  |  |  |  |
| HDL-Total | ($F_{1.2}$ 0-9) | 228±51.8 | 207±43.3 | -21.3±40.8* |
| HDL2b | ($F_{1.2}$ 3.5-9) | 37.1±34.1 | 24.7±24.3 | -12.4±22.1* |
| HDL2a | ($F_{1.2}$ 2.5-3.5) | 50.5±14.6 | 45.1±14.3 | -5.34±12.8* |
| HDL3a | ($F_{1.2}$ 1.5-2.5) | 84.1±14.0 | 80.8±13.8 | -3.35±11.9† |
| HDL3b+c | ($F_{1.2}$ 0-1.5) | 56.2±13.8 | 56.0±13.7 | -0.18±13.9 |

Difference significant * p<0.0001  † p<0.01

Diet-induced changes in HDL parameters showed no significant correlations with change in LDL-cholesterol (results not shown). However, HDL components were found to correlate significantly with changes in subclasses of apoB-containing lipoproteins as measured by analytic ultracentrifugation (Table 3). Change in HDL-C was strongly positively correlated with change in LDL-I, and negatively correlated with changes in LDL-III and VLDL. Stepwise regression analysis (results not shown), indicated that LDL-I and VLDL changes contributed independently to variation in HDL-C, while the correlation with LDL-III was not independent of these variables.

Interestingly, change in HDL2b mass exhibited reciprocal relationships with changes in LDL-I and LDL-III similar to those observed for HDL-C, but there was no correlation with change in VLDL or with plasma triglyceride levels (results not shown). Furthermore, stepwise regression analysis indicated that change in LDL-III but not LDL-I was an independent predictor of HDL2b change.

The results in Table 3 also show significant positive correlations of HDL2a with LDL-I change, and inverse correlations of HDL2a change with change in LDL-III and LDL-IV. Among the HDL3 fractions, change in

HDL$_{3a}$ was positively correlated with change in LDL-II, and change in HDL$_{3b+c}$ was correlated with changes in both LDL-III and IDL.

**TABLE 3**

Spearman Correlations of Diet-Induced Changes in HDL Measurements

| Lipoprotein Mass* | HDL Chol | ApoAI | HDL - Mass* Total | HDL $_{2b}$ | HDL$_{2a}$ | HDL$_{3a}$ | HDL$_{3b+c}$ |
|---|---|---|---|---|---|---|---|
| VLDL | -0.28** | -0.04 | 0.08 | 0.01 | -0.02 | 0.09 | 0.22 |
| IDL | -0.11 | -0.02 | 0.13 | -0.06 | -0.01 | 0.22 | 0.29** |
| LDL-I | 0.44†† | 0.23 | 0.18 | 0.30** | 0.31** | 0.14 | -0.14 |
| LDL-II | 0.01 | 0.00 | 0.15 | -0.11 | 0.19 | 0.32* | 0.11 |
| LDL-III | -0.35† | -0.17 | -0.13 | -0.34† | -0.31* | -0.03 | 0.31** |
| LDL-IV | -0.19 | -0.14 | -0.09 | -0.07 | -0.28** | -0.17 | 0.24 |

*Mass of lipoprotein subfractions defined by flotation rate invervals as for Table 2. Correlation coefficient significant: **p<0.01, †p<0.001, ††p<0.0001.

## DISCUSSION

The findings in the present report are consistent with previous evidence from our laboratory that changes in plasma levels of HDL and LDL subclasses are strongly intercorrelated (2, 3). They further indicate that in men on low fat diets, reductions in HDL-C primarily reflect decreases in the HDL$_{2b}$ subclass. However, the results indicate that there may be multiple metabolic determinants of the diet-induced changes in HDL-C. Both increases in VLDL and reductions in LDL-I contributed independently to the lowering of HDL-C on the low fat diet, but VLDL change was not correlated with change in HDL$_{2b}$ mass. This suggests that changes in triglyceride metabolism, possibly induced by increased carbohydrate intake (24-28), altered HDL composition without changing HDL total mass. One possible mechanism for such an effect is an equivalent exchange of VLDL triglyceride for HDL-C (29) without significant changes in overall metabolism of HDL particles.

There is as yet no explanation for the concordant changes of LDL-I, HDL-C and HDL$_{2b}$ mass. Recent metabolic turnover studies have indicated that reductions in HDL-C on low-fat low-cholesterol diets are related to reduced transport rates of apoA-I (30). Therefore it has been proposed that on such diets, reduced HDL-C may result from reduced apoA-I synthesis (30). If this mechanism were operative in the current study, this would suggest a possible linkage of apoA-I production with increased synthesis or reduced clearance of LDL-I. An alternative hypothesis is that LDL-I or a metabolic precursor might be a preferential acceptor of cholesterol from HDL, and thus diet-induced variations in LDL-I metabolism may contribute significantly to changes in HDL-C levels.

Previous studies from our laboratory (2, 3) have indicated reciprocal changes in levels of LDL-I and LDL-III, consistent with the findings in the present report. As discussed elsewhere (31, 32), this reciprocity may result from a direct precursor-product relationship between these species, or from coordinate regulation of their production or clearance.

While changes in HDL$_{2b}$ and HDL$_{2a}$ were correlated with changes in levels of the largest LDL particles, changes in HDL$_{3a}$ and HDL$_{3b+c}$ species were correlated with changes in smaller, denser LDL-II and LDL-III, respectively. Again consistent with previous reports (2, 3), these changes were also correlated with changes in levels of IDL. The mechanisms underlying these changes are not known.

It is possible that the concordant relationships of changes in progressively smaller and denser HDL and LDL species are due to a common metabolic mechanism operating in individuals with differing distributions of HDL and LDL subclasses. In particular, we have described a common heritable trait characterized by a predominance of small,dense LDL-III particles, increases in VLDL and IDL, reductions in HDL2, and a relative increase in coronary disease risk (33, 34). Individuals with this trait, designated LDL subclass pattern B, or the atherogenic lipoprotein phenotype (35) have recently been found to have increased plasma levels of HDL$_{3b}$ which are correlated with increased levels of LDL-III, IDL, and VLDL (4). In the present study population, 18 men (17%) were found to have LDL subclass pattern B on both high-and low-fat diets, and in these men, but not in the remaining subjects, there were diet-induced reductions in both LDL-III and HDL$_{3b+c}$ (Krauss, R., Dreon, D., Miller, B. unpublished). Thus, an individual's lipoprotein subclass response to reduced fat intake may be strongly influenced by underlying genetic or metabolic factors responsible for that individual's plasma lipoprotein subclass profile. In the case of subjects with LDL subclass pattern B, these factors may be of particular importance, since in these subjects, but not in the remaining group, the low-fat diet resulted in a significant decrease in ratio of LDL- to HDL-C (36).

## SUMMARY

Measurements of subclasses of plasma HDL and LDL have revealed interrelationships among these lipoproteins that are not apparent from measurements of total HDL- or LDL-cholesterol. In the present report, we have investigated whether reductions in levels of HDL and LDL that have been observed on low fat diets involve selective changes in specific lipoprotein subclasses, and whether these changes, in turn, are interrelated. Subjects consisted of 105 healthy men who were randomly assigned to outpatient treatment with diets containing high (46%) and low (24%) fat content for six weeks each in a double cross-over design. Dietary fat content was changed by substitution of carbohydrate without significant change in other major dietary variables. Measurements of lipoprotein mass by analytic ultracentrifugation revealed significant reductions on the low-fat diet for larger, more buoyant LDL subclasses (LDL-I and LDL-II), and significant increases in mass of smaller, denser LDL particles (LDL-III and LDL-IV). Within the HDL spectrum, the major reduction was in the largest, most buoyant $HDL_{2b}$ subclass, with smaller reductions in particles of progressively higher density. Changes in HDL components were found to correlate significantly with changes in subclasses of apoB-containing lipoproteins  Change in HDL-C was strongly positively correlated with change in LDL-I, and negatively correlated with changes in LDL-III and VLDL.  Both increases in VLDL and reductions in LDL-I contributed independently to the lowering of HDL-C on the low fat diet, but VLDL change was not correlated with change in $HDL_{2b}$ mass. This suggests that changes in triglyceride metabolism, possibly induced by increased carbohydrate intake, resulted in lower HDL cholesterol content, perhaps via cholesterol-triglyceride exchange, without changing HDL total mass. Diet-induced variations in $HDL_{2b}$ may thus be more closely related to factors regulating concentrations of LDL-I than to changes in plasma VLDL levels. While changes in $HDL_{2b}$ and $HDL_{2a}$ were correlated with changes in levels of the largest LDL particles, changes in $HDL_{3a}$ and $HDL_{3b+c}$ species were correlated with changes in LDL-II and LDL-III, respectively. It is possible that the concordant relationships of changes in progressively smaller and denser HDL and LDL species are due to a common metabolic mechanism operating in individuals with differing distributions of HDL and LDL subclasses.

## ACKNOWLEDGEMENTS

This work was supported by the National Dairy Promotion and Research Board and by the National Institutes of Health Grant HL18574 and was conducted at the Lawrence Berkeley Laboratory (Department of Energy Contract DE-AC03-76SF00098 to the University of California).

## REFERENCES

1    The Lipid Research Clinics Coronary Primary Prevention Trial results. II. JAMA 1984; 251(3): 365-74.
2    Krauss RM, Lindgren FT, Ray RM   Clin. Chim. Acta 1980; 104(3): 275-90.
3    Krauss RM, Williams PT, Lindgren FT, Wood PD.   Arteriosclerosis 1988; 8(2): 155-62.
4    Williams PT, Krauss RM, Vranizan KM, Stefanick ML, Wood PDS, Lindgren FT. Atherosclerosis and Thrombosis 1992; 12: 332-340.
5    Deckelbaum RJ, Granot E, Oschry Y, Rose L, Eisenberg S. Arteriosclerosis 1984; 4: 225-231.
6    Fisher WR. Metabolism 1983; 32: 283-291.

232

7    Patsch, JR, Prasad, S, Gotto, AM, Jr, Patsch, W, J Clin Invest 1987; 80: 341-347.
8    Vega GL, Grundy SM. Arteriosclerosis 1986; 6: 395-406.
9    Crouse JR, Parks JS, Schey HM, Kohl FR. J. Lipid Res. 1985; 26: 566-574.
10   National Cholesterol Education Program Expert Panel. National Heart, Lung, and Blood Institute. Arch Intern Med 1988; 148: 36-69.
11   Kris-Etherton PM, Krummel D, Russell ME, et al. J Am Diet Assoc 1988; 88: 1373-1400.
12   Grundy SM, Denke MA. J Lipid Res 1990; 31: 1149-1172.
13   Srinivasan SR, Radhakrishnamurthy B, Foster TA, Berneson GS. Metabolism 1983; 32: 777-786.
14   Srinivasan SR, Radhakrishnamurthy B, Foster TA, Berneson GS. Am. J. Clin. Nutr. 1984; 40: 485-495.
15   Jackson B, Dujovne CA, DeCoursey S, Beyer P, Brown EF, Hassanein K. J. Am. Diet. Assoc. 1986; 86: 1531-1535.
16   Feskanich D, Buzzard IM, Welch BT, et al. J Am Diet Assoc 1988; 88: 1263-1267.
17   Feskanich D, Sielaff BH, Chong K, Buzzard IM. Comput Methods Programs Biomed 1989; 30: 47-57.
18   Schakel SF, Sievert YA, Buzzard IM. J Am Diet Assoc 1988; 88: 1268-1271.
19   Warnick GR, Nguyen T, Albers JJ. Clin. Chem. 1985; 31: 217-222.
20   Friedewald WT, Levy RI, Fredrickson DS. Clin. Chem. 1972; 18: 499-502.
21   Cheung MC, Albers JJ. J. Clin. Invest. 1977; 60: 43-50.
22   Oucherony O, Nilsson L-Q. In: Weir DM, ed. Handbook of Experimental Immunology. Oxford, England: Blackwell Scientific Publications, 1978: 19: 10-19.13.
23   Lindgren FT, Jensen LC, Hatch FT. In: Nelson GJ, ed. Blood Lipids and Lipoproteins: Quantitation, Composition, and Metabolism. New York: John Wiley and Sons, 1972: 181-274.
24   Nichols AV, Dobbin V, Gofman JW. Geriatrics 1957; 12: 7-17.
25   Ahrens EH Jr., Hirsch J, Oette K, Farquhar JW, Stein Y. Trans. Assoc. Am. Physicians 1961; 74: 134.
26   Ruderman NB, Jones AL, Krauss RM, Shafrir E. J Clin Invest 1971; 50(6): 1355-1368.
27   Ginsberg H, Olefsky JM, Kimmerling G, Crapo P, Reaven GM. J Clin Endocrinol Metab 1976; 42(4): 729-35.
28   Gonen B, Patsch W, Kuisk I, Schonfeld G. Metabolism 1981; 30: 1125-1129.
29   Nichols AV, Smith L. J. Lipid Res. 1965; 6: 206-210.
30   Brinton EA, Eisenberg S, Breslow JL. J Clin Invest 1990; 85: 144-151.
31   Krauss RM. Am Heart J 1987; 113: 578-582.
32   Krauss RM. Curr Opin Lipidol 1991; 2: 248-252.
33   Austin MA, Breslow JL, Hennekens CH, Buring JE, Willett WC, Krauss RM. JAMA 1988; 260: 1917-1921.
34   Austin MA, King MC,, Vranizan, KM, Newman, B, Krauss RM. Am J Hum Genet 1988; 43: 838-846.

35    Austin MA, King MC, Vranizan KM, Krauss RM.   Circulation 1990;
      82(2): 495-506.
36    Dreon DM, Krauss RM.   Circulation 1991; 84: II-681.

Diagnosis and Management of High Density Lipoprotein Deficiency States

E.J. Schaefer and J.M. Ordovas

Lipid Metabolism Laboratory, USDA Human Nutrition Research Center on Aging at Tufts University, and Lipid Division, New England Medical Center, Boston, MA

## I.    INTRODUCTION

The recent National Institutes of Health Consensus Development Conference on Triglyceride, High Density Lipoprotein, and Coronary Heart Disease (February 26-28, 1992) concluded that a decreased high density lipoprotein (HDL) cholesterol (< 35 mg/dl) is a significant independent coronary heart disease (CHD) risk factor, and that HDL cholesterol should be measured whenever total cholesterol is measured for CHD risk assessment. Moreover, panel members of the conference concluded that efforts should be made to increase low HDL cholesterol to reduce CHD risk by diet, exercise, weight reduction and smoking cessation.

## II.    APPROACH TO THE PATIENT

An initial step in the diagnosis of HDL deficiency is to measure serum cholesterol, triglyceride, and HDL cholesterol after an overnight 12 hour fast by accurate and standardized assays (1,2). If plasma is used, the values obtained should be multiplied by 1.03. Serum cholesterol and HDL cholesterol can be measured in the non-fasting state, as well, but HDL cholesterol can be as much as 7% lower in the non-fasting state than in the fasting state (3,4). The advantage of measuring cholesterol, triglyceride, and HDL cholesterol after an overnight fast is that low density lipoprotein (LDL) cholesterol can be calculated if triglyceride values are less than 400 mg/dl by the Friedewald formula: LDL cholesterol = total cholesterol - HDL cholesterol - triglycerides/5 (5,6). If triglyceride values are over 400 mg/dl, then ultracentrifugation of plasma at its own density of 1.006 g/ml, and the measurement of cholesterol in the infranatant fraction is essential for an adequate evaluation of plasma lipoprotein. In this circumstance HDL cholesterol is subtracted from the cholesterol in this fraction to estimate LDL cholesterol. A classification of lipid values is provided in Table 1.

### TABLE 1:  CLASSIFICATION OF SERUM LIPID VALUES IN mg/dl

|  | OPTIMAL | BORDERLINE | HIGH RISK* |
|---|---|---|---|
| Total cholesterol | <200 mg/dl | 200-239 mg/dl | ≥240 mg/dl |
| LDL cholesterol | <130 mg/dl | 130-159 mg/dl | ≥160 mg/dl |
| HDL cholesterol | ≥ 50 mg/dl | 35 - 49 mg/dl | <35 mg/dl |
| Triglycerides | <250 mg/dl | 250-500 mg/dl | >500 mg/dl |

*High risk refers to increased risk for CHD. Elevated triglyceride has not clearly been shown to be an independent CHD risk factor after multivariate analysis, but is a risk factor by univariate analysis.

The classification of lipid values as shown in Table 1 is based on recommendations of the Adult Treatment Panel of the National Cholesterol Education Program (NCEP) as well as the recent Consensus Conference on Triglyceride, HDL and CHD (1). Significant independent CHD risk factors include: male $\geq$45 years, female $\geq$55 years, LDL cholesterol $\geq$160 mg/dl, HDL cholesterol < 35 mg/dl, cigarette smoking, hypertension, diabetes mellitus, and a family history of CHD in a male parent or sibling < 55 years or in a female parent or sibling < 65 years. A risk factor should be subtracted if HDL cholesterol $\geq$50 mg/dl (7).

Current NCEP CHD risk factors in addition to an LDL cholesterol $\geq$ 160 mg/dl, are: male gender, family history of myocardial infarction or sudden-death in a parent or a sibling prior to age 55, cigarette smoking, hypertension, HDL cholesterol <35 mg/dl, diabetes mellitus, cerebrovascular or peripheral vascular disease, and obesity (>30% above ideal body weight).

## III.  SECONDARY CAUSES OF HDL DEFICIENCY

In addition to assessing lipids and the presence of CHD risk factors in a patient, it is important to consider secondary causes of decreased HDL cholesterol as shown in Table 4 (8-13). Secondary causes include: hypertriglyceridemia, male gender, obesity, diabetes mellitus, lack of exercise, cigarette smoking, anabolic steroids, progestins, beta blockers, probucol, and liver disease.

It is well known that hypertriglyceridemia is associated with decreased HDL cholesterol levels (14,15). It is also known that in the setting of hypertriglyceridemia, there is replacement of cholesterol ester by triglyceride within the core of the HDL particle (16,17). In both men and women the fractional catabolic rate is the major determinant of plasma apoA-I levels, and this in turn is correlated with plasma triglyceride levels and the triglyceride content of HDL (16,17). However, the gender differences in HDL cholesterol and apoA-I levels are related to increased apoA-I synthesis and decreased post-heparin hepatic lipase activity in women as compared to men (16). This effect is enhanced when women receive estrogen therapy (18,19).

It has also been reported that hypertriglyceridemic patients, as observed in diabetic subjects with type V hyperlipoproteinemia or non-diabetic subjects with type I hyperlipoproteinemia and homozygous familial lipoprotein lipase deficiency have decreased plasma apoA-I levels due to enhanced fractional catabolism (17). More recently it has been reported that apoA-I fractional catabolism is enhanced in subjects with HDL deficiency with or without hypertriglyceridemia (20). However, some patients with decreased HDL cholesterol and apoA-I levels have decreased apoA-I production (21). The data are most consistent with the view that hypertriglyceridemia and states associated with hypertriglyceridemia (obesity, diabetes, lack of exercise, beta blockers) have decreased HDL due to enhanced fractional catabolism of apoA-I, while in other situations such as with probucol administration, HDL cholesterol and apoA-I levels are decreased because of decreased production (22). Conversely, gemfibrozil has been reported to increase apoA-I production (23). Liver disease can cause HDL deficiency due to the lecithin:cholesterol acyltransferase (LCAT) deficiency associated with advanced hepatocellular liver disease (24). From family studies and twin studies it is known that HDL cholesterol and apoA-I levels are strongly affected by environmental factors, and are only modestly affected by genetic factors (25,26).

## III.  RARE GENETIC CAUSES OF HDL DEFICIENCY

Rare familial disorders associated with HDL deficiency include: Tangier disease, ApoA-I, C-III, and A-IV deficiency, ApoA-I and C-III deficiency, ApoA-I deficiency, ApoA-I variants, Lecithin:Cholesterol Acyl Transferase deficiency, and Fish Eye disease. These disorders are discussed below.

IIIA. Tangier Disease: This disorder is a rare autosomal codominant disease, in which homozygotes generally have HDL cholesterol and apoA-I levels less than 5 mg/dl, (normal apoA-I are over 100 mg/dl), mild hypertriglyceridemia, and LDL cholesterol levels below the 10th percentile of normal (27-31). ApoA-I is present in plasma with an increased amount of pro apoA-I. These patients have markedly enhanced fractional catabolism of apoA-I and apoA-II, and the molecular defect causing this disorder is not known (28-31). These patients have cholesterol ester laden macrophages in their tonsils, liver, spleen, lymph nodes, bone marrow, gastrointestinal tract, and Schwann cells, resulting in lymph adenopathy, orange tonsils, orange GI mucosa, hepatosplenomegaly, and often peripheral neuropathy and thrombocytopenia (27-32). Splenectomy appears to worsen the process (32). Homozygotes have mild corneal opacification due to cholesterol deposition (33). Both the apoA-I and apoA-II genes are normal in these patients. There has been debate as to whether these patients have premature CHD. Some authorities have suggested that they do not. However, when we reviewed all available data on homozygotes between the ages of 40 and 60, 40% had evidence of CHD, as compared to 5% in the general population (29). This survey was based on 27 homozygotes. Recently we have reviewed the literature again. Of 55 homozygotes reported, 17 were between the ages of 40 and 60, and of these 13 (76%) have evidence of CHD. These data are consistent with the view that patients with homozygous Tangier disease are at increased risk of CHD in the fifth and sixth decades of life. They may be protected from CHD earlier because of their low LDL levels (29). Tangier heterozygotes have HDL cholesterol levels that are about 50% of normal.

IIIB. ApoA-I, C-III, A-IV Deficiency: The proband in this kindred from northern Alabama, USA, died of coronary atherosclerosis documented at autopsy in her early forties (34-36). Neither apoA-I or apoC-III was detectable in her plasma. ApoA-IV was not measured. Her HDL cholesterol was less than 5 mg/dl, her LDL cholesterol level was normal, and her triglyceride level was low (34-36). She had mild corneal opacification, and also had evidence of mild intestinal fat malabsorption. No xanthomas were noted. Heterozygotes had plasma HDL cholesterol, apoA-I, apoC-III, and apoA-IV levels that were 50% of normal (37). The molecular defect was found to be due to a complete deletion of the entire apoA-I, C-III, A-IV gene complex (37).

IIIC. ApoA-I,C-III Deficiency: The two female homozygous probands in this kindred developed CHD in their twenties, and subsequently required coronary artery bypass surgery. They had planar xanthomas, mild corneal opacification, and no evidence of fat malabsorption (38,39). HDL cholesterol levels were very low, and apoA-I and apoC-III were undetectable in plasma. LDL cholesterol levels were normal and triglyceride levels were decreased. Heterozygotes had HDL cholesterol, apoA-I, and apoC-III levels that were about 50% of normal. The defect was shown to be a DNA rearrangement affecting the adjacent apoA-I and apoC-III genes (40).

IIID. ApoA-I Deficiency: A number of different kindreds have recently been reported in which the proband had marked HDL deficiency and undetectable apoA-I levels due to mutations within the apoA-I gene (41-43). These mutations have included a single nucleotide insertion in codon 3-5 associated with marked HDL deficiency, xanthomatosis, and CHD, a truncated form of apoA-I at codon 32 due to an aberrant stop codon, a deletion of amino acid residues 146-160, a single nucleotide deletion in codon 202 that results in a shift of the reading frame and premature termination in codon 230, and a codon 84 nonsense mutation (41-43).

IIIE.   ApoA-I Variants:   ApoA-I variants have been largely detected in asymptomatic subjects whose plasma was analyzed for the presence of apoA-I of abnormal molecular weight or isoelectric focusing pattern (44-48). The initial kindred described had an abnormal cysteine containing apoA-I known as apoA-I Milano (cysteine for arginine at residue 173) with reduced LCAT activation by apoA-I (44).    Other apoA-I variants associated with reduced LCAT activation include a deletion of lysine at residue 107, a replacement of arginine for proline at residue 143, and a replacement of arginine for proline at residue 165 (45-47). All subjects had a greater deficiency of HDL cholesterol than apoA-I, and all were heterozygotes for the abnormality.   None have been reported to have premature CHD.

Mutations at residue 3 (substitution of either arginine or histidine for proline) have been reported to impair the conversion of proapoA-I to apoA-I (45). The replacement of glycine by arginine at residue 26 within apoA-I (apoA-I Iowa) in the heterozygous state has been associated with HDL deficiency and familial amyloidotic polyneuropathy (48). Other mutations within the apoA-I sequence in the heterozygous state have been reported at residues 4 (proline), 10 (arginine), 13 (asparagine), 89 (asparagine), 103 (asparagine), 107 (lysine), 110 (glutamine), 136 (glutamine), 139 (glutamine), 147 (glutamine), 158 (alanine), 169 (glutamine), 177 (arginine), 198 (glutamine), and 213 (asparagine).    None of these mutations have been associated with any functional abnormalities of apoA-I or any clinical disease (45-49).

IIIF.   Familial Lecithin:Cholesterol Acyl Transferase Deficiency:   These subjects have a marked impairment of the ability to transfer a fatty acid (usually linoleic acid) from phosphatidyl choline or lecithin to cholesterol to form cholesterol ester on all lipoprotein particles (50).   The mutations causing this disorder are well described elsewhere in this monograph. These patients have increased triglyceride rich lipoproteins, abnormal LDL rich in free cholesterol known as Lp-X, and marked HDL deficiency with a greater depletion of HDL by the finding that most of the cholesterol in plasma is in the free form (in contrast to normal subjects where 70% is in the esterified form). The most common cause of this abnormality is endstage liver disease with cirrhosis (24).  However, rare patients have this genetic disorder in the absence of liver disease. These patients have a deficiency of both alpha and beta LCAT activity (50).   Such patients develop marked corneal opacification, anemia, and may develop renal failure (50).

IIIG.   Fish Eye Disease:   These patients develop marked corneal opacification and have HDL deficiency. Their HDL cholesterol is much more greatly reduced than their apoA-I levels. They do not develop premature atherosclerosis. These patients lack alpha LCAT activity, so that only HDL particles have free cholesterol enrichment (51,52).

IIIH.   Familial ApoA-II Deficiency:   A Japanese kindred has been reported in which the female proband was noted to have undetectable plasma apoA-II levels, but had normal levels of apoA-I and HDL cholesterol, and no evidence of CHD in their 50's. The defect was found to be a point mutation in position 1 of intron 3 of the apoA-II gene causing abnormal splicing of the apoA-II gene (53).

III I.   Summary of Rare Genetic HDL Deficiency States:   These data indicate: 1) that apoA-I is essential for HDL formation, but not for LCAT activation; 2) that apoA-II is not necessary for normal HDL formation; 3) that apoC-III may cause hypertriglyceridemia, and its lack is associated with low triglycerides; and 4) that apoA-IV may play a role in intestinal fat absorption. Most of the rare HDL deficiency states have been associated with premature CAD. An exception to this rule may be those disorders in which the conversion of free cholesterol to cholesterol ester within HDL is impaired due to a selective deficiency of alpha LCAT activity as in Fish Eye Disease, or due to the presence of an abnormal form of apoA-I that is less effective than normal in activating LCAT as in apoA-I Milano. It does appear that HDL deficiency whether it is due to decreased production as in the apoA-I, C-III deficiency sates or enhanced catabolism as in Tangier disease or hypertriglyceridemia is associated with premature CHD. However how premature the CHD is it also appears to be modulated by circulating levels of LDL. It should be noted that in our studies of those subjects within the Framingham Offspring Study (n=3671) who had HDL cholesterol and apoA-I below the 5th percentile of normal (n=184), none were noted to have any of the above mentioned disorders as determined by genomic blotting analysis of the apoA-I, C-III, A-IV gene complex, isoelectric focusing with immunoblotting for apoA-I variants, and measurement of free and esterified cholesterol within plasma and HDL. Therefore such disorders are very infrequent causes of HDL deficiency.

## IV.    COMMON FAMILIAL HDL DEFICIENCY STATES

After male gender, age and cigarette smoking, HDL deficiency is the most common risk factor present in patients with premature CHD in our society (54). In our recent studies, HDL deficiency defined as a plasma HDL cholesterol level below the 10th percentile of age and gender adjusted norms is observed in three familial lipid disorders: familial dyslipidemia, familial combined hyperlipidemia and familial hypoalphalipoproteinemia (54-56).

IVA. Familial Dyslipidemia:    This disorder is a variant of familial hypertriglyceridemia (57). Our definition of this disorder is the finding of both plasma triglycerides above the 90th percentile and HDL cholesterol levels below the 10th percentile within the same kindred (56). However, individuals within the kindred do not need to have both abnormalities. This disorder is present in approximately 15% of patients with CHD below the age of 60. Probands for this disorder also have elevated LpB:E particles (58). This disorder appears to differ from familial hypertriglyceridemia because of the HDL deficiency, the increase in LpB:E particles, and the degree of CHD risk.

IVB. Familial Combined Hyperlipidemia: This disorder was originally defined as the finding of both an elevated cholesterol level above the 95th percentile and an elevated triglyceride above the 95th percentile within the same kindred (57). However, individuals within the kindred did not need to have both abnormalities. Approximately 10% of myocardial infarction survivors under age 60 had this familial disorder, which has been associated with increased very low density lipoprotein apoB production (57,59,60). In our family studies we defined familial combined hyperlipidemia as the finding of elevations of both triglyceride and LDL cholesterol levels above the 90th percentile within the same kindred. We noted this disorder to be present in approximately 15% of CHD patients under age 60 (56). Moreover, in most kindreds HDL deficiency was also present in affected family members, as were elevated LpB:E levels (58).

IVC. Familial Hypoalphalipoproteinemia: This disorder is characterized by the finding of HDL cholesterol levels below the 10th percentile of normal in affected family members (61,62). In our own studies this disorder was present in approximately 5% of patients with CHD prior to age 60 (56). Moreover, affected family members often had elevated LpB:E levels (58).

IVD. Association of Lipid Disorders with LDL Particle Size: In our studies decreased LDL particle size is highly correlated with increased plasma triglyceride levels, and decreased HDL cholesterol values (63-68). Moreover, females have significantly larger LDL particle sizes than do males. Based on our analysis in contrast to those of Dr. Krauss' group, LDL size is not very heritable when this parameter is not dichotomized into large and small LDL. Moreover, our data indicate that LDL size is not an independent risk factor, but CHD patients do have smaller LDL particles than controls (68).

IVE. Summary of Common HDL Deficiency States: Common familial lipid disorders associated with premature CHD include familial dyslipidemia, familial combined hyperlipidemia, and familial hypoalphalipoproteinemia (56,57). We have not been able to associate these disorders with any restriction fragment length polymorphisms of the apoA-I, C-III, A-IV gene complex, the apoB gene, or the apoA-II gene (69-71). Others have also found no consistent associations in this regard. A common feature of these disorders is an increase in LpB:E particles and decreases in both LpA-I and LpA-I/A-II (58). In our view these disorders may represent a spectrum of abnormalities associated with hepatic overproduction of apoB containing lipoproteins and enhanced fractional catabolism of apoA-I containing lipoproteins. Other common familial disorders associated with premature CHD include familial hyperhomocysteinemia, which can be treated with folate, and familial Lp(a) excess which can be treated with niacin (72-74). These latter two disorders were observed in 14% and 17%, respectively of kindreds with premature CHD (72-74).

## V.    TREATMENT

Elevated LDL cholesterol has been shown to be an independent CHD risk factor and lowering LDL cholesterol levels in hypercholesterolemic and in some cases in normocholesterolemic patients with diet, with clofibrate, with cholestyramine, with niacin, with gemfibrozil, with niacin and colestipol, with lovastatin and colestipol, and with ileal bypass surgery has been shown to reduce CHD risk and CHD progression in prospective, randomized studies (75-113). For these reasons the Adult Treatment Panel of the National Cholesterol Education Program formulated guidelines for the treatment of hypercholesterolemia (1).

Current NCEP recommendations with regard to the initiation of diet and drug therapy based on LDL cholesterol values are shown in Table 2. Guidelines for dietary therapy are shown in Table 3. While dietary restriction of saturated fat and cholesterol as part of an NCEP Step 2 diet lowers LDL cholesterol by 10-20%, it also lowers HDL cholesterol by 5-10%. However, such reductions may be offset by the weight reduction that often accompanies dietary fat restriction in the free living state. As part of a diet low in total fat (<30% of calories) no great benefit of monounsaturated fat versus polyunsaturated fat is observed with regard to minimizing HDL reduction. It should be noted that fat is a rich source of calories, and both fat restriction and exercise are an excellent way to minimize age related weight gain.

**TABLE 2: LDL CHOLESTEROL DECISION VALUES**

| | INITIATE DIET THERAPY | INITIATE DRUG THERAPY AFTER DIET | GOAL OF THERAPY |
|---|---|---|---|
| <2 CHD risk factors | ≥160 mg/dl | ≥190 mg/dl | <160 mg/dl |
| CHD or 2 or more CHD risk factors | ≥130 mg/dl | ≥160 mg/dl | <130 mg/dl |

**TABLE 3: DIETARY THERAPY***

| Nutrient | Average US Diet | Step One Diet | Step Two Diet |
|---|---|---|---|
| Total Fat | 36% | <30% | <30% |
| Saturated Fat | 15% | <10% | < 7% |
| Polyunsaturated fat | 6% | 6-10% | 6-10% |
| Monounsaturated fat | 15% | 10-15% | 10-15% |
| Cholesterol (mg/day) | 400-500 | <300 | <200 |
| Total Calories | To achieve and maintain desired weight | | |

* % indicates percentage of total calories

Medications used for LDL cholesterol lowering are shown in Table 4. Since a low HDL cholesterol is considered as a risk factor, its presence increases the aggressiveness with which one treats elevated LDL cholesterol. Moreover, if medication is indicated after diet therapy for an elevated LDL cholesterol, and a low HDL cholesterol is also present, it has been recommended that an agent be selected that has a beneficial effect on HDL cholesterol levels (1).

## TABLE 4:  MEDICATIONS

| | RESINS | NIACIN | GEMFIBROZIL | HMG CoA REDUCTASE INHIBITORS* | PROBUCOL |
|---|---|---|---|---|---|
| Patient Acceptance and Compliance | Often Poor | Often Poor | Generally Excellent | Generally Excellent | Generally Excellent |
| Side Effects | Constipation Bloating Decreased absorption of certain medicines | Flushing Itching Gastritis Hepatotoxicity Hyperuricemia Hyperglycemia | Myositis Hepatotoxicity GI Side Effects Coumadin interaction | Hepatotoxicity Myositis Headaches Insomnia | GI side effects |
| Usual Dose | 8-10 gm po BID | 1 g po BID with food | 600 mg po BID | 20 mg po BID | 500 mg po BID |
| LDL Reduction | 10-20% | 10-20% | 0-15% | 25-35% | 10-15% |
| Triglyceride Reduction | ** | 30% | 35% | 20% | 0% |
| HDL Increase | 3% | 15-25% | 5-20% | 5-10% | *** |
| CHD Risk Reduction Documented | Yes 19% 7 yr. | Yes 27% 5 yr. | Yes 34% 5 yr. | No | No |
| Long Term Safety Documented | Yes | Yes | Yes | No | No |

*Not all HMGCoA reductase inhibitors have the same side effect profile.
**May increase triglycerides
***Lowers HDL cholesterol 15-25%, both resins and niacins should be started at low doses and gradually increased.

Specific strategies for HDL raising include an exercise program consisting of vigorous aerobic exercise for at least 30 minutes at least three times per week.  In addition, weight reduction via fat restriction and calorie control can also increase HDL cholesterol, as can smoking cessation.  Such strategies can increase HDL cholesterol by 10-20%.  Alcohol increases HDL cholesterol and decreases CHD risk, but one cannot recommend its use in non-drinkers with low HDL levels for CHD prevention because of known adverse effects of alcohol.  Estrogen administration can be considered in post-menopausal women because it lowers LDL cholesterol and raises HDL cholesterol levels, and reduces CHD risk (166,167).  However, beneficial effects on lipids may be somewhat counteracted by the effects of progestins which must be used in women with an intact uterus.  Better control of diabetes when present can also increase HDL cholesterol levels.

The question that remains is should a drug be used specifically for HDL cholesterol raising. It is well known that a decreased HDL cholesterol level is a potent CHD risk factor. Moreover, data from both the Lipid Research Clinics (LRC) Study with cholestyramine and the Helsinki Heart Study with gemfibrozil support the concept that raising HDL cholesterol is of significant benefit in CHD risk reduction (95,116). For every 1% increase in HDL cholesterol, there appears to be a 1-2% decrease in CHD risk. Interestingly in the LRC study the greatest benefit in CHD risk reduction with cholestyramine was observed in hypercholesterolemic subjects with normal or increased HDL cholesterol levels. In contrast, in the Helsinki Heart Study the greatest benefit in CHD risk reduction with gemfibrozil was noted in hypercholesterolemic subjects with decreased HDL cholesterol, especially those with hypertriglyceridemia and an LDL cholesterol/HDL cholesterol ratio >5.0 (116,117). However, no prospective intervention study has been carried out specifically in subjects selected for HDL deficiency. For this reason only lifestyle changes can be recommended for HDL raising. However, recent data from angiographic regression studies in CHD patients clearly suggests that the goal of therapy in CHD patients, especially those with HDL deficiency, is to reduce LDL cholesterol to less than 100 mg/dl, with an agent that also has a beneficial effect on HDL cholesterol.

## CONCLUSIONS

Decreased HDL cholesterol has clearly been shown to be an independent risk factor for CHD, and this parameter should be measured in all subjects being assessed for CHD risk. The presence of a decreased HDL cholesterol should alert the practicing physician to be aggressive in lowering LDL cholesterol levels by dietary, and if necessary, by pharmacologic means. Moreover, if drugs are used, agents should be selected that not only lower LDL cholesterol, but also lower triglyceride levels, and raise HDL cholesterol in this setting. Future research needs identified by the NIH Consensus Conferences on Triglyceride, HDL and CHD include: 1) precise identification of atherogenic and anti-atherogenic fractions of VLDL and HDL, 2) a better definition of relationships between lipids and thrombosis, 3) studies on the relationship between lipoproteins and CHD in minorities, 4) primary and secondary prevention studies to assess benefit of lowering triglycerides and raising HDL in CHD risk reduction, 5) transgenic mouse models overexpressing apoA-I, 6) effects of estrogens on lipid and CHD risk in women and 7) the development of effective hygienic intervention programs for populations to lower triglycerides, LDL cholesterol, and raise HDL cholesterol levels.

## REFERENCES

1.   The Expert Panel. Report of the National Cholesterol Education Expert Panel on detection, evaluation and treatment of high blood cholesterol in adults. Arch Intern Med 148:36-69, 1988.
2.   McNamara JR, Schaefer EJ. Automated enzymatic standardized lipid analyses for plasma and lipoprotein fractions. Clin Chim Acta 166:1-8, 1987.
3.   Cohn JS, McNamara JR, Cohn SD, Ordovas JM, Schaefer EJ. Postprandial plasma lipoprotein changes in human subjects of different ages. J Lipid Res 29:469-478, 1988.

4.  Cohn JS, McNamara JR, Schaefer EJ. Lipoprotein concentrations in the plasma of human subjects as measured in the fed and fasted states. Clin Chem 34:2456-2459, 1988.

5.  Friedewald WT, Levy RI, Fredrickson DS. Estimation of the concentration of low density lipoprotein cholesterol in plasma without use of the preparative ultracentrifuge. Clin Chem 18:499-502, 1972.

6.  McNamara JR, Cohn JS, Wilson PWF, Schaefer EJ. Calculated values for low density lipoprotein cholesterol in the assessment of lipid abnormalities and coronary disease risk. Clin Chem 36:36-42, 1990.

7.  Anderson KM, Wilson PW, Odell PM, Kannel WB. An updated coronary risk profile. A statement for health professionals. AHA medical/scientific statement science advisory. Circulation 83:356-62, 1991.

8.  Taggart HM, Applebaum-Boweden D, Haffner S, et al. Reduction in high density lipoproteins by anabolic steroid (stanzolol) therapy for postmenopausal osteoporosis. Metabolism 31:1147-1152, 1982.

9.  Wolfe RN, Grundy SM. Influence of weight reduction on plasma lipoproteins in obese patients. Arteriosclerosis 3:160-168, 1983.

10. Criqui MH, Wallace RB, Heiss G, Mishkel M, Schonfeld G, Jones GTL. Cigarette smoking and plasma high density lipoprotein cholesterol. The Lipid Research Clinics Program Prevalence Study. Circulation 62(suppl IV):70-76, 1980.

11. Wood PD, Klein H, Lewis S, Haskell WL. The distribution of plasma lipoprotiens in middle aged male runners. Metabolism 25:1249-1254, 1976.

12. Fager G, Berglund G, Bondjers F, et al. Effects of antihypertensive therapy on serum lipoproteins: treatment with metoprolol, propranolol, and hydrochlorothiazide. Artery 11:283-296,1983.

13. Kennedy AL, Lappin TRJ, Lavery TD, Hadden DR, Weaver JA, Montgomery DAD. Relation of high density lipoprotein cholesterol concentration to type of diabetes and its control. Br Med J 2:1191-1194, 1978.

14. Schaefer, E.J., R.I. Levy, D.W. Anderson, R.N. Danner, H.B. Brewer, Jr., W.C. Blackwelder: Plasma-triglycerides in regulation of HDL-cholesterol levels. Lancet 2:391-393, 1978.

15. Davis CE, Gordon D, LaRosa J, et al. Correlations of plasma high density lipoprotein cholesterol levels with other plasma lipid and lipoprotein concentrations. Circulation 62(suppl IV):IV24-IV30, 1980.

16. Schaefer, E.J., L.A. Zech, L.L. Jenkins, R.A. Aamodt, T.J. Bronzert, E.A. Rubalcaba, F.T. Lindgren, H.B. Brewer, Jr.: Human apolipoprotein A-I and A-II metabolism. J. Lipid Res. 23:850-862, 1982.

17. Schaefer, E.J., J.M. Ordovas: Metabolism of the apolipoproteins A-I, A-II, and A-IV. In Methods in Enzymology, Plasma Lipoproteins, Part B: Characterization, Cell Biology and Metabolism (J. Segrest, J. Albers, eds.). Academic Press. 129:420-442, 1986.*

18. Schaefer, E.J., D.A. Foster, L.A. Zech, H.B. Brewer, Jr., R.I. Levy: The effect of estrogen administration on plasma lipoprotein metabolism in premenopausal females. J. Clin. Endocr. Metab. 57:262-270, 1983.

19. Granfone, A., H. Campos, J.R. McNamara, M.M. Schaefer, J.M. Ordovas, E.J. Schaefer. Effects of estrogen replacement on plasma lipoproteins and

apolipoproteins in dyslipidemic postmenopausal women. Metabolism (submitted).

20. Brinton EA, Eisenberg S, Breslow JL. Increased apoA-I and apoA-II fractional catabolic rate in patients with low high density lipoprotein cholesterol levels with or without hypertriglyceridemia. J Clin Invest 87:536-44, 1991.

21. Le AN, Ginzberg HN. Heterogeneity of apolipoprotein A-I turnover with reduced concentrations of plasma high density lipoprotein cholesterol. Metabolism 37:614-617, 1988

22. Nestel PJ, Billington T. Effects of probucol on low density lipoprotein removal and high density lipoprotein synthesis. Atherosclerosis 88:203-209, 1981.

23. Saku K, Gartside PS, Hynd BA, Kashyap ML. Mechanism of action of gemfibrozil on lipoprotein metabolism. J Clin Invest 75:1702-1712, 1985.

24. Jahn, C.E., E.J. Schaefer, L. Taam, J. Hoofnagle, E.A. Jones, H.B. Brewer, Jr.: Lipoprotein abnormalities in primary biliary cirrhosis: association with hepatic lipase inhibition as well as altered cholesterol esterification. Gastroenterology 89:1266-1278, 1985.

25. Christian JC, Carmelli D, Castelli WP, Fabsitz R, Grim CE, Meaney FJ, Norton JA Jr, Reed T, William CJ, Wood PD. High density lipoprotein cholesterol. A 16 year longitudinal study in aging male twins. Arteriosclerosis 10:1020-1025, 1990.

26. Lamon-Fava S, Jimenez D, Christian JC, Fabsitz RR, Reed T, Carmelli D, Castelli WP, Ordovas JM, Wilson PWF, Schaefer EJ. The NHLBI Twin Study: Heritability of apolipoprotein A-I, B, and low density lipoprotein subclasses and concordance for lipoprotein(a). Atherosclerosis 91:97-106, 1991.

27. Fredrickson DS, Altrocchi PH, Avioli LC. Tangier Disease: combined clinical staff conference at the National Institutes of Health. Ann Intern Med 55:1016-1031, 1961.

28. Schaefer, E.J., C.B. Blum, R.I. Levy, L.L. Jenkins, P. Alaupovic, D.M. Foster, H.B. Brewer, Jr.: Metabolism of high density lipoprotein apolipoproteins in Tangier disease. N. Eng. J. Med. 299:905-910, 1978.

29. Schaefer, E.J., L.A. Zech, D.S. Schwartz, H.B. Brewer, Jr.: Coronary heart disease prevalence and other clinical features in familial high density lipoprotein deficiency (Tangier disease). Ann. Int. Med. 93:261-266, 1980.

30. Schaefer, E.J., D.W. Anderson, L.A. Zech, F.T. Lindgren, T.J. Bronzert, E.A. Rubalcaba, H.B. Brewer, Jr.: Metabolism of high density lipoprotein subfractions and constituents in Tangier disease following the infusion of high density lipoproteins. J. Lipid Res. 22:217-226, 1981.

31. Alaupovic, P., E.J. Schaefer, W.J. McConathy, J.D. Fesmire, H.B. Brewer, Jr.: Plasma apolipoprotein concentrations in familial apolipoprotein A-I and A-II deficiency (Tangier disease). Metabolism 30:805-809, 1981.

32. Schaefer, E.J., T.J. Triche, L.A. Zech, L.A. Stein, M.M. Kemeny, M.F. Brennan, H.B. Brewer, Jr.: Massive omental reticuloendothelial cell lipid uptake in Tangier disease following splenectomy. Am. J. Med. 75:521-526, 1983.

33. Chu, F.C., T. Kuwabara, P.G. Cogan, E.J. Schaefer, H.B. Brewer, Jr.: Ocular manifestations of familial high density lipoprotein deficiency (Tangier disease). Arch. Opthalmol. 97:1926-1928, 1979.

34. Schaefer, E.J., W.H. Heaton, M.G. Wetzel, H.B. Brewer, Jr.: Plasma apolipoprotein A-I absence associated with marked reduction of high density lipoproteins and premature coronary artery disease. Arteriosclerosis 2:16-26, 1982.

35. Schaefer, E.J.: The clinical, biochemical, and genetic features in familial disorders of high density lipoprotein deficiency. Arteriosclerosis 4:303-322, 1984.

36. Schaefer, E.J., J.M. Ordovas, S. Law, G. Ghiselli, M.L. Kashyap, L.S. Srivastava, W.H. Heaton, J.J. Albers, W.E. Connor, Y. Lemeshev, J. Segrest, H.B. Brewer, Jr.: Familial apolipoprotein A-I and C-III deficiency, variant II. J. Lipid Res. 26:1089-1101, 1985.

37. Ordovas, J.M., D.K. Cassidy, F. Civeira, C.L. Bisgaier, E.J. Schaefer. Familial apolipoprotein A-I, C-III, and A-IV deficiency with marked high density lipoprotein deficiency and premature atherosclerosis due to a deletion of the apolipoprotein A-I, C-III, and A-IV gene complex. J. Biol. Chem 264:16339-16342, 1989.

38. Norum RA, Lakier JB, Goldstein S, et al. Familial deficiency of apolipoproteins A-I and C-III and precocious coronary artery disease. N Engl J Med 306:1513-1519, 1982.

39. Norum RA, Forte TM, Alaupovic P, Ginsberg HN. Clinical syndrome and lipid metabolism in hereditary deficiency of apolipoproteins A-I and C-III, variant I. Adv Exp Med Biol 201:137-149, 1986.

40. Karathanasis SK, Haddad I. DNA inversion within the apolipoprotein A-I/C-III/A-IV encoding gene cluster of certain patients with premature atherosclerosis. Proc Natl Acad Sci USA 84:7198-7202, 1987.

41. Matsunaga T, Hiasa Y, Yanagi H, Maeda T, Hattori N, Yamakawa K, Yamanouchi Y, Tanaka I, Obara T, Hamaguchi H. Apolipoprotein A-I deficiency due to a codon 84 nonsense mutation of the apolipoprotein A-I gene. Proc Natl Acad Sci USA 88:2793-7, 1991.

42. Deeb SS, Cheung MC, Peng RL, Wolf AC, Stern R, Albers JJ, Knopp RH. A mutation in the human apolipoprotein A-I gene. Dominant effect on the level and characteristics of plasma high density lipoproteins. J Biol Chem 266:13654-60, 1991.

43. Funke H, von Eckardstein A, Pritchard PH, Karas M, Albers JJ, Assmann G. A frameshift mutation in the human apolipoprotein A-I gene causes high density lipoprotein deficiency, partial lecithin:cholesterol-acyltransferase deficiency, and corneal opacities. J Clin Invest 87:371-6, 1991.

44. Weisgraber KH, Bersot TP, Mahley RW, Francheschini G, Sirtori CR. A-I Milano apoprotein: Isolation and characterization of a cysteine-containing variant of the A-I apoprotein from human high density lipoproteins. J Clin Invest 66:901-909, 1980.

45. von Eckardestein A, Funke H, Walter M, Altland K, Benninghoven A, Assmann G. Structural analysis of human apolipoprotein A-I variants. Amino acid substitutions are nonrandomly distributed throughout the apolipoprotein A-I primary strucutre. J Biol Chem 265:8610-7, 1990.

46. von Eckardstein A, Funke H, Henke A, Altland K, Benninghoven A, Assmann G. Apolipoprotein A-I variants. Naturally occurring substitutions of proline residues affect plasma concentration of apolipoprotein A-I. J Clin Invest 84:1722-30, 1989.

47. Nichols WC, Gregg RE, Brewer HB Jr, Benson MD. A mutation in apolipoprotein A-I in the Iowa type of familial amyloidotic polyneuropathy. Genomics 8:318-23, 1990.

48. Ladias JA, Kwiterovich PO Jr, Smith HH, Karathanasis SK, Antonarakis SE. Apolipoprotein A1 Baltimore (Arg10----Leu), a new apoA1 variant. Human Genetics 84:439-45, 1990.

49. Strobl W, Jabs HU, Hayde M, Holzinger T, Assmann G, Widhalm K. Apolipoprotein A-I (Glu 198---Lys): a mutant of the major apolipoprotein of high-density lipoproteins occurring in a family with dyslipoproteinemia. Pediatric Research. 24:222-8, 1988.

50. Glomset JA, Norum KR, Gjone E. Familial lecithin:cholesterol acyltransferase deficiency. In: The Metabolic Basis of Inherited Disease, 5th ed. Stanbury JB, Wyngaarden JB, Fredrickson DS, Goldstein JL, Brown MS ed. McGraw-Hill, New York, 1983, 643-654.

51. Carlson LA. Fish-eye disease: a new familial condition with massive corneal opacities and dyslipoproteinemia. Eur J Clin Invest 12:41-53, 1982.

52. Carlson LA, Holmquist. Evidence for deficiency of high density lipoprotein lecithin:cholesterol acyltransferase activity (LCAT) in fish eye disease. Acta Med Scand 218:189-196, 1985.

53. Deeb SS, Takata K, Peng RL, Kajiyama G, Albers JJ. A splice-junction mutation responsible for familial apolipoprotein A-II deficiency. Am J Hum Genetics 46:822-7, 1990.

54. Genest, J.J., J.R. McNamara, D.N. Salem, E.J. Schaefer. Prevalence of risk factors in men with premature coronary artery disease. Am J Cardiol 67:1185-1189, 1991.

55. Genest, J.J., J.R. McNamara, J.M. Ordovas, J.L. Jenner, J.S. Millar, S.R. Silberman, K.M. Anderson, P.W.F. Wilson, D.N. Salem, E.J. Schaefer. Prevalence of lipoprotein cholesterol and apolipoprotein A-I, B and Lp(a) abnormalities in men with premature coronary artery disease. J Am Coll Cardiol (in press).

56. Genest, J.J., S. Martin-Munley, J.R. McNamara, J.M. Ordovas, J. Jenner, R. Meyers, P.W.F. Wilson, E.J. Schaefer. Prevalence of familial lipoprotein disorders in patients with premature coronary artery disease. Circulation (in press).

57. Goldstein JL, Schrott HG, Hazzard WR, Bierman EL, Motulsky AG. Hyperlipidemia in coronary heart disease. II. Genetic analysis of lipid levels in 176 families and delineation of a new inherited disorder, combined hyperlipidemia. J Clin Invest 52:1544-1568, 1973.

58. Genest JJ, Bard JM, Fruchart JC, Ordovas JM, Wilson PWF, Schaefer EJ. Plasma apolipoproteins (a), A-I, A-II, B, E, and C-III containing particles in men with premature coronary artery disease. Atherosclerosis 90:149-157, 1991.

59. Janus ED, Nicoll AM, Turner PR, Magill P, Lewis B. Kinetic bases of the primary hyperlipidemias:studies of apolipoprotein B turnover in genetically defined subjects. Eur J Clin Invest 10:161-172, 1980.

60. Chait A, Albers JJ, Brunzell JD. Very low density lipoprotein overproduction in genetic forms of hypertriglyceridemia. Eur J Clin Invest 10:17-22, 1980.

61. Vergani C, Bettale A. Familial hypoalphalipoproteinemia. Clin Chem Acta 114:45-52, 1981.

62. Third JLHC, Montag J, Flynn M, Freidel J, Laskarzewski P, Glueck CJ. Primary and familial hypoalphalipoproteinemia. Metabolism 33:136-146, 1984

63. McNamara J.R., H. Campos, J.M. Ordovas, J. Peterson, P.W.F. Wilson, E.J. Effect of gender, age, and lipid status on low density lipoprotein subfraction distribution: results from the Framingham Offspring Study. Arteriosclerosis 7:483-490, 1987.

64. Campos, H., J.R. McNamara, P.W.F. Wilson, J.M. Ordovas, E.J. Schaefer. Differences in low density lipoprotein subfractions and apolipoproteins in

premenopausal and postmenopausal women. J Clin. Endocr. Metab. 67: 30-35, 1988.

65. Lamon-Fava, S., E.C. Fisher, M.E. Nelson, W.E. Evans, J.S. Millar, J.M. Ordovas, E.J. Schaefer. Effect of exercise and menstrual cycle status on plasma lipids, low density lipoprotein particle size, and apolipoproteins. J. Clin. Endocr. Metab. 68:17-21, 1989.

66. Campos, H., P.W.F. Wilson, D. Jimenez, J.R. McNamara, J.M. Ordovas, E.J. Schaefer. Differences in apolipoproteins and low density lipoprotein subfractions in postmenopausal women on and off estrogen therapy: Results from the Framingham Study. Metabolism 39:1033-1038, 1990.

67. Campos H, Willet WC, Peterson RM, Siles X, Bailey SM, Wilson PWF, Posner BM, Ordovas JM, Schaefer EJ. Nutrient intake comparisons between Framingham and rural and urban Puriscal, Costa Rica: associations with lipoproteins, apolipoproteins, and LDL particle size. Arteriosclerosis 11:1089-1099, 1991.

68. Campos H, Genest JJ, Blijlevens E, McNamara JR, Jenner J, Ordovas JM, Wilson PWF, Schaefer EJ. Low density lipoprotein particle size and coronary artery disease. Arteriosclerosis & Thrombosis 12:187-195, 1992.

69. Ordovas, J.M., F. Civeira, J. Genest, A.H. Robbins, T. Meade, M. Pocovi, P.M. Frossard, U. Masharani, P.W.F. Wilson, D.N. Salem, R.H. Ward, E.J. Schaefer. Restriction fragment length polymorphisms of the apolipoprotein A-I, C-III, A-IV gene locus: Relationships with lipids, apolipoproteins, and coronary artery disease. Atherosclerosis 87:75-86, 1991.

70. Genest, J.M., J.M. Ordovas, J.R. McNamara, A.M. Robbins, T. Meade, S.D. Cohn, D.N. Salem, P.W.F. Wilson, U. Masharani, P.M. Frossard, E.J. Schaefer. DNA polymorphisms of the apolipoprotein B gene in patients with premature coronary artery disease. Atherosclerosis 82:7-17, 1990.

71. Civeira F, Genest J, Pocovi M, Salem DN, Herbert PN, Wilson PWF, Schaefer EJ, Ordovas, JM. The MspI restriction fragment length polymorphism 3' to the apolipoprotein A-II gene: relationships with lipids, apolipoproteins, and premature coronary artery disease. Atherosclerosis (in press).

72. Genest, J.J., J.R. McNamara, D.N. Salem, P.W.F. Wilson, E.J. Schaefer, M.R. Malinow. Plasma homocyst(e)ine levels in men with premature coronary artery disease. J. Am. Coll. Cardiol. 16:1114-1119, 1990.

73. Genest JJ Jr, McNamara JR, Upson B, Salem DN, Ordovas JM, Schaefer EJ, Malinow MR. Prevalence of familial hyperhomocysteinemia in men with premature coronary artery disease. Arteriosclerosis and Thrombosis 11:1129-1136, 1991.

74. Genest J, JL Jenner, JR McNamara, JM Ordovas, SR Silberman, PWF Wilson, EJ Schaefer. Prevalence of lipoprotein (a) [Lp(a)] excess in coronary artery disease. Am J Cardiol 67:1039-1045, 1991.

75. Research Committee to the Medical Research Council. Low-fat diet in myocardial infarction: a controlled diet. Lancet 2(411):501-4, 1965.

76. Research Committee to the Medical Research Council. Controlled trial of soya-bean oil in myocardial infarction. Lancet 2(570):693-9, 1968.

77. Leren P. The effect of plasma cholesterol lowering diet in male survivors of myocardial infarction. Acta Med Scand 466(suppl):92, 1966.

78. Dayton S, Pearce ML, Hashimoto S, Dixon WJ, Tomiyasu U. A controlled clinical trial of a diet high in unsaturated fat in preventing complications of atherosclerosis.

Circulation 40(suppl II):11-1-11-63, 1969.

79. Miettinen M, Karvonen MJ, Turpeinen O, Elosuo R, Paavilainen E. Effect of cholesterol-lowering diet on mortality from coronary heart disease and other causes. A twelve year clinical trial in men and women. Lancet 2(782):835-8, 1972.

80. Research Committee of the Scottish Society of Physicians. Ischaemic heart disease: a secondary prevention trial using clofibrate. Br Med J 4:775-84, 1971.

81. Geizerova H, Green KG, Gyarfas I, et al. A summary report: primary prevention of ischaemic heart disease: WHO coordinated cooperative trial. Bull World Health Organ 5:801-5, 1979.

82. World Health Organization European Collaborative Group. Multifactorial trial in the prevention of coronary heart disease: 3. Incidence of mortality results. Eur Heart J 4:141-7, 1983.

83. Group of Physicians of the Newcastle-upon-Tyne Region. Trial of clofibrate in the treatment of ischaemic heart disease. Br Med J 4:767-75, 1971.

84. Coronary Drug Project Research Group. Clofibrate and niacin in coronary heart disease. JAMA 231:360-81, 1975.

85. Canner PL, Berge KG, Wenger NK, et al. Fifteen year mortality in coronary drug project patiens: long-term benefit with niacin. J Am Coll Health 8:1245-1255, 1986.

86. Carlson LA, Rosenhamer G. Reduction of mortality in the Stockholm Ischaemic Heart Disease Secondary Prevention Study by combined treatment with clofibrate and nicotinic acid. Acta Med Scand 223:405-18, 1988.

87. Carlson LA, Danielson M, Ekberg I, Klintemar B, Rosenhamer G. Reduction of myocardial reinfarction by the combined treatment with clofibrate and nicotinic acid. Atherosclerosis 28:81-6, 1977.

88. Woodhill JM, Palmer AJ, Leelarthaepin B, McGilchrist C, Blacket RB. Low fat, low cholesterol diet in secondary prevention of coronary heart disease. Adv Exp Med Biol 109:317-30, 1978.

89. Dorr AE, Gundersen K, Schneider JC Jr, Spencer TW, Martin WB. Colestipol hydrochloride in hypercholesterolemic patients -- effect on serum cholesterol and mortality. J Chronic dise 31:5-14, 1978.

90. Hjermann I, Holme I, Byre KV, Leren P. Effect of diet and smoking intervention on the incidence of coronary heart disease. Lancet 2:1303-10, 1981.

91. Holme I, Hjermann I, Helgeland A, Leren P. The Oslo Study: diet and antismoking advice:additional results from a 5-year primary preventiv trial in middle-aged men. Prev Med 14:279-92, 1985.

92. Multiple Risk Factor Intervention Trial Research Group. Multiple Risk Factor Intervention Trial: risk factor changes and mortality results. JAMA 248:1465-77, 1982.

93. Lipid Research Clinics Program. The Lipid Research Clinics Coronary Primary Prevention Trial results: II. The relationship of reduction in incidence of coronary heart disease to cholesterol lowering. JAMA 251:365-74, 1984.

94. Lipid Research Clinics Program. The Lipid Research Clinics Coronary Primary Prevention Trial results: I. Reduction in incidence of coronary heart disease. JAMA 251:351-64, 1984.

95. Gordon DJ, Knoke J, Probstfield JL, Superko R, Tyroler HA. High density lipoprotein cholesterol and coronary heart disease in hypercholesterolemic men: the

Lipid Research Clinics Coronary Primary Prevention Trial. Circulation 74:1217-25, 1986.

96. Miettinen TA, Huttunen JK, Naukkarinen V, et al. Multifactorial primary prevention of cardiovascular diseases in middle-aged men: risk factor changes, incidence, and mortality. JAMA 254:2097-102, 1985.

97. Strandberg TE, Salomaa VV, Naukkarinen VA, Vanhanen HT, Sarna SJ, Miettinen TA. Long-term mortality after 5-year multifactorial primary prevention of cardiovascular diseases in middle-aged men. JAMA 266:1225-9, 1991.

98. Frick MH, Elo O, Haapa K, et al. Helsinki Heart Study: a primary-prevention trial with gemfibrozil in middle-aged men with dyslipidemia: safety of treatment, changes in risk factors, and incidence of coronary heart disease. N Engl J Med 317:1237-45, 1987.

99. Brensike JF, Levy RI, Kelsey SF, et al. Effects of therapy with cholestyramine on progression of coronary arteriosclerosis: results of the NHLBI Type II Coronary Intervention Study. Circulation 69:313, 1984.

100. Levy RI, Brensike JF, Epstein SE, et al. The influence of changes in lipid values induced by cholestyramine and diet on progression of coronary atherosclerosis: results of the NHLBI Type II Coronary Intervention Study. Circulation 69:325, 1984.

101. Blankenhorn DH, Nessim SA, Johnson RL, Sanmarco ME, Azen SP, Cashin-Hemphill L. Beneficial effects of combined colestipol-niacin therapy on coronary atherosclerosis and coronary venous bypass grafts. JAMA 257:3233, 1987.

102. Blankenhorn DH, Alaupovic P, Wickham E, Chin HP, Azen SP. Prediction of angiographic change in native human coronary arteries and aortocoronary bypass grafts. Circulation 81:470, 1990.

103. Ornish D, Brown SE, Scherwitz L, et al. Can lifestyle changes reverse coronary heart disease? Lancet 336:129, 1990.

104. Buchwald H, Varco RL, Matts J et al. Effect of partialileal bypass surgery on mortality and morbidity from coronary heart disease in patients with hypercholesterolemia. N Engl J Med 232:946, 1990.

105. Brown G, Albers JJ, Fisher LD, et al. Regression of coronary artery disease as a result of intensive lipid-lowering therapy in men with high levels of apolipoprotein B. N Engl J Med 323:1289, 1990.

106. Kane JP, Malloy NJ, Ports TA, Phillips NR, Diehl, JC, Havel RJ. Regression of coronary atherosclerosis during treatment of familial hypercholesterolemia with combined drug regimens. JAMA 264:3007, 1990.

107. Lewis B, et al. The St Thomas' Hospital Atheroma Regression Study. Presented at NHLBI Workshop on Stabilization and Regression of Coronary Atherosclerosis. Bethesda, June 19-20, 1991.

108. Cohn K, Sakai FJ, Langston MF. Effect of clofibrate on progression of coronary disease: a prospective angiographic study in man. Am Heart J 89:591, 1975.

109. Kuo PT, Hayase H, Kostis JB, Moreyra AE. Use of combined diet and colestipol in long-term (7-71/2 years) treatment of patients with type II hyperlipoproteinemia. Circulation 59:199, 1979.

110. Nash DT, Gensini G, Esente P. Effect of lipid-lowering therapy on the progression of coronary atherosclerosis assessed by scheduled repetitive coronary arteriography. Int J Cardiol 2:43, 1982.

111. Nikkila EA, Viikinkoski P, Valle M, Frick MH. Prevention of progression of coronary atherosclerosis by treatment of hyperlipidemia: a seven-year prospective angiographic study. Br Med J 289:220, 1984.

112. Arntzenius AC, Kromhout D, Barth JD, et al. Diet, lipoproteins, and the progression of coronary atheroscleosis: the Leiden Intervention Trial. N Engl J Med 312:805, 1985.

113. Hahmann HW, Bunte T, Hellwig N, et al. Progression and regression of minor coronary arterial narrowings by quantitative angiography after fenofibrate therapy. Am J Cardiol 67:957, 1991.

114. Bush TL,Cowan LD, Barrett CE, et al. Estrogen use and all-cause mortality. Preliminary results from the Lipid Research Clinics program followup. JAMA 249:903-911, 1983.

115. Stampfer MJ, Willett WC, Colditz GA, Rosner B, Speizer FE, Hennekens CH. A prospective study of postmenopausal estrogen use and coronary heart disease. N Engl J Med 313:1044-1049, 1985.

116. Manninen V, Elo O, Frick MH, Haapa K, Heinonen OP, Heinsalmi P, Helo P, Huttunen JK, Kaitaniemi P, Koskinen P, Maenpaa H, Malkonen M, Mantari M, Norola S, Pasternak A, Pikkaranen J, Romo , Sjomblom T, Nikkila E. Lipid alterations and decline in the incidence of coronary heart disease in the Helsinki Heart Study. JAMA 260:641-651, 1988.

117. Manninen V, Tenkaner L, Koskinen P, Huttinen JK, Manttari M, Heinonen OP, Frick MH. Joint effects of serum triglyceride and LDL cholesterol and HDL cholesterol concentrations on coronary heart disease risk in the Helsinki Heart Study. implications for Treatment. Circulation 85:37-45, 1992.

High density lipoproteins and atherosclerosis III.
N.E. Miller and A.R. Tall, editors.

Low HDL cholesterol and coronary heart disease risk: Helsinki Heart Study experience

M. Heikki Frick[a], Olli P. Heinonen[b], Jussi K Huttunen[c], Pekka Koskinen[a],
Matti Mänttäri[a], Leena Tenkanen[a] and Vesa Manninen[a]

[a]First Department of Medicine, University Central Hospital, Helsinki, Finland

[b]Department of Public Health, University of Helsinki, Finland

[c]National Public Health Institute, Helsinki, Finland

## INTRODUCTION

The initial observations, some 40 years ago (1-2), on the adverse effect of low serum high density lipoprotein cholesterol (HDL cholesterol) on the occurrence of coronary heart disease (CHD) have been amply confirmed by a series of both longitudinal and cross-sectional studies (3-7). The placebo group of the Helsinki Heart Study has also been used to demosntrate the HDL cholesterol/CHD interrelationships (8-9). The present report is based on a number of subgroup analyses on the importance of low HDL cholesterol.

## SUBJECTS AND METHODS

The participants of the Helsinki Heart Study were selected from 23531 men aged 40 - 55 years. The primary screening and selection process (10) and the main outcome of the study (11-12) have been reported in detail. Briefly, the eligible men had to exhibit a non-HDL cholesterol (total cholesterol - HDL cholesterol) of $\geq$ 5.2 mmol/l on two successive determinations. Individuals with a history or any sign of heart disease or other major illnesses were excluded.

The trial participants were randomly allocated either to gemfibrozil therapy (n = 2046) or placebo (n = 2035), and were followed for 5 years. Analysis of the event rate in the placebo group is appropriate to demonstrate the effect of low HDL cholesterol.

HDL cholesterol was measured after precipition of very low density (VLDL) and low density lipoprotein (LDL) cholesterol with dextran sulfate magnesium chloride by an enzymatic method (Boehringer Mannheim kit No. 236691). The triglycerides (TG) were measured as glycerol after enzymatic hydrolysis with lipase/esterase (Boehringer Mannheim kit No. 124966). The LDL cholesterol was derived with the formula: LDL cholesterol = total cholesterol - HDL cholesterol - TG/2.2 (13). When the distribution of baseline HDL cholesterol of the study participants (n = 4081) was compared with the distribution of screened men (n = 18966) they were identical (8-9) revealing that data on the HDL cholesterol/CHD relationships are applicable to middle-aged caucasian males in general. The distribution of total cholesterol of the study participants, as compared to the screened individuals, was shifted to the right classifying the individuals as hypercholesterolemic. When the seasonal variation of HDL cholesterol was eliminated by calculating yearly mean values the HDL cholesterol remained very stable in the placebo group during the whole 5-year follow-up period.

Baseline lipid values are used in the present analyses. The HDL cholesterol tertiles were < 1.08, 1.08-1.32, and > 1.32 mmol/l. The LDL cholesterol tertiles were < 4.5, 4.5-5.2, and > 5.2 mmol/l. In some analyses the lipid values were dichotomized. The cut-off points were: LDL cholesterol 5.0 mmol/l, TG 2.3 mmol/l, HDL cholesterol 1.08 mmol/l, and LDL/HDL cholesterol ratio 5. The smokers were cathegorized as non-smokers + past smokers/current smokers, age as below and above the median age (47 years). Blood pressure was dichotomized using 130/90 as the cut-off value. The risk patterns were also studied using Cox proportional hazard models (14) with age, smoking and systolic blood pressure as covariates.

## RESULTS

In this selected dyslipidemic population both total cholesterol and LDL cholesterol were unsatisfactory indicators of CHD risk whereas low HDL cholesterol and high TG were much better predictors (Table 1). The CHD risk was significantly increased in both groups of individuals.

Table 1
Relative risk of CHD in relation to baseline HDL cholesterol and TG

|  |  | Risk |
|---|---|---|
| HDL cholesterol |  |  |
|  | ≥ 1.08 mmol/l | 1 |
|  | n = 1384 |  |
|  | < 1.08 mmol/l | 1.73 |
|  | n = 651 | (1.12-2.66) |
| TG |  |  |
|  | ≤ 2.3 mmol/l | 1 |
|  | n = 1529 |  |
|  | > 2.3 mmol/l | 1.81 |
|  | n = 506 | (1.16-2.81) |

Estimations with Cox regression models with age, smoking, and systolic blood pressure as covariates. Risk was set at 1 in high HDL cholesterol and low TG individulas. 95% confidence intervals in parenthesis.

HDL cholesterol/LDL cholesterol interrelationships demonstrate that the CHD risk is low in the highest HDL tertile irrespective of the LDL cholesterol (Fig. 1). The impact of increased LDL cholesterol is most clearcut in the lowest HDL cholesterol tertile. Relationships with CHD incidence and HDL cholesterol and LDL cholesterol showed much clearer gradients in the respective tertiles of HDL cholesterol when analysed with respect to age, smoking and blood pressure.

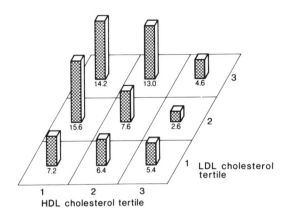

Figure 1. Crude CHD incidence rates (per 1000 person-years) in relation to HDL cholesterol and LDL cholesterol tertiles. From reference No. 8 with permission.

Table 2
Relative risk of CHD in relation to baseline HDL cholesterol and TG combined and LDL/HDL ratio and TG combined

|  | Risk |
| --- | --- |
| HDL cholesterol ≥ 1.08 mmol/l and TG ≤ 2.3 mmol/l n= 1166 | 1 |
| HDL cholesterol < 1.08 mmol/l and TG > 2.3 mmol/l n= 218 | 2.43 (1.43-4.12) |
| LDL/HDL ratio ≤ 5.0 and TG ≤ 2.3 mmol/l n= 1262 | 1 |
| LDL/HDL ratio > 5.0 and TG > 2.3 mmol/l n= 138 | 3.82 (2.20-6.63) |

The lipid combinations with lowest CHD risk were set at 1. Cox regression models with age, smoking and systolic blood pressure as covariates. 95% confidence intervals in parenthesis.

Analyses of the joint effects of LDL cholesterol, HDL cholesterol and TG reveal a significantly vulnerable subgroup consisting of individuals with a LDL cholesterol/ HDL cholesterol ratio above 5 and TG above 2.3 mmol/l (Table 2).

## DISCUSSION

The selected Helsinki Heart Study population is not ideally suited for a risk factor analysis over the whole range of total cholesterol and LDL cholesterol distribution since the participants represent a high cholesterol population with a limited number of individuals at the lower end of the distribution curve. On the other hand, it is ideally amenable for the analysis of the importance of low HDL cholesterol. Both the univariate and joint-effect analyses amply illustrate the deleterious effect of low HDL cholesterol. There seems to be an especially vulnerable subgroup consisting of individuals with a LDL/HDL cholesterol ratio above 5 and TG above 2.3 mmol/l. In this subgroup gemfibrozil therapy resulted in a marked (75%) reduction in CHD incidence, as reported in detail recently (15). It is evident that the currently used recommendations for initiating therapy in lipid disorders (16) do not sufficiently take into account the importance of low HDL cholesterol. Even the limit of "low HDL cholesterol" is arbitrarily set at below 35 mg% while much higher values seem to be assosiated with increased risk of CHD. Th lowest tertile in our population was below 1.08 mmol/l (42 mg%) representing a markedly increased risk as compared to the higher tertiles (Table 1) and when analysed jointly with LDL and TG (Table 2) its impact was even more clearly discernible. The adverse effect of increased LDL cholesterol became evident only in the two lowest tertiles of HDL cholesterol distribution (Fig. 1). In the highest HDL cholesterol tertile LDL cholesterol did not play any role in the CHD incidence. Hence the LDL/HDL cholesterol ratio seems to be the most valid criterion for CHD risk assessment. Our recent data on the  joint effects of various lipid fractions (15) indicate that TG should be added to the calculations.

## REFERENCES

1   Barr DP, Russ EM, Eder HA. Am J Med 1951; 11: 480-485.

2   Nikkilä E. Scand J Clin Lab Invest 1953; 5: Suppl. 8.

3   Miller GJ, Miller NE. Lancet 1975; 1: 16-19.

4   Berg K, Borresen A-L, Frick MH, Dahlen G. Lancet 1976; 1: 1014.

5   Pearson TA, Bulkley BH, Achuff SC, Kwiterovich PO, et al. Am J Epidemiol 1979; 109: 285-295.

6   Heiss G, Johnson NJ, Reiland S, Davis CE, et al. Circulation 1980; 62: Suppl. IV: 116-136.

7   Abbott RD, Wilson PWF, Kannel WB, Castelli WP. Arteriosclerosis 1988; 8: 207-211.

8   Manninen V, Huttunen JK, Tenkanen L, Heinonen OP, et al. In: Miller NE, ed. High Density Lipoproteins and Atherosclerosis II. Amsterdam: Elsevier, 1989; 35-42.

9   Frick MH, Manninen V, Huttunen JK, Heinonen OP, et al. Drugs 1990; 40: Suppl. 1: 7-12.

10  Mänttäri M, Elo O, Frick MH, Haapa K, et al. Eur Heart J 1987; 8: Suppl. 1: 1-29.

11  Frick MH, Elo O, Haapa K, Heinonen OP, et al. N Engl J Med 1987; 317: 1237-1245.

12  Manninen V, Elo O, Frick MH, Haapa K, et al. JAMA 1988; 260: 641-651.

13  Friedewald WT, Levy RI, Fredrickson DS. Clin Chem 1972; 18: 499-502.

14  Cox DR, Oakes D. In: Monographs on Statistics and Applied Propability. London: Chapman & Hall Ltd, 1984.

15  Manninen V, Tenkanen L, Koskinen P, Huttunen JK, et al. Circulation 1992; 85: 37-45.

16  National Cholesterol Education Program. National Heart, Lung, and Blood Institute publication No (NIH) 1988; 88-2925.

# ALTERATIONS IN PLASMA HIGH DENSITY LIPOPROTEIN LEVELS WITH GEMFIBROZIL TREATMENT

Roger S. Newton and Brian R. Krause

Atherosclerosis Pharmacology, Parke-Davis Pharmaceutical Research Division, Warner-Lambert Company, Ann Arbor, Michigan 48105 USA

## INTRODUCTION

Gemfibrozil (Lopid®) (5-(2,5-dimethylphenoxy)-2,2-dimethylpentanoic acid) is a fibric acid derivative which has been shown to beneficially alter plasma lipids and reduce cardiac endpoints in men at risk for coronary heart disease (1-6). The primary pharmacologic action of this agent has not been elucidated, but the plasma lipid regulating effects generally occurring in dyslipidemic animal models and human subjects are a reduction in total and low density lipoprotein (LDL) cholesterol, an increase in high density lipoprotein (HDL) cholesterol and a lowering of plasma triglycerides. The mechanisms by which gemfibrozil produces these changes in plasma lipoprotein levels and their composition include the following: 1) increased postheparin lipolytic activity (7-9); 2) decreased hepatic synthesis and secretion of very low density lipoprotein (VLDL) triglycerides, cholesterol and apolipoprotein (apo) B (10-12); 3) increased fractional catabolic rate of VLDL triglycerides and apo B (12-14); and 4) enhanced synthesis of apo A-I and A-II (9,15-18). For the purposes of this short review, the focus will be on how gemfibrozil affects HDL metabolism and thereby produces alterations in HDL cholesterol levels, HDL subfractions and HDL apolipoprotein (apo) composition in rats and man. How the resulting changes may be important in preventing atherosclerosis and promoting reverse cholesterol transport will also be discussed.

## PHARMACOLOGIC EFFECTS IN NORMAL AND DYSLIPIDEMIC RATS

Gemfibrozil was first screened in chow-fed rats to evaluate its hypotriglyceridemic activity (19). When compared with other fibrates (clofibrate, bezafibrate and fenofibrate) for its effects on plasma triglyceride reduction, gemfibrozil was found to be 15x more potent than clofibrate and more efficacious than the other fibrates at higher doses (19-21). Gel filtration chromatography revealed the expected reduction in VLDL triglycerides. The hypotriglyceridemic activity of gemfibrozil and the members of its chemical series have been attributed to structure activity relationships that allow for a variety of substitutions in the aryl portion of the molecule, the chain spacing between the phenoxy and the isobutyric acid portions as well as the substitution pattern on the $\alpha$-carbon (22,23).

Although the gemfibrozil dose-response curve for plasma cholesterol reduction in chow-fed rats is somewhat flat, changes in cholesterol distribution among the lipoproteins are different as compared to those for other fibrates (20). Gemfibrozil lowers plasma total cholesterol in normal rats by lowering non-HDL cholesterol, while HDL cholesterol is unchanged. In contrast, the reduction in total cholesterol by fenofibrate, and to a lesser extent clofibrate and bezafibrate, is due to the lowering of HDL cholesterol. Therefore, gemfibrozil was the only fibrate which did not lower HDL cholesterol in adult Sprague-Dawley rats treated with different fibrates by oral gavage for two weeks (2.5-125 mg/kg).

Table I. EFFECTS OF FIBRATES IN NORMAL, CHOW-FED RATS*

| Fibrate | Total Chol | Apo AI | | | Apo E | |
|---------|------------|--------|-------|-------|--------|-------|
| | | Plasma | LmRNA | ImRNA | Plasma | LmRNA |
| fenofibrate | ↑ | ↓ | ↓ | NE | ↓↓ | ↓ |
| clofibrate | ↓ | ↓ | ↓ | NE | ↓ | NE |
| gemfibrozil | ↑ | NE | ↓ | NE | ↑↑ | NE |

*From Staels, et al, 1992 (Ref. 24)
L =Liver, I =Intestine, NE =No Effect

Others have recently described fibrate-induced changes in plasma cholesterol, plasma apolipoproteins and apolipoprotein gene expression in a different rat strain (Wistar) using diet-admix drug administration (Table I)(24). These changes included a dose-dependent decrease in liver apo A-I mRNA levels by all fibrates tested. In contrast, only fenofibrate lowered liver apo E mRNA. The response to gemfibrozil treatment was very different in that it increased plasma cholesterol and apo E, but did not lower plasma apo A-I levels. No change was observed in the liver mRNA for apo E, suggesting post-transcriptional effects. Although HDL cholesterol was not measured in this study, the results are consistent with the changes in HDL cholesterol in chow-fed rats discussed above (20). Unlike other fibrates, it is also interesting that gemfibrozil treatment of normal rats results in an increase of liver cholesterol concentrations (20). It is possible that this increase in cholesterol mass represents cholesterol transported to the liver in HDL particles. Since gemfibrozil is the only fibrate that inhibits cholesterol synthesis ex vivo in chow-fed rats ($ED_{50}$ = 19.7 mg/kg), some of this HDL derived cholesterol could enter the regulatory free sterol pool, thereby decreasing de novo cholesterol biosynthesis (25).

The effects of gemfibrozil in rats fed high fat/high cholesterol diets have been extensively evaluated in both euthyroid and hypothyroid animals (26-28). Such diets produce an abnormal lipoprotein pattern characterized by an increase in VLDL and intermediate density lipoprotein (IDL) particles and a lowering of plasma HDL (29-31). These abnormal lipoproteins (d<1.063g/ml) are thought to be of hepatic and intestinal origin (32-35). The diet-induced alterations in plasma apo A-I, apo B, apo E and apo A-IV have also been previously described (36-39). In these high fat/high cholesterol rat models gemfibrozil lowered the total plasma cholesterol, altered the distribution of cholesterol in the lipoprotein fractions to that resembling a chow-fed rat and changed the composition of the apolipoproteins associated with the different lipoprotein fractions. This lowering of non-HDL cholesterol and the redistribution of cholesterol into the HDL fraction (26) has been substantiated using precipitation methods, sequential and density gradient ultracentrifugation, agarose gel filtration, and most recently, with automated Superose HPGC using an on-line cholesterol reagent (40) (see Figure 1). The HDL elevating activity in this high fat/high cholesterol-fed rat model has been extensively used in structure activity relationship studies to optimize the pharmacologic effect of compounds. From these studies, the 2,5-dimethyl substitution on the phenoxy portion of the molecule and the trismethylene spacer between the phenoxy ring and the isobutyric acid side chain are required structural components for HDL elevation (22,23). No other fibrate drugs tested in this model have produced qualitatively similar results (27).

FIGURE 1*

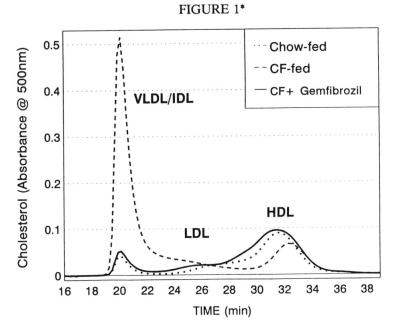

*Experimental conditions as described by Krause and Newton, 1985 (Ref. 26)

A more detailed discussion of the pharmacologic action of gemfibrozil in this animal model and its impact on HDL metabolism is important for better understanding its role in altering human lipoprotein and apolipoprotein metabolism. With the high fat/high cholesterol diet, plasma apo E and A-I were reduced by 60% and 15%, respectively, while the apo B concentrations were increased two-fold (26). Gemfibrozil treatment tended to normalize the concentrations and distribution of these apolipoproteins. More specifically, gemfibrozil increased the amount of apo E in HDL and decreased the amount in VLDL and IDL. Thus, gemfibrozil prevented the loss of apo E from HDL and its redistribution to apo B containing particles (26). It has been hypothesized that apo E may be important both in the blood and peripheral lymph for directing cholesterol to the liver for removal via the bile (34,42,43). If under conditions of a high fat/high cholesterol diet the apo E is shifted away from HDL towards chylomicrons, VLDL and IDL for their eventual removal via hepatic receptors, it is not surprising that there is a reduction in total plasma apo E and HDL apo E during cholesterol feeding. The possibility also exists that under these conditions the livers of these animals overproduce VLDL and IDL, thereby providing a sink for any available apo E from HDL. Gemfibrozil treatment may reduce the production of these apo B-containing lipoproteins so that less apo E is transferred from HDL to VLDL and IDL. Thus, gemfibrozil normalizes the plasma levels of apo E and its distribution into HDL, primarily represented in the rat by the $HDL_1$ subfraction (d = 1.063-1.080g/ml) (37).

We further explored the increase in plasma and HDL apo E in high fat/high cholesterol-fed rats treated with gemfibrozil by isolating and culturing primary hepatocytes from these animals and measuring apo E secretion using [3]H-leucine (41). The rate of [3]H-leucine incorporated into apo E secreted into the media VLDL was increased 3-fold, while comparatively little radiolabeled apo E appeared in the d = 1.006-1.21g/ml lipoproteins. Therefore, it is possible that gemfibrozil increases apo E synthesis in cholesterol-fed rats as mentioned above for chow-fed animals. This would imply modulation by gemfibrozil at post-transcriptional events (24). These results, together with the in vivo effects of gemfibrozil in this animal model, suggest that gemfibrozil increases the production of hepatic apo E, in the form of VLDL, which is rapidly transferred to the HDL fraction upon the intravascular hydrolysis. Thus, the ability of gemfibrozil to decrease VLDL and increase HDL lipids may be related to its ability to modulate the synthesis, transfer and ultimate distribution of apo E. Whether gemfibrozil induces an enhanced synthesis and secretion of apo E in other tissues/cells besides liver parenchymal cells remains to be determined. If apo E synthesis and secretion is increased by gemfibrozil in monocyte-macrophage foam cells of the arterial wall, cholesterol efflux from these cells may be enhanced, thereby facilitating reverse cholesterol transport. In additional rat hepatocyte studies an increase in the incorporation of newly synthesized sterols into d > 1.006-1.21g/ml lipoproteins was observed (10). Since rat hepatocytes do not normally secrete IDL or LDL particles into the media, the above result suggests that gemfibrozil increases newly synthesized sterol into native HDL particles. More recent studies indicate that in HepG2 and Hep 3B cells exposed to gemfibrozil (40 ug/ml) there is a two-fold induction in apo A-I mRNA, a one third reduction in apo B mRNA and no significant effect on apo E mRNA levels (17). Pulse-chase experiments further substantiated that gemfibrozil selectively alters the rates of apo A-I and B production at the level of synthesis. No alteration was seen on apo E synthesis. Therefore, there are differences with respect to gemfibrozil's influence on apo E metabolism as measured ex vivo in whole animals (24), in cultured rat hepatocytes (41) and following in vitro addition to human hepatoma cell lines (17).

## PLASMA LIPOPROTEIN AND APOLIPOPROTEIN ALTERATIONS IN CLINICAL STUDIES EMPLOYING GEMFIBROZIL

Numerous clinical studies have reported that gemfibrozil's major plasma lipid regulating effects in humans are characterized by a reduction in plasma triglycerides (40-60%) and an increase in HDL cholesterol (10-25%) (1-6,44-53). Depending upon the extent of the hypertriglyceridemia, there may or may not be an associated decrease in LDL cholesterol (44,48,49). Even in moderate hypertriglyceridemic subjects, the LDL subfractions are characterized by a composition of triglyceride-rich, cholesteryl ester-poor particles, which may adversely limit their ability to carry cholesterol (54,55). These small, dense, LDL particles of hypertriglyceridemic subjects are thought to be atherogenic (56-58). Gemfibrozil treatment alters their composition so that they become more normal in their cholesterol/apo B ratios and in their cholesterol/triglyceride ratios (14,44,48,60,61). Furthermore, HDL cholesterol is also often increased in these subjects.

Although it was observed in the Helsinki Heart Study that there was a reduction in coronary heart disease for all treatment groups, the Type IIb hyperlipoproteinemic individuals derived the most benefit from gemfibrozil treatment (1-6). In a subgroup analysis of the Helsinki Heart Study population, it was shown that the lower the HDL cholesterol at baseline, the greater the pharmacologic response to gemfibrozil and the greater the impact for reducing cardic endpoints relative to placebo (4-6). In a further analysis of the effects of gemfibrozil on the concentration and composition of serum lipoproteins, it was determined that gemfibrozil not only changed the absolute amounts of the lipoprotein lipids, but also normalized the qualitative abnormalities associated with hypertriglyceridemia (44). The drug-induced changes included alterations in the HDL, LDL and VLDL cholesterol to triglyceride molar ratios, resulting in an enrichment in both HDL and LDL cholesterol and a reduction in VLDL cholesterol. Only the LDL cholesterol was dependent upon the initial plasma triglyceride levels. Gemfibrozil enriched primarily the $HDL_3$ subfraction with a lesser effect on the $HDL_2$, consistent with previous reports observed in smaller studies (7,9,18,45,48,51-53,59). It is interesting to note that the most recent analysis of the Helsinki Heart Study database indicates that those individuals with a LDL/HDL cholesterol ratio of >5 and triglycerides >2.3 mmol/l(200 mg/dl) had an almost four-fold greater incidence of coronary heart disease relative to those with a ratio <5 and triglycerides <2.3mmol/l(200 mg/dl) (5). Gemfibrozil treatment in the high risk group reduced the incidence of coronary heart disease events by 71% as compared to the corresponding placebo subgroup. It is this dyslipidemic population that is often associated with the small, dense LDL particles, which have been shown to be atherogenic (54-58). Gemfibrozil's pharmacologic action of altering the composition of these and other lipoprotein fractions is therefore tied to a beneficial effect on coronary heart disease (4-6).

Lipoprotein kinetic studies performed with gemfibrozil not only confirm quantitatively the alteration in plasma lipids and lipoprotein mass, but provide evidence as to the mechanism of these changes. Investigations using radiolabeled glycerol and apo B in hypertriglyceridemic individuals have indicated that gemfibrozil reduced the production rate of VLDL triglycerides and apo B in both Type II and IV individuals and also altered their fractional catabolic rate towards normal (12-14,60,61). In subjects with HDL deficiency (HDL cholesterol values of 22 mg/dl) and characterized with familial endogenous hypertriglyceridemia, gemfibrozil treatment resulted in elevations in apo A-I (29%) and apo A-II (38%) mass and an increase in HDL cholesterol of 36% (9,15,16). Based on the decay curves following injection of autologous $^{125}$I-HDL, there was no change in the fractional catabolic rate, suggesting increased rates of synthesis for both Apo A-I (27%) and apo A-II (34%). Since the HDL particles found in the plasma after gemfibrozil treatment were smaller and denser, this supports an enhancement in newly synthesized HDL in the blood and possibly a greater availability of the particles to promote cholesterol efflux and reverse cholesterol transport (18,62). Other studies confirm the compositional changes in the lipid components of plasma lipoproteins discussed previously; however, more inconsistent results have been reported with respect to alterations in apo A-I and A-II (9,45,47,51-53). Additional studies have also evaluated changes in other apolipoproteins including apo C-II, C-III and apo E (48,51,52). Gemfibrozil administration was associated with a reduction of these apolipoproteins since a large proportion of them are associated with triglyceride-rich lipoproteins.

A recent study with a strong correlate to the previously described rat studies (26-28) focused on serum apo E and its distribution in both Type IIa and IIb subjects treated with gemfibrozil. The results from this study suggest that the redistribution of apo E into HDL particles in cholesterol-fed rats may also occur in humans (Figure 2) (50). The total apo E and HDL apo E in the Type IIa group were increased, while the non-HDL fraction was unchanged. In contrast, the Type IIb individuals who had elevated serum apo E levels at baseline, reduced their serum and non-HDL levels of apo E, while also increasing the apo E in the HDL fraction HDL apo E has been reported to be significantly lower in normolipidemic survivors of myocardial infarctions compared to control subjects (63). Thus, the amount of apo E in HDL may be a marker for the efficiency of reverse cholesterol transport; that is, a low amount indicates impairment and a high amount reflects enhancement.

This hypothesis is supported by recent studies in transgenic mice in which apo E was overexpressed (64). In these animals which proved to be resistant to dietary-induced hypercholesterolemia, all plasma lipoproteins were reduced with the exception of HDL. Furthermore, intravenous apo E administration to Watanabe rabbits prevented the progression of atherosclerosis by reducing cholesteryl ester

FIGURE 2*

## EFFECT OF GEMFIBROZIL TREATMENT
## ON SERUM APO E DISTRIBUTION

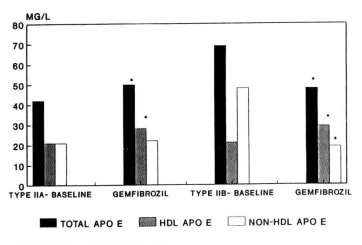

P. GAMBERT ET AL, ATHERO. 89:267, 1991

*From Gambert, et al, 1991 (Ref. 50)

accumulation in the aorta and decreasing the percentage of surface area covered by macroscopic plaques (65). Lastly, individuals with familial cholesteryl ester transfer protein deficiency have enlarged, apo E-rich HDL particles and are not susceptible to atherosclerosis (66). Additional studies are therefore warranted to determine whether the reduction in cardiac endpoints associated with the Helsinki Heart Study may in part be associated with changes in the distribution of apo E from non-HDL particles to HDL particles, thereby promoting reverse cholesterol transport and beneficially affecting atherosclerotic disease.

1. Manninen V, Malkonen M, Eisalo O, et al. Acta Med. Scand. (Suppl) 1982; 668:82-87.
2. Frick MH, Elo O, Haapa K, et al. N. Engl J. Med. 1987; 317:1237-1245.
3. Manninen V, Elo, O, Haapa K, et al. J. Amer. Med. Assoc. 1988; 260:641-651.
4. Manninen V, Huttunen JK, Heinonen O, et al. Am. J. Cardiol. 1989; 63:42H-47H.

5. Manninen V, Tenkanen L, Koskinen P, et al. Circulation 1992; 85:37-45.
6. Huttunen JK, Manninen V, Tenkanen L, et al. In Miller NE, ed. High Density Lipoproteins and Atherosclerosis II. New York: Excerpta Medica, 1989; 191-198.
7. Nikkila EA, Ylikahri R, Huttunen JK. Proc. Roy. Soc. Med. (Suppl 2) 1976; 69:58-62.
8. Vessby B, Lithell H, Boberg J, et al. Proc. Roy. Soc. Med. (Suppl 2) 1976; 69:32-37.
9. Saku K, Gartside PS, Hynd BA, Kashyap ML. J. Clin. Invest. 1985; 75:1702-1712.
10. Newton RS. Today's Therapeutic Trends (Suppl) 1985; I:13-21.
11. Newton RS, Krause BR, Cutter CS, et al. Arteriosclerosis 1984; 4:552a.
12. Kesaniemi YA, Grundy SM. J. Amer. Med. Assoc. 1984; 251:2241-2246.
13. Kissebah, AH, Alfarsi S, Adams PW, et al. Atherosclerosis 1976; 24:199-218.
14. Vega GL, Grundy SM. J. Amer. Med. Assoc. 1985; 253:2394-2403.
15. Kashyap ML Saku K. In Paoletti R, et al., eds. Drugs Affecting Lipid Metabolism. Berlin: Springer-Verlag, 1987; 367-371.
16. Kashyap ML. In Miller NE, ed. High Density Lipoproteins and Atherosclerosis II. New York: Excerpta Medica 1989; 199-207.
17. Tam, SP. Atherosclerosis 1991; 91:51-61.
18. Bard, JM, Farnier M, Buxtorf JC, et al. 9th International Symposium on Atherosclerosis 1991; 128.
19. Rodney G, Uhlendorf P, Maxwell RE. Proc. Roy. Soc. Med. (Suppl 2) 1976; 69:6-9.
20. Newton RS, Krause BR. In Miller NE, ed. High Density Lipoproteins and Atherosclerosis II. New York: Excerpta Medica 1989; 209-216.
21. Newton RS, Krause BR. In Fear R, ed. Pharmacologic Control of Hyperlipidaemia. Barcelona: JR Prous, 1986; 171-186.
22. Creger PL, Moersch GW, Neuklis WA. Proc. Roy. Soc. Med. (Suppl 2) 1976; 69:3-5.
23. Roth BD, Newton RS. In Witiak D, et al. eds. Antilipidemic Drugs-Medicinal, Chemical and Biochemical Aspects. New York: Elsevier, 1991; 225-255.
24. Staels B, van Tol A, Andreu T, Auwerx J. Arteriosclerosis and Thrombosis 1992; 12:286-294.
25. Krause BR, Kieft K, Bennett MK, Stanfield R, Newton RS. FASEB J. 1988; 2:7689.
26. Krause BR, Newton, RS. J. Lipid Res. 1985; 26:940-949.
27. Krause, BR, Newton, RS. Atherosclerosis 1986; 59:95-98.
28. Krause, BR, Newton, RS. Atherosclerosis 1986; 61:245-248.
29. Lasser NL, Roheim PS, Edelstein D, Eder HA. J. Lipid Res. 1973; 14:1-8.
30. Frnka J, Reiser R. Biochim. Biophys. Acta 1974; 360:322-338.
31. Calandra S, Pasquali-Ronchetti I, Gherardi C, et al. Atherosclerosis 1977; 22:369-387.
32. Davis RA, McNeal MM, Moses RL. J. Biol. Chem. 1982; 257: 2635-2640.

33. Riley JW, Glickman RM, Green PHR, Tall AR. J. Lipid Res. 1980; 21:942-952.
34. Mahley RW. Med. Clin. N. Amer. 1982; 66:375-402.
35. DeLamatre, JG, Roheim PS. J. Lipid Res. 1981; 22:297-306.
36. Dory L, Roheim PS. J. Lipid Res. 1981; 22:287-296.
37. Roheim PS, DeLamatre JG. In Nutritional Diseases: Research Directions in Comparative Pathobiology. New York: Alan R. Liss, 1986; 475-500.
38. DeLamatre JP Hoffmeier CA, Lacko AG, Roheim PS. J. Lipid Res. 1983; 24:1578-1585.
39. DeLamatre JP, Krause BR, Roheim PS. Proc. Natl. Acad. Sci. USA 1982; 79:1282-1285.
40. Kieft KA, Bocan TMA, Krause BR. J. Lipid REs. 1991; 32:859-866.
41. Krause, BR, Newton, RS, Cutter CS, et al. Arteriosclerosis 1984; 4:521a.
42. Sloop CH, Dory L, Hamilton R, et al. J. Lipid Res. 1983; 24:1429-1440.
43. Dory L, Sloop CH, Boquet LM, et al. Proc. Natl. Acad. Sci USA 1983; 80:1282-1285.
44. Mantari M, Koskinen P, Manninen V, et al. Atherosclerosis 1990; 81:11-17.
45. Odman B, Ericsson S, Lindmark M, et al. Eur. J. Clin. Invest. 1991; 21:344-349.
46. Averna MR, Barbgallo CM, Pata G, et al. Curr. Therap. Res. 1991; 49:47-53.
47. Klosiewicz-Laroszek L, Szostak WB. Eur. J. Clin. Pharmacol. 1991; 40:33-41.
48. Cominacini L, Garbin U, Bosello O, et al. Curr. Therap. Res. 1989; 46:1045-1058.
49. Tilly-Kiesi M, Tikkanen MJ. J. Intern. Med. 1991; 229:427-434.
50. Gambert P, Farnier M, Girardot G, et al. Atherosclerosis 1991; 89:267-269.
51. Kloer, HU, Luley C. Athero. Cardiovasc. Diseases 1987; 3:1121-1126.
52. Gnasso A, Lehner B, Haberbosch W, et al. Metabolism 1986; 35:387-393.
53. Sirtori CR, Franceshini G, Gianfranceshi G, et al. J. Lab. Clin. Med. 1987; 110:279-286.
54. Deckelbaum RJ, Granot E, Oschry Y, et al. Arteriosclerosis 1984; 4:225-231.
55. Packard CJ, Shepherd J, Joerns S, et al. Biochim Biohys Acta 1979; 572:269-282.
56. Austin MA, Breslow, Hennekens CH, et al. J. Amer. Med. Assoc. 1988; 260:1917- 1921.
57. Austin MA, King MC, Vranizan KM, Krauss RM. Circulation 1990; 82:495-506.
58. Grundy SM, Vega GL. Arch. Intern. Med. 1992; 152: 28-34.
59. Sorisky A, Ooi TC, Simo IE, et al. Atherosclerosis 1987; 67:181-189.
60. Kissebah AH, Alfarsi S, Evans DJ. Arteriosclerosis 1984; 4:614-624.
61. Turner PR, Cortese C, Wootton, R, et al. Eur. J. Clin. Invest. 1985; 15:100-112.
62. Puchois P, Kandoussi A, Fievet P et al. Atherosclerosis 1987; 67:35-40.
63. Bittolo Bon G, Cazzalato G, Saccardi M, et al. Atherosclerosis 1984; 53:69-75.
64. Shimano H, Yamada N, Katsuki M, et al. Proc. Natl. Acad. Sci. USA 1992; 89:1750-1754.
65. Yamada N, Inoue I, Kawamura M, et al. J. Clin. Invest. 1992; 89:706-711.
66. Bisgaier CL, Siebenkas MV, Brown MA, et al. J. Lipid Res. 1991; 32:21-33.

# INDEX OF AUTHORS